Anita Marie Fleury
M C H

An Introduction to
Public Health

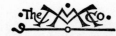

THE MACMILLAN COMPANY
NEW YORK • CHICAGO
DALLAS • ATLANTA • SAN FRANCISCO
LONDON • MANILA

IN CANADA
BRETT-MACMILLAN LTD.
GALT, ONTARIO

An Introduction to Public Health

fourth edition

Harry S. Mustard, M.D., LL.D.

Professor Emeritus of Public Health Practice,
Columbia University

Ernest L. Stebbins, M.D.

Dean of the Johns Hopkins School
of Hygiene and Public Health

THE MACMILLAN COMPANY
NEW YORK

Previous editions, copyright, 1935, 1944, and 1953, by The Macmillan Company

Library of Congress catalog card number: 59–5639

The Macmillan Company, New York
Brett-Macmillan Ltd., Galt, Ontario

Printed in the United States of America

To Sarah Haile Mustard
and
Helen Ross Stebbins

Foreword to Fourth Edition

PUBLIC HEALTH MEANS different things to different people but there seems to be complete agreement that whatever is included in the definition it represents a changing, and we trust progressive, area of human activity. In the quarter of a century since the first edition there have been major changes in the generally accepted scope of public health. New scientific discoveries are almost constantly adding to the potential prevention of disease, prolongation of life and improvement of physical and mental well being.

In the six and one half years since the third edition there have been major changes in public health organization in the United States and in the world. Active immunization against poliomyelitis has been developed, tried and found effective. Artificial fluoridation for public water supplies has been clearly established as a safe and effective means of preventing dental caries. The treatment of tuberculosis has been dramatically changed with impressive results. Community mental health programs have blossomed and borne fruit. The concept of world-wide eradication of diseases such as malaria has gained general acceptance as within range of possibility. Protection against radiological health hazards has assumed major importance. The association between excessive cigarette smoking and lung cancer has been generally accepted.

These and many other developments make revision of the text necessary, but the credit for the basic concept goes to the original author. Thanks are due him also for inspiration and help throughout the revision. Dr. Mustard generously, however reluctantly, interrupted the delightful leisure of his retirement to read text, check figures, and give wise counsel at all times. Thanks are also due to my efficient secretaries, Mrs. Josephine Feder and Mrs. Nancy Petersen, for long hours of work on the manuscript, and to Mrs. Hermine E. Bird for preparing the index.

E. L. S.

April, 1959

Foreword to First Edition

THIS VOLUME IS designed mainly to orient the student in the field of public health. It furnishes a background of information and, in one way or another, tends to develop a philosophy and perspective. It is purposely brief and does not concern itself with the details of public health administration; nor does it presume to offer suggestions for classroom or field instruction in any of the specialized phases of public health practice. It therefore provides information rather than direction.

Judgment as to selection of material included in the text rests upon a number of years' experience in public health organization and practice, and in teaching graduate students in public health, medical students, and nurses. The subjects covered and the details furnished are those which observation indicates as necessary for the groups for which the book is designed.

The factual material presented is, of course, not new. Similar information may be found in most texts on the various basic subjects covered. But, because such material is scattered through a number of volumes, and is not infrequently masked by detail, the student encounters difficulty in finding the facts desired. It is hoped that the basic information collected in this text, supplemented as it is by analysis of problems and interpretation of public health programs and practices, may prove useful. However, it should be remembered that the whole field of public health is in a fluid stage, and a non-frozen perspective and an elasticity of attitude are essentials. For these reasons, when in the following pages one encounters what are quite obviously the writer's opinions, they should be taken for only what they are: opinions.

H. S. M.

Jan., 1935

Contents

Foreword to Fourth Edition   vii

Foreword to First Edition   ix

Chapter 1. The Background and Associations of Hygiene and
             Public Health   1

Chapter 2. Vital Statistics   19

Chapter 3. Organization and Administration of Public Health
             Work   47

Chapter 4. Health Education and Related Activities   75

Chapter 5. The Acute Communicable Diseases   89

Chapter 6. Tuberculosis as a Public Health Problem   125

Chapter 7. The Venereal Diseases   149

Chapter 8. Mental Health   165

Chapter 9. Environmental Health   184

Chapter 10. The Individual and His Hygiene   222

Chapter 11. Childbearing and Its Relation to the Public Health   236

Chapter 12. The Hygiene of Infancy and Young Childhood   248

Chapter 13. School Health Service   263

Chapter 14. Chronic Diseases   288

Chapter 15. Medical Care   299

Index   315

An Introduction to
Public Health

chapter 1

The Background and Associations of Hygiene and Public Health

THE GREAT AND never-ending problem which each species faces is the struggle for survival, for perpetuation of its kind. This means that the species must successfully meet its environment—its enemies, its food problems, the hazards to its young; otherwise it perishes. The species continues its existence through two major efforts: by adaptation to the conditions in which it finds itself, and by reproduction far in excess of the need for replacement of adults removed by death.

Sometimes offsetting, sometimes aiding the survival efforts of any given species are the forces in nature, which act continuingly, impartially, unerring, and inevitably. They hew to the line, are neither cruel nor merciful, pitying nor pitiless. They see neither virtue nor vice, health nor disease. One individual's loss, by nature, becomes another's gain; one species' extinction may mean another's ascendancy; a death from typhoid fever is but an unbalanced parasitism.

With what appears to be his higher intelligence man relies but slightly on overproduction and more upon adaptation to his environment in the preservation of the species. Actually, the more his civilization advances the lower goes the birth rate and the higher goes his success in adapting himself to his environment. He wears warm cloth-

1

ing to keep him comfortable in the winter and protective clothing to offset the harmful effects of heat or other hazards in his environment. He builds more and more complex shelters which he heats in the winter and cools in the summer, and devises intricate protective equipment to permit him to function in unnatural environments. He makes his kill via the slaughterhouse, without danger to himself, and employs policemen to protect him from predatory humans who might do him physical harm, or steal his goods. To a great extent he relies upon the skill of others for the rearing of his young. He frequently utilizes natural forces to save him labor, time, or danger: by creating an environment inimical to typhoid bacilli, he brings about their destruction; through interference in the life cycle of his insect enemies he prevents the transmission of disease and the destruction of his food supply; by vaccinating an individual, he causes the natural process of antibody formation to go into play. Such protective procedures, in common with all social measures, must have unremitting direction of the human mind. At best they are imperfect and intermittent in accomplishment, not comparable with the forces of nature which operate with the simplicity, directness, and certainty of cause and effect.

Out of these considerations there might well arise, in fact there has arisen, a question as to the ultimate benefit of measures for conservation of life and health. It may be asked if such efforts are not "antibiological," if they do not but tend to save the weaklings. It is difficult to answer such a question categorically, particularly as there is no satisfactory definition of what is meant by "weakling" or unfit. One might define a weakling on a physical basis. But big-muscled people are no more immune to infection, or the degenerative diseases, than are the slender; and big brains and a sound nervous system, themselves evidence of strength, are no more frequent in the physically strong than in the less strong.

In a broad sense, in terms of the human species as a whole, and its status a million years hence, perhaps public health work and medical and nursing care save lives and promote health in the "weak" as well as in the strong. But so does kindness to the aged, and laws, customs, and conventions which restrict the strong, crafty, or ruthless from destroying their competitors; thus all social forces, including those which frown upon promiscuity and forbid rape, could be said to be as antibiological as are public health measures.

Man has been so successful in reducing the ravages of disease in a large part of the world that even with a slight overproduction, with a rapidly declining mortality rate, serious problems of overpopulation have been created. In certain parts of the world serious question has been raised as to whether further protection of man against his natural enemies will not merely produce another and more serious problem of food supply for the increasing population. In some quarters, question has seriously been raised as to whether it is better to die of starvation than from malaria or cholera.

Society, however, is organized for today rather than for the distant future, and makes more or less effective efforts to counteract so-called primitive impulses on the one hand and the impact of natural forces on the other. And although it could be argued, from a cold-blooded standpoint, that it might be better to let each individual either succumb or survive disease, in order that the ten-thousandth generation might be more resistant to these diseases, that generation is too remote to permit a sacrifice of present lives for its benefit.

Properly speaking, public health work, including medical care, is but one of many social measures: a manifestation of man's conscious effort to overcome a particular group of hazards or hardships. The relation between what may be called the part, public health work, and the whole, social betterment, may be summarized briefly as follows:

1. As health is an essential factor in human welfare, its maintenance and protection are necessarily of social importance.

2. The extent and manner in which society concerns itself as to the public health depend upon the social philosophy which prevails.

3. Under a system where individualism obtains, society tends to take only those public health measures which are beyond the scope of individual action: organization for the prevention and control of epidemics, the provision of public water supplies, sewer systems, milk sanitation, research, hospital facilities, etc.

4. Since, for generations, the social philosophy in the United States was largely one of individualism, quite naturally health problems have been left to the individual, public health work assuming responsibility only for those measures which the citizen, alone, could not institute.

5. Within recent years, society has shown a tendency to assume an increasing responsibility for the individual as an individual: for his education, his employment, his general welfare.

6. Out of this evolution there has come a tendency to broaden and intensify public health work; and in this expansion government, representing society, appears more and more inclined to regard provision of adequate public health and medical care as society's responsibility to each individual if he cannot himself procure such service.

In spite of these relationships wherein public health work would appear to be one of society's tools for human betterment, there is a wide gap between the available knowledge in medicine and hygiene, on the one hand, and its practical application, on the other. Society is slow to utilize such knowledge and probably always will be, because of a number of factors. These may be listed as follows:

1. The knowledge is in possession of relatively a few: its existence and importance are not generally recognized by the people as a whole.

2. Even when there is widespread information, prejudice and lethargy tend to delay its general application.

3. Assuming that society is convinced as to the efficacy of a procedure in the abstract, practically there must be assurance that application of the new knowledge will return benefits in proportion to the cost in effort and dollars.

4. With knowledge at hand, with conviction that it should be applied, there still remains an obstacle: the cupidity of man. If the new knowledge conflicts with the ego, the security, or the gain of some powerful individual or interest, its acceptance and benefits may be long delayed.

Hygiene, Medicine, and the Scientific Method. In common with the exact sciences, hygiene and medicine are indebted to those influences which, in the sixteenth century, culminated in the scientific method.

Essentially, the scientific method separates beliefs and assumptions from facts. It demands precision and accuracy in observation. It insists that observations be made, classified, and studied qualitatively and quantitatively. It permits interpretation and conclusion only if substantiable by facts. It buttresses itself by experimentation. It prohibits wishes from fathering thoughts. It outlaws rule of thumb.

The scientific method of approach was not born without having gone through a period of incubation, nor was it born full grown. Hippocrates and many of his contemporaries manifested it. Roger Bacon, a thinking friar of the thirteenth century, urged exact and careful observation of natural objects; he advocated experimentation, he forecast the necessity and invention of new instruments of precision in measurement and analysis. Then came Copernicus, Galileo, Boyle, Newton, Descartes, who, in astronomy, chemistry, physics, mathematics, overthrew the citadels of tradition, assumption, and prejudice. Such men, their intellectual heirs and their interpreters, opened the way for the more specialized investigators in the field of medicine.

Contributors to Basic Public Health Knowledge. Aside from the very essential contributions in the fields of general science, there has come from medicine much of that body of knowledge and of those techniques upon which the public health practice of today is based. There follows below the briefest sort of identification of some who have made important contributions. Not all of these were physicians.

Much of the material used in these summaries was obtained from Garrison's *Introduction to the History of Medicine,** to which grateful acknowledgment is made.

Aesculapius. The mythical son of the god Apollo and the nymph Coronis. Among the Greeks his reputation as a physician was held in reverence. To him were attributed curative powers far beyond the scope of mortal ability, and in temples dedicated to him, his miraculous aid was besought. According to tradition, his popularity aroused jealousy among the gods, and Zeus destroyed him. Hygeia and Panacea were daughters of Aesculapius.

* Garrison, Fielding H.: *Introduction to the History of Medicine,* 4th ed. W. B. Saunders Company, Philadelphia. 1929.

Hippocrates (ca. 460–377 B.C.). A physician of ancient Greece, who lived in the golden age of Socrates and Plato. He did much to separate medicine from mysticism, and emphasized the necessity for observation and interpretation of the events of nature and the illness of people. His was the scientific spirit in ancient medicine. After him, European medicine was in darkness for many centuries. The works of Hippocrates, often referred to in medical literature, are really the collected writings of Hippocrates and a number of other physicians of, or shortly after, his time.

Girolamo Fracastoro (1483–1553). A Veronese physicist and geologist as well as physician. In a poem entitled *Syphilis sive Morbus Gallicus,* he presents as a character a shepherd named *Syphilus.* It is from this poem that the name of the disease is derived.

Thomas Sydenham (1624–1689). An English physician. An important part of his contribution to medicine and public health came through his insistence upon the need for diagnosis of illness in terms of specific disease entities. He did much to make possible a differentiation of the various communicable diseases, one from the other.

Anton van Leeuwenhoek (1632–1723). A Dutch brewer whose hobbies were natural history and lenses. The microscopes which he developed made it possible to view organisms and structures never before seen.

Edward Jenner (1749–1823). A country practitioner in Gloucestershire, England, credited formally as the discoverer of smallpox vaccination. The results of his experiments and observations were published in 1798. Jenner's work opened up a new field in the development of artificial, active immunity, and has changed the occurrence of smallpox from pandemics to relatively mild and occasional local incidence.

Thomas Robert Malthus (1766–1834). An English clergyman, but also an economist and sociologist, who made intensive studies of populations: their tendency to increase or decrease, and especially as to their relationship to food supply. While his conclusions are not today accepted without qualification, Malthus was a pioneer in the scientific study of population problems.

Pierre Bretonneau (1778–1862). A pathologist, of Tours, France.

Bretonneau was an early authority on diphtheria, to which he gave its present name. In 1825 he performed the first tracheotomy for croup. His classical monograph on diphtheria was published in 1826.

René T. H. Laennec (1781–1826). A French physician, who not only gave to medicine masterly descriptions of diseases of the chest, but also is a famous historical figure as the inventor of the stethoscope. Many of the words used today to describe sounds heard in auscultation (e.g., "rales") were coined by Laennec.

Lemuel Shattuck (1793–1859). A publisher and bookseller of Boston. As chairman of the Massachusetts Sanitary Commission, he published, in 1850, a report entitled *Sanitary Survey of the State of Massachusetts*. This document is recognized as a public health classic.

William Farr (1807–1883). An Englishman whose principal contribution to public health was in the field of vital statistics. His analysis, utilization, and interpretation of material coming to the office of the Registrar General in England established the pattern largely followed in treatment of vital statistics today.

Oliver Wendell Holmes (1809–1894). A prominent American physician, although now known best as an author. In 1843 he published his paper on the "Contagiousness of Puerperal Fever," in which he drew the conclusion that the condition could be transmitted to patients by the contaminated hands of attendants. He laid down excellent rules for the prevention of such transmission. This very important contribution to medical literature can be found reprinted in the *Harvard Classics*.

William Budd (1811–1880). An English physician. He demonstrated the fact that typhoid fever is communicable, and the manner in which it is transmitted. His monograph, *Typhoid Fever, Its Nature, Mode of Spreading and Prevention*, published in 1873, is a classic in public health literature.

John Snow (1813–1858). A London practitioner, recognized as the outstanding anesthetist of his day, Snow also demonstrated water as an important factor in the dissemination of cholera. His epidemiological analysis of the London cholera epidemic of 1854 was outstanding, and his report of this work, published in 1855, is a landmark in the science of epidemiology.

Ignaz Philipp Semmelweis (1818–1865). A pioneer in the prevention of puerperal septicemia, who was born in Budapest and educated
in Vienna. Observing the results of tragic puerperal septicemia in
lying-in hospitals, noting its especial frequency in cases delivered by
medical students fresh from the dissecting room, Semmelweis instituted in his wards hand disinfection by chloride of lime. Against
violent opposition and spurred on by the fanaticism of a psychopathic
personality, he, almost coincident with Oliver Wendell Holmes, laid
the foundation for clean obstetrics.

Gregor Mendel (1822–1884). An Austrian monk and naturalist.
Science is indebted to him for his painstaking observations in heredity
and for his sound interpretations of his findings. Through his recognition of "dominant" and "recessive" characters in offsprings of various
matings, he clarified much that had been confusing in genetics.

Louis Pasteur (1822–1895). A French chemist, physicist, and bacteriologist, who pushed forward the frontier of bacteriology and
established it in the domain of science. Noting the relationship
between fermentation and microorganisms, Pasteur opened the field
of bacteriology. The specific things for which he is best remembered
in medicine and public health are (1) the demonstration, in sheep, of
the effectiveness of an attenuated virus against anthrax (1881); (2)
the development of the Pasteur prophylaxis against rabies (1885);
and (3) the process of pasteurization. He developed the latter about
1863–1865.

Joseph Lister (1827–1912). An English physician, who revolutionized surgery through application of Pasteur's discoveries. His col-
leagues accepted suppuration in surgical wounds as inevitable, but
Lister questioned this assumption. He strove for antisepsis and out
of it, and dependent upon it, has come asepsis. In his day, case fatality
in surgery was sufficiently high to make the need for safe surgery a
public health problem; and in decreasing illness and deaths, Lister's
work may be truly regarded as an important contribution in the field
of public health.

Carlos Juan Finlay (1833–1915). A physician in Cuba, who sug-
gested in 1881 the transmission of yellow fever by the mosquito. He

identified the particular mosquito concerned (now known as *Aëdes aegypti*) and provided Walter Reed and his party with specimens. Finlay even attempted and perhaps succeeded in infecting humans with yellow fever through the bite of the mosquito. His work, however, was not controlled, and the actual proof of mosquito transmission had to await demonstration by Reed. In medical history in the United States there is an unfortunate tendency to overlook Finlay's important contributions to the solving of the yellow fever puzzle.

T. A. Edwin Klebs (1834–1913). A Prussian pathologist, who was a pioneer in the then new field of bacteriology. His contributions were extensive, but he is best remembered in connection with the Klebs-Loeffler bacillus, *Corynebacterium diphtheriae*, to which he called attention in 1883.

Karl Joseph Eberth (1835–1926). A German physician, who in 1880 demonstrated the typhoid bacillus. Although Eberth's name was for a long time associated with this organism, Klebs actually deserves some of the credit, since his description was published a few months before Eberth's. Neither was exactly correct in his description.

Robert Koch (1843–1910). A German physician, who may be called the logician of bacteriology. After a series of most important contributions in this field, he demonstrated the tubercle bacillus in 1882. Koch's postulates for determining whether or not a given organism is actually the cause of a particular disease still form the basis for such a decision.

C. L. Alphonse Laveran (1845–1922). A French army surgeon, who in 1880 discovered malarial parasites in blood cells. This discovery made possible a more scientific approach to diagnosis, epidemiology, and treatment of this disease.

William H. Welch (1850–1934). A Connecticut-born American. Aside from specific contributions in the fields of pathology and bacteriology, he exercised a world-wide and inspiring influence in the fields of medical education and research. He was the first professor of pathology of the Johns Hopkins Medical School (1884) and organized (1916) and directed for many years the School of Hygiene and Public Health of the Johns Hopkins University. Dr. Welch's pupils are scattered throughout the world, and his influence and stimulation still live through them.

Walter Reed (1851–1902). An American, a major in the Medical Corps, U.S. Army. In 1901 Reed proved that yellow fever is transmitted by the *Aëdes aegypti* mosquito. This work, done in Havana, was most dramatic and convincing. Members of the board for study of yellow fever made not only a scientific but a most courageous approach to the subject. The noninfectiousness of bodily discharges, sheets, furniture, etc., was proved when, without harm, volunteers lived in (screened) rooms and slept in beds recently occupied by persons who had died of yellow fever. To prove mosquito transmission, they permitted themselves to be bitten by mosquitoes they believed to be infected—and some of them developed yellow fever.

Paul Ehrlich (1854–1915). A German scientist and physician whose fame rests upon discoveries of the relationship of dyes to tissues. Out of his interest in this subject he greatly improved laboratory methods of staining tissues, developed the side-chain theory of immunity, and discovered arsphenamine (Salvarsan).

Emil von Behring (1854–1917). A German physician. During the period 1890–1893 von Behring noted that the blood serum of an animal which had received mild doses of diphtheria toxin was effective in the prevention and treatment of that disease in others. In a year or two, diphtheria antitoxin was made available to the medical profession. His associate in this work was Kitasato, a Japanese.

William C. Gorgas (1854–1920). An American, Surgeon General of the U.S. Army, 1914–1918. Gorgas' great contribution was in demonstrating the practical application of measures for control of yellow fever in Havana and in the Panama Canal Zone.

William T. Sedgwick (1855–1921). An American public health engineer and teacher. The outstanding contributions of Sedgwick are that he brought about widespread acceptance of the importance of knowledge of sciences basic to environmental control of disease, that in epidemiological practice and teaching he pioneered in what may be termed the biological approach, and that the proficiency of his students tended to establish the place of the public health engineer in modern health organizations.

Charles V. Chapin (1856–1941). An American public health officer. For nearly half a century Dr. Chapin served as superintendent of health of Providence, Rhode Island. During that time, concepts and practice in public health were undergoing marked changes and great expansion. Perhaps more than any of his brother epidemiologists and administrators, he interpreted, applied, and contributed to this newer knowledge. He exhibited an unusual ability to question the apparent and to re-express the residue in terms of the real. He forced routinism and precedent to justify themselves or give way to common sense. His writings reflect his precision of thought. His was a most salutary influence in evaluating and elevating public health procedures.

Ronald Ross (1857–1932). An English pathologist and parasitologist, in the Indian Medical Service. In 1895 Ross gave the first clue as to the mosquito's role in the transmission of malaria. He further contributed knowledge as to prevention of the disease by devising methods for destruction of mosquitoes in their larval stage.

Arthur Newsholme (1857–1943). An English medical officer of health. Newsholme lived through that period when public health practice, previously concerned mainly with sanitary reform, was incorporating into itself programs for improving personal hygiene and care of the individual. Newsholme's vision and ability did much to establish a sound national system of public health in Great Britain; and through his writings and visits to the United States, he influenced American concepts and practices.

Hermann M. Biggs (1859–1923). A physician of unusual administrative ability and vision. He made provision in New York City for free distribution of diphtheria antitoxin, established a public health laboratory for free Wassermann examinations, and made obligatory the reporting of tuberculosis (1897). These provisions and requirements are basic in the public health practice of today.

Theobald Smith (1859–1934). An eminent American pathologist and bacteriologist, who made lasting contributions to knowledge of infectious diseases in man and animals. His work in connection with diphtheria, Texas fever, and tuberculosis has been of vast importance in bacteriology and public health.

Almroth Wright (1861–1947). An Irish pathologist. In 1896 he demonstrated the practicability of typhoid vaccine and aroused a new interest in the artificial production of active immunity.

G. Fernand Widal (1862–1929). A French physician. His contribution to public health is in connection with the diagnosis of typhoid fever. He demonstrated (1896) that blood serum of typhoid cases would agglutinate typhoid bacilli—the Widal reaction.

August von Wassermann (1866–1925). A German to whom the public health field is indebted for the development of a serological test for syphilis—the Wassermann reaction (1906). Many modifications of the test have since been made.

Fritz Schaudinn (1871–1906). A German biologist whose great contribution to medicine and public health was the demonstration (1905) of the *Treponema pallidum* as the cause of syphilis.

Wade Hampton Frost (1880–1938). An American, professor of epidemiology, the Johns Hopkins University. As Koch was the logician of bacteriology, Frost was the logician of epidemiology. His approach to problems was an exemplification of the scientific method; his writings are models of incisive thought. The influence of his teaching is world-wide.

Alexander Fleming (1881–1955). A British physician, particularly interested in research. Fleming discovered penicillin in 1928–1929. He thus established the basis for a new era in medicine, and placed humanity deeply and permanently in debt to him. Under the impetus of this discovery, other workers developed additional antibiotics and solved the problem of mass production of these materials.

Jonas E. Salk (1914–   ). A young American virologist. Supported by research grants from the National Foundation for Infantile Paralysis, and utilizing the tissue culture technique developed by John Enders for the production of poliomyelitis virus as well as the techniques of Howard A. Howe and others for inactivation with formalin, Salk developed a successful antipoliomyelitis vaccine. In one of the most extensive, scientifically controlled field trials ever undertaken, this vaccine, in 1954, was demonstrated to be effective in the prevention of paralytic disease due to poliomyelitis virus.

Othmar Zeidler. A German student of chemistry. In 1874 Zeidler synthesized dichlorodiphenyltrichloroethane, commonly known as DDT. However, this was just another interesting organic chemical until 1939, when the Swiss firm of J. R. Geigy tested it and many other compounds for mothproofing ability. This chemical showed unusual insecticidal properties, and a sample was sent to the U.S. Bureau of Entomology and Plant Quarantine where E. F. Knipling demonstrated its remarkable properties in the destruction of lice. DDT has become recognized as the most potent weapon available to man in the eradication of many insect-borne diseases, particularly louse-borne typhus and malaria.

Nursing as a Development in the Public Health Field. Extremely important among those measures inaugurated for the betterment of community health is public health nursing. This professional service has come to be an essential in the modern public health program. Its development has been evolutionary, probably the result of a number of different forces. The most influential of these perhaps were: (1) the more or less neighborly and ancient practice of visting the sick, (2) sick visitation as a part of the work of monasteries and religious orders, (3) as a form of charity, (4) as a business, closely related to midwifery, (5) the development of the hospital trained nurse, (6) the obvious need in the home for more skillful service and better instruction than could be furnished by lay workers, and (7) the adaptation of the trained nurse to the various phases of public health work.

From a historical standpoint, the following are important in the development of public health nursing:

Sairy Gamp. A fictional character, thoroughly dissolute, a sort of neighborhood nurse, portrayed by Charles Dickens. She was ignorant, dirty, a thief, and a drunkard. She staggered through the pages of *Martin Chuzzlewit* as an ugly index of the plight of the poor in London. It should be remembered that not only was she fictional, but a caricature. Her type was no more a nurse than is the quack healer a physician.

St. Vincent de Paul. Founded the Order of the Sisters of Charity in the seventeenth century. These Sisters were organized for visiting the homes of the sick. They had more liberty of movement than the nuns, who were cloistered.

Florence Nightingale. The outstanding individual in the history of nursing. Aside from the very practical work which she did, it was she who insisted upon and gained public recognition of the fact that nursing required special training and experience. Modern conception of nursing rests largely upon the foundation laid by Florence Nightingale.

Fliedner of Kaiserswerth. A Lutheran pastor who organized a school for deaconesses at Kaiserswerth, Germany, in 1836. Here definite training and experience in nursing were given, and here, too, Florence Nightingale attended and gained inspiration.

William Rathbone. An Englishman who founded in Liverpool, in 1859, the first district nursing association.

Among the important organizations which tended to extend nursing on a community basis were these:

1. *The Order of St. John of Jerusalem.* This military nursing order came into existence in the eleventh century, incident to the Crusades. In 1874 the Order undertook an investigation of district nursing in England. The facts obtained led to the conclusion that the existing situation was deplorable in every way, and, in turn, definite provisions were made for a better type of district nursing.

2. *The Queen's Institute, in London.* Founded by Queen Victoria in 1887, the institute laid down strict requirements for visiting nursing; gave special training to qualified graduate nurses, and extended its work and influence throughout the British Empire.

3. *The Ladies Benevolent Society of Charleston, South Carolina.* Founded in 1813, this was perhaps the first organized secular effort to provide for visitation of the sick. Members of the society made regular visits to the sick poor and provided nurses when it appeared necessary.

4. *The New York City Mission.* This organization was the first (1877) in this country which systematically provided trained nurses for home care of the sick poor.

Material for these summaries was obtained largely from Mary S. Gardner's *Public Health Nursing.* *

Other Professions from Which Public Health Draws. From the preceding discussions it is obvious that public health work draws from the general field of science, from medicine and its subsidiary techniques, from dentistry, and from nursing.

Engineers make their contribution in sanitation: in water supplies, sewage disposal, those parts of milk control which involve mechanical apparatus, in drainage for mosquito eradication, in industrial hygiene, in housing, heating, ventilation, and lighting. Veterinarians come into the public health picture particularly in connection with those diseases of animals which may affect man: especially in bovine tuberculosis, brucellosis, rabies, anthrax, glanders, tularemia; and in the inspection of foods derived from meat. Upon the entomologist public health practice is dependent for expert knowledge as to the natural history of disease-bearing insects: lice, fleas, flies, ticks, mosquitoes. From mathematics are drawn formulas and procedures useful in testing the soundness of hypotheses which seem to interpret numerical data. To all these, and in special circumstances to others, public health turns for guidance and assistance. But as said above, it is with the field of medicine that hygiene is most closely allied. Between the two there are a number of similar objectives so closely alike that there is no clearly defined dividing line; and because of this zone of mutual responsibility, there is some confusion and occasionally conflict.

The Characteristics or Qualities of Problems Which Are of Public Health Significance. Opinions and conclusions as to the scope of the public health field are undergoing change. There are as many perspectives as there are interests concerned, and one's opinion is almost inevitably influenced by his own particular interests and background. Bearing in mind that the writers are necessarily influenced by such factors, the following definition may be considered: *A health problem becomes a public responsibility if or when it is of such char-*

* Gardner, Mary S.: *Public Health Nursing*, 3rd ed. The Macmillan Company, New York, 1936.

acter or extent as to be amenable to solution only through system-
atized social action. Its relative importance varies with the hazard
to the population exposed. This hazard may be qualitative, in terms
of disability or death; quantitative, in terms of proportion of popula-
tion affected; it may be actual or potential.

It will be noted that the definition given above sets forth what
constitutes a public health problem. It is *not* a definition of "public
health." It is necessary, however, to define the latter term, but it is
not easy. Many persons tend to use the phrases "public health" and
"preventive medicine" as synonyms. They consider the *prevention* of
disease as the sole responsibility of the health department, disavow-
ing any official interest in "curative medicine." Thus, the operation
of a venereal disease clinic or a tuberculosis clinic is explained as but
a means of discovering and eliminating foci of these diseases and so
preventing their transmission to others.

It is obvious, of course, that a part of public health practice is
preventive in character, but it is also apparent that prevention forms
no small part of the service rendered by the private physician to his
private patient: in pediatrics, in obstetrics, in nutrition, in vaccination against one disease or another. It would not, therefore, be sound
either in theory or practice to consider that all preventive work done
is a part of public health work. Further, public health is concerned
not only with prevention of disease but with any health hazard or
disability which threatens or affects any considerable proportion of
the public. These considerations, it would seem, lead logically to the
following definitions of preventive medicine and public health.

Preventive medicine may be regarded as that body of knowledge
and those practices that contribute to the maintenance of health and
the prevention of disease either in the individual or the aggregate.

Public health may be regarded as that body of knowledge and
those practices that contribute to health in the aggregate either
through preventive or curative measures, or both.

This does not mean that all problems of public health must necessarily be handled by a public health agency as such. In the United
States in recent years the voluntary health movement has developed
very markedly, and the voluntary health agencies have assumed

In a narrower sense, the term "vital statistics" refers to statistics of (1) births, (2) deaths, (3) population. Statistics of sickness in the population are frequently classified separately as "morbidity statistics." Although some health departments procure information as to numbers of marriages, such figures are seldom subjected to critical analysis. Divorce statistics have heretofore been considered more by social agencies than by health departments, but the proposed Uniform Vital Statistics Law includes the collection and analysis of statistics on marriage and divorce as essential in public health practice. Federal vital statistics now contain such data.

It is upon reports of physicians, midwives, undertakers, and, occasionally, others that tables of births and deaths are based. These figures, when expressed in proportion to the number of persons (population) residing in the area in which these events occurred, are designated "rates." See pages 36 and 37.

Requirements as to Reports of Births and Deaths. Each state has a law requiring, in general, the following:

Births. That any physician or midwife who attends a birth shall report it to an official, commonly called a "registrar." Ordinarily, the registrar has an office in the health department, although in rural areas, the storekeeper, a schoolteacher, or some other responsible person may serve as registrar. If a birth occurs without either doctor or midwife present, the head of the family is usually the one responsible for reporting.

Deaths. If his patient dies, the doctor must give a certificate as to *cause of death,* date of death, etc. With this certificate, the undertaker obtains from the local registrar a burial permit. If no physician was in attendance, the death certificate may, in most places, be signed by the health officer. In any situation where death was from accident or violence, or if there is reason to suspect foul play, only the coroner or medical examiner may sign the death certificate. He may insist upon an autopsy or a coroner's jury. The place and function of the coroner vary from state to state and from county to county. The office is a political one.

The Federal Government and Vital Statistics. All vital statistic laws requiring reporting of births and deaths are *state* laws, and the federal government exercises no direct authority in this connection. In other words, if a physician failed or refused to report births or deaths, the federal government would have no power to take legal action against him. The state has such authority, but the extent to which it is used varies from state to state, and varies to some extent in different places in the same state. The federal government, however, does participate in the collection and utilization of vital statistics, along the following lines:

1. Through the Bureau of the Census, Department of Commerce, which makes a nationwide census of population and publishes results every 10 years.

2. Through the National Office of Vital Statistics, U.S. Public Health Service, which collects from the various states transcripts of each birth and death certificate and publishes summaries of these facts in a volume entitled *Vital Statistics of the United States*. The U.S. Public Health Service also collects from the states weekly reports of the more important communicable diseases and publishes these findings from time to time.

Population Data. The federal censuses are made by listing certain information for every person resident in the United States at a given time. The first census was taken in 1790, and there has been one each 10 years since that time. Information is obtained by "enumerators" who visit every home and obtain records as to name, age, sex, occupation, color, nativity, etc., of each inhabitant. Other important economic and sociological data are obtained at the same time.

Data obtained in the census are tabulated, separated, and assembled in such a way that anyone interested may find details as to population for the country as a whole or for any particular place. One can obtain information as to numbers of males, numbers of females, whites, nonwhites, foreign-born, native-born, numbers in each age group and separated by age and sex, numbers engaged in the various occupations, etc. All of this information is published by the Bureau of the Census as quickly as possible after the completion of each census: about two or three years.

Population data obtained by censuses are of great importance in public health, because in drawing conclusions as to the significance of the number of births, deaths, or communicable diseases it is absolutely essential that one have knowledge as to the size and make-up of the population under consideration. Example: A hundred deaths a year from tuberculosis would be far more significant in a city of 50,000 population than in one with 200,000; a greater number of deaths per year would be expected in a place with a large proportion of Negroes than in practically an all-white population of the same size. In a community where males largely predominate, fewer births would be expected than if the sexes were fairly evenly balanced. Without known populations, it is not practicable to compare public health problems in various places, or in the same place from year to year.

Libraries contain the census reports, and hospitals, health departments, similar agencies, and interested individuals may obtain copies free or for a minimum charge. For purposes of reference, certain population data, for the United States, are given in Table 1.

TABLE 1

POPULATION OF THE UNITED STATES (ESTIMATED), 1957,* SEPARATED AS TO SEX, AND BY WHITE, NONWHITE†

Race	Total	Male	%	Female	%
All races	171,229,000	84,858,000	49.56	86,371,000	50.44
White	152,464,000	75,688,000	49.64	76,776,000	50.36
Nonwhite	18,765,000	9,170,000	48.87	9,595,000	51.13

* It should be noted that the figures here used are estimates. In this table and in others where data are based upon estimated population, due precaution should be observed before conclusions are drawn. Estimates of population, made toward the latter part of an intercensal period, are particularly subject to error. In this case data of the 1960 census should be consulted as soon as possible.

† U.S. Bureau of the Census, Current Population Reports, Population Estimates. Series P-25, No. 170, December 18, 1957.

The Estimation of Populations between Census Years. Health departments each year study the significance of the number of births and deaths of the previous 12 months in relation to the total population, and by age, sex, color, and in some instances by other subdivisions. In addition, it is necessary in studying mortality to consider the causes from which deaths occurred. In such studies one must know the size and character of the population in which the various events took place. Population, however, is ordinarily obtained by a census every 10 years,* and if one wished to study the vital statistics of 1951 or 1952 it would be necessary to estimate the population for the inter-censal year in question. There are two methods commonly employed in these estimations of population.

The Census Method. The number in a population at any given time is obviously the net result of increases by births and immigration, minus the decreases from deaths and emigration. It is, therefore, theoretically possible to estimate population by adding to the last census figure the increases and subtracting the decreases which occurred since that census.

For the United States, data on incoming immigrants are available, and emigration is somewhat incidental and temporary; and while there are some deficiencies in birth and death reporting, the addition and subtraction of these increases and decreases in a given period plus the population at the beginning of that period will give an approximate figure as to the population of the nation. This method of calculation may be used for the whole country; and some of the individual states, which believe that their experience is about the same as for the nation, apply the per cent of increase since the last census (calculated for continental United States) to the last census of the state. It must be borne in mind, however, that this "census method" may not be applied safely in small localities, not only because there is no record of how many new people have come in and how many have left, but also because the ratio of births to deaths and the completeness of reporting in that particular place may be quite unusual. If one leaves New York City to spend his old age in Florida, there is no one to whom, under the law, he must report either his going or his coming; and it may not be assumed that arrivals and departures will offset each other: they may or may not.

Arithmetic Method. This method of estimating population in inter-censal years is the one usually followed for small population units.

---

* The last three censuses of the United States were taken as of April 1, 1930, 1940, and 1950. Great Britain and its associated countries generally use the first year in the decade—1931, 1941, 1951.

Essentially what one does is to subtract, from the population figure obtained at the last census, the population figure obtained by the census preceding the last one. The figure obtained represents the population increase or decrease in that 10–year period. This is divided by 10 in order to obtain the average increase or decrease per year. Thus, if one wishes to find the population of 1952, he would proceed as indicated above, and would multiply the average increase per year between 1940 and 1950 by 2 and add this to the 1950 population figure.

For example, a given city, as of April 1, 1940, had a population of 50,000. In 1950, as of April first, the population was 60,000. What is the population as of April 1, 1952? It is apparent here that in the 10 years between 1940 and 1950 the population increased by 10,000, or at the rate of 1000 per year. Assuming that this same increase of 1000 per year continued evenly from 1950, the 1952 population would be 60,000 plus 2000.

For public health purposes the midyear population, that is, population as of July first, is usually calculated. In the above example, because the 1950 census was taken as of April first, it would be necessary to include the 3 months from April 1, 1952, to July 1, 1952. Thus, 250 (a fourth of a year and a fourth of the yearly increase) would have to be added to obtain the midyear population of 1952.

Geometric Method. A third method of estimating population in intercensal years is by the geometric method. This procedure gives recognition to the fact that population increase or decrease does not necessarily proceed arithmetically, but, as in compound interest, the increase itself increases. Those particularly interested, who have a table of logarithms at hand, may find the formula for this calculation in any good book on algebra or in standard statistical texts.

The Registration Areas of the Federal Government. In publications relating to vital statistics, one frequently encounters references to the "Registration Area for Births" and the "Registration Area for Deaths." Both of these, since 1933, have included all states in the Union, and are, therefore, coterminous. The purpose of the registration areas is to provide the federal government with a mechanism for collecting, through the several states, data reflecting the occurrence of births and deaths. Behind the idea of these areas, too, was the hope that by setting high standards for definiteness, completeness, and promptness of reporting, state and local performance would be improved. These goals have been partially but not completely attained. In most urban areas, reporting of both births and deaths is good. In rural areas, reporting of deaths is fairly good, but also, in many of them, birth reporting is not all that could be desired. As a result of this, an individual desiring to obtain a certified copy of a birth certificate sometimes finds that his or her birth is not a matter of record.

Annual collection of birth statistics was authorized by the federal government in 1902, but the Birth Registration Area was not established until 1915. To qualify for recognition in this area a state must have sound and workable laws for the collection of records of births, and must be able to prove the collection of reports of at least 90 per cent of all births occurring. The area at first contained only 10 states and the District of Columbia.

Every state in the Birth Registration Area* sends to the National Office of Vital Statistics, U.S. Public Health Service, a transcript or microfilm of each birth certificate received. On the basis of these reports the U.S. Public Health Service publishes birth statistics annually. The volume formerly carried the title, *Birth, Stillbirth and Infant Mortality Statistics for the Birth Registration Area of the United States*. At present, data on births are published in the volume, *Vital Statistics of the United States*.

The Registration Area for Deaths was provided for in 1880 by the federal Bureau of the Census, but it was not until 1902 that data as to deaths were obtained currently for each year. At first it contained but few states and certain selected cities, where registration of deaths was reasonably complete.

To be admitted into or remain in the Registration Area for Deaths* a state must have had sound and workable vital statistics laws and be able to prove registration of at least 90 per cent of deaths. Tests and studies as to completeness of reporting are made by officials of the National Office of Vital Statistics.

* Since all the states are now included in what were originally designated as registration areas, the term is of academic interest, except in the use of U.S. data representing vital statistics before 1933. Data on Hawaii, Puerto Rico, and the Virgin Islands are carried as supplements to *Vital Statistics of the United States*.

Transcripts or microfilms of all death certificates received in the states are forwarded to the National Office of Vital Statistics. On the basis of these reports this office of the U.S. Public Health Service publishes death statistics annually. The volume formerly carried the title, *Mortality Statistics.* At present they are to be found in *Vital Statistics of the United States.*

The "Model Law" for Vital Statistics. This is not really a law, but is a pattern recommended to states for their adoption in vital statistics laws. It was developed about 1907 with the endorsement of practically all agencies and organizations interested in this matter. The general requirements of the "Model Law" are contained in the vital statistics laws of most of the states, with some changes in provisions and phraseology to meet local needs and customs. Experience, however, indicates that this is not enough. New demands arising from the complex and changing social structure of the nation make it desirable to bring up to date the requirements and provisions of the vital statistics laws of the 49 states. To meet this need, the Bureau of the Census, in 1941, published an argument for, and the outline of, a proposed new model "Act for Vital Statistics," which it hoped would be submitted to the several state legislatures through proper channels. The proposed act would carefully safeguard the confidential aspects of birth certificates (illegitimacy, adoption), providing such information only on court order. It would further provide for delayed registration of births and for collection and preservation of records of marriages, divorces, and annulment of marriages. Of no small importance, too, the new model law would ensure the status and value of vital statistics records in legal matters. Some of the states have incorporated these new proposals into their respective laws, but the change is only gradual.

The Essentials in a Good Vital Statistics Law. Experience in the collection of reports of births and deaths indicates that the following provisions are essential:

1. That all births and deaths shall be reported by the physician in attendance (or by midwife, in case of births).
2. That these reports be made promptly to local officials designated to receive them.

3. That these local officials be required to transmit the original certificates to the state or local department of health, keeping a copy locally. As an exception, a large city may keep the originals and forward copies.

4. That death certificates contain reasonably complete information as to the age, sex, race, nativity, occupation of the deceased, with statement as to place and date of burial.

5. That physicians certify as to cause of death, length of illness, length of attendance, date physician last saw person alive, and date of death.

6. That no body may be interred, transported, or otherwise disposed of without a permit for disposal (burial, cremation, other disposal, transportation).

7. That local registrars (persons authorized to carry out the details of the law) be forbidden to issue such a disposal permit unless a properly executed death certificate be furnished them.

8. That no sexton or manager of a cemetery permit any burial or cremation unless the undertaker presents a properly signed burial permit.

9. That coffin manufacturers and dealers report all sales of coffins.

10. That details as to parentage, sex, color, date and place of birth be included in all birth reports.

11. That death and birth certificates and documents as to marital status be carefully filed, indexed, and preserved in fireproof vaults.

12. That definite provision be made for the official and permanent registration of records of births which should have been reported but were not—delayed registration of births.

13. That persons proven guilty of violating the law be subject to penalty.

The Usual Sequence of Events in the Preparation and Handling of a Death Certificate. The step-by-step procedure is generally as follows:

1. The patient dies, and an undertaker is called.

2. The undertaker fills in that part of the death certificate dealing with age, sex, race, place of birth, occupation, place of death, place for

burial, and similar data, on the basis of information given by some-one, usually a member of the family, who has had close association with the deceased.

3. The undertaker then presents the certificate to the physician concerned, who fills in data as to length of illness, length of time he attended, the date he last saw patient alive, the date and hour of death, and cause of death.

4. The undertaker then presents the completed certificate to a registrar of vital statistics who, if everything is in order, issues a burial or transportation permit. In most places the burial permit is endorsed by the sexton of the cemetery and returned to the vital statistics registrar, after the burial has taken place.

5. The death certificate goes from the local registrar to the state health department, preferably through the local health department, where it is examined for completeness, and, in accordance with the *International Statistical Classification of Diseases, Injuries, and Causes of Death,* the number on the list corresponding to the cause of death as set forth is entered on the certificate.

6. The certificate is filed in the state health department, with necessary indexing for future reference.

7. Copies or microfilms of certificates are made and forwarded to the National Office of Vital Statistics. (For this the federal government pays a small fee to offset costs to states.)

8. In future study of certificates, data from death certificates are separated as to cause, age, sex, race, place of death, place of usual residence, occupation; and from these figures and from combinations of them, tables and graphs are made.

9. Most state and city health departments prepare a "punch card" for each certificate so that all separations and counts are done mechanically, by placing the punch cards in a tabulating machine.

Stillbirths. There does not exist among the several states any commonly accepted definition of stillbirths. In one state the criterion is "no evidence of life after birth." In another, "no evidence of life after 28th week of gestation," and in still another, "no pulmonary respiration after 28th week of gestation." There is a general tendency, however, to center on the criterion, "no evidence of life after 5th month." The federal Bureau of the Census and the American Public Health Association some years ago adopted the following definition of still-birth: "A fetus showing no evidence of life after complete birth (no action of heart, breathing, or movement of voluntary muscle), if the 20th week of gestation has been reached, should be registered as a stillbirth."

The League of Nations and the International Institute of Statistics recommended the following definition: "A dead-birth (stillbirth) is the birth of a (viable) foetus, after at least 28 weeks pregnancy, in which pulmonary respiration does not occur; such a foetus may die either: (a) before, (b) during or (c) after birth, but before it has breathed."

Another aspect in the use and interpretation of the term "stillbirths" is to be noted. This term, as ordinarily defined, is concerned with an infant who had advanced sufficiently in development to have lived on being born, but was dead. However, from the standpoint of what has been called "pregnancy wastage," it is also important to know the number or per cent of pregnancies in which the fetus died or was ex-pelled before extrauterine survival is possible. As a contribution to at-taining such knowledge, the World Health Organization has sug-gested gathering data on fetal deaths, on a form that perhaps would replace the stillbirth report. Under this recommendation, the term "fetal death" would replace the term "stillbirth," and data would be separated into (1) those of less than 20 weeks of gestation, (2) those of 20 weeks and more of gestation, but less than 28 weeks, (3) those of 28 weeks and more of gestation.

Although it is obviously desirable that there be a commonly ob-served definition of fetal deaths or stillbirths among the different states and internationally, it must be remembered that in the United States the acceptance or rejection of such a definition is a state prerogative. It is not something that may be brought about overnight by a federal law. But there is, among the state health authorities, a strong tendency to accept federal leadership directed toward coordi-nation of procedures in vital statistics and in the establishment of uniform definitions. It seems likely, therefore, that as time passes, a greater proportion of the states will accept the federal definition of stillbirth. The development of a common international definition of stillbirth might come about suddenly or may remain in abeyance indefinitely.

The forms used in reporting stillbirths in the several states also lack uniformity. The U.S. Public Health Service recommends that for purposes of reporting stillbirths a special standard certificate of stillbirth be used. Heretofore the practice in many states has been to issue a birth certificate and, at the same time, a death certificate. While the greater number of state health authorities agree that the special certificate of stillbirth is preferable to the utilization of separate birth and death certificates in stillbirths, comparatively few of the states have adopted the special form. Extensive adoption is inhibited to some extent by the fact that a change in procedure in the individual state would require that the vital statistics law be resubmitted to the legislature for amendment. Ordinarily this takes some time.

Nomenclature as to Causes of Death. It is quite obvious that it would be possible to use thousands of terms to describe causes of death. It is also apparent that two persons, or a hundred, might use different terminology to describe the same cause or, in some instances, similar terms to describe different causes. What is now called intestinal obstruction once had the homely title "twisting of the guts"; and suicide was literally translated and recorded as "self-murder." Even now, some physicians use such vague terms as "worn out," "weakness," "heart stopped beating." When it is further realized that, in various countries, practitioners are reporting causes of death in that country's language and idiom, it needs no argument to prove the desirability of some standard international nomenclature. This need is met to as great an extent as is immediately practicable by an international list of causes of death. This in the United States was formerly published by the Bureau of the Census, Department of Commerce, under the title, *Manual of the International List of Causes of Death and Joint Causes of Death*. It is now published by the World

Health Organization, under the title (so far as concerns English-speaking nations), *International Statistical Classification of Diseases, Injuries, and Causes of Death.*

This manual is designed to establish international usage of comparable terms and is used routinely by health departments. The list is revised every 10 years through an international congress. A smaller booklet entitled *Physicians' Handbook on Birth and Death Registration* is also published in the United States. Most physicians may obtain this without cost. Anyone may obtain it from the Superintendent of Documents, Washington, D.C., for a small amount.

It must be borne in mind that not infrequently there are elements of error in deciding, in a given instance, what disease caused death. These arise because of: (1) limitations of medical science; facilities for diagnosis are not infallible as regards accuracy or comprehensiveness; (2) inevitable errors of judgment on the part of the physician in attendance; these vary with his competence and opportunity for study of the case; (3) deaths occurring without medical attendance and sudden deaths where, without autopsy, a probable cause of death is assigned; (4) occasional instances when the physician feels that he must protect the family of the deceased from stigma, and may avoid certifying that death was due to syphilis, cancer, tuberculosis, etc. Because of these various factors, many of which influence or limit the decision of the attending physician in ascribing death as due to this cause or that, data based upon autopsy findings furnish much more exact information than figures that arise from clinical judgment.

The Usual Sequence of Events from the Time a Birth Certificate Is Made Out by a Physician to the Time When It Is Permanently Filed. The step-by-step procedure is generally as follows:

1. The physician mails the certificate, usually within 10 days, to the local registrar.

2. The local registrar copies, retains copy, and sends original to the state health department, preferably through the local health department. As an exception, a large city may keep the originals and forward copies.

3. The certificate is checked for completeness in the local and state departments of health.

4. If incomplete in any detail, the local health department, or the state health department if the certificate is sent there directly by the local registrar, sends an inquiry blank to the physician, asking for the missing information.

5. This supplementary information is added to the original certificate, but in such a way as to show that it was added subsequent to the time the certificate was originally filed.

6. In some states or localities parents are furnished with a formal, written statement that the birth of the child has been recorded in the state or local health department. This document is not, however, a certified copy of the birth certificate.

7. Copies or microfilms of certificates are made and forwarded to the National Office of Vital Statistics. (For this the federal government pays a small fee to offset costs to states.)

8. The original birth certificate is bound into a volume, indexed, and stored in a fireproof vault in the state health department.

9. Certificates are subsequently used for statistical study.

The "Certified Copy" of a Birth or of a Death Certificate. This is an exact copy of the original certificate, properly signed, and stamped with the seal of the state. As a rule, only a state health department may issue a certified copy of a birth or death certificate, as this usually is the place where the original certificate is filed. A true certified copy cannot be made from a copy of the original.

The Value of Birth and Death Certificates. Aside from furnishing necessary and valuable material for statistical study, as indicated above and presented in more detail below, birth and death certificates are of considerable value to those concerned or their families.

Some of the more important values of the birth certificate are the following:

1. To establish record of parentage, race, and the right to inheritance.

2. To establish proof of age in connection with school attendance, work, voting, military service, public office, marriage, pension.

3. To establish proof of citizenship, passports, right to hold office, to receive public benefits, to vote, to certain types of employment.

The death certificate is of importance on the following counts:

1. It is evidence of the fact that death did occur on a given date, from a given cause, in given circumstances, at a given place.

2. It is necessary in connection with insurance policies and similar benefits.

3. It is of interest for future reference as to descent.

Delayed Registration of Births. As previously indicated, the reporting of births is quite poor in some places and nowhere is it perfect as regards accuracy, promptness, and completeness. In the best circumstances there will be errors, delays, and occasionally omissions. As a result, an individual having reason to obtain a copy of his birth certificate may find that the record of his birth is not officially registered in the archives of his community or state. Heretofore in such circumstances, state and city departments of vital statistics have tended to be quite passive. If a given birth was not recorded it was no affair of theirs; and state laws had made but little provision for an individual to register his birth on finding that it was not previously recorded. A person in need of proving age, parentage, and citizenship then had to gather such substantiating documents as the particular agency he was dealing with might demand. He might be able to obtain a statement from the physician who was present at birth, or submit a certified copy of entry in the family Bible, or of a baptismal record, or get a photostatic copy of an earlier census of his household.

None of these things was completely satisfactory, and although they might meet the particular needs of the moment they did not, as a rule, eventuate in a final, permanent, and official registration of the record of birth, from which the individual might at any time in the future obtain a certified copy of birth certificate.

In recent years, demands for substantial data as to age, parentage, and place of birth have become more exacting, and an increasing number of individuals have found need of proof as to these data. As a result, many state health departments have undertaken to provide a means for delayed registration of births, setting forth exactly the procedure to be followed, and stating specifically what will and what will not be considered satisfactory evidence. These procedures and requirements will vary from state to state, as it is the individual state and not the federal government which enacts legislation or promulgates regulations in relation to vital statistics.

But the federal Bureau of the Census, through its division of Vital Statistics, made an important contribution in this connection when in April, 1941, it recommended, to the several states, procedures for registration of delayed certificates of birth and for standards to be observed. This document recommended that births registered after age 4 be considered as delayed in registration; that, in establishing the facts of birth in delayed registration, genuine documentary evidence be required in support of statements as to age, birthplace, and parentage; that these items must each be proved by two records established before the individual became 4 years of age or by three records executed after that age. In the latter case the three substantiating records must themselves have been executed at least 5 years previously.

Thus, an individual of 25 attempting to establish facts of birth could not use as evidence records that were established after he became 20 years of age. The Bureau of the Census sets forth the type of evidence recommended as acceptable in order of preference. This is presented in detail, under nine general headings, the first of which is the baptismal, cradle roll, or other church record, the last an affidavit from a person who presumably knows and remembers the date, place of birth, and parentage of the individual concerned. Between these two extremes in value as evidence are listed seven other kinds of documents which might also be submitted. The Bureau of the Census further recommended, and some states have adopted, a uniform "delayed certificate of birth" form which once having been registered could serve as a basis for further certified copies.

The Presentation of Vital Statistics. Such data are most frequently presented as, or are converted into, "rates": birth rates; death rates; death rates from particular causes, such as tuberculosis, diphtheria, cancer, heart disease; death rates of persons in various age groups; death rates for males or females, for whites or Negroes; death rates by occupation; and combinations of these various elements, such as death rate of children under three years of age from diphtheria, or of white females over 50 from cancer, or unskilled laborers from tuberculosis.

In vital statistics, the term *rate* means the number of times an event occurs in proportion to a given number of persons, in a given time (usually one year). If in a village with 500 persons there were 6 deaths in 1952, the rate would be 12 per 1000 population; if, in a state with 3,000,000 population, there were 30,000 deaths, the rate would be 10 per 1000 persons.

Rates are used in vital statistics in order to provide a common denominator for populations of various sizes. If they were not used, it would be difficult to compare the inroads of disease and death or the proportion of the births of one population with another, or in the same area in succeeding years. Thus, to say that one city had 8000 deaths in 1950 and that another had 5500 deaths in the same year does not convey much information unless the population of each is known. With the knowledge that the first city had a population of 700,000 and the second 600,000, it is easy to calculate for the former a rate of 11.4 deaths per 1000 population, and for the latter a rate of 9.2 deaths per 1000 persons.

The Conventional Bases Used in Expressing Rates. One does not need to remember verbatim definitions of the various rates used in vital statistics. Instead, the principle involved and the method of derivation should be understood clearly, and then there is no longer a need of definitions. However, in the interest of uniformity and precision the following definitions, modified from a publication of the Bureau of the Census, are presented. It will be noted that the bases, or denominators, from which the different rates are established are not necessarily the same, either in size or character.

Crude Birth Rate. The number of live births reported in the calendar year per 1000 actual or estimated population at the middle of the year.

Crude Death Rate. The number of deaths reported in the calendar year per 1000 actual or estimated population at the middle of the year.

Stillbirth (or Fetal Death) Ratio. The number of stillbirths or fetal deaths per 1000 live births.

Age-specific Birth Rate. The number of births to women in a specified age group per 1000 women in the same specified age group of the population. (For certain purposes, the number of married women in each age group is used, instead of the total number of women.)

Age-specific Death Rate. The number of deaths in a specified age group per 1000 population in the same specified age group.

Specific-cause-of-death Rate. The number of deaths from a specific disease (e.g., measles, pneumonia, etc.) per 100,000 population.

Maternal Mortality Rate. The number of deaths from deliveries and complications of pregnancy, childbirth, and the puerperum, per 10,000 live births. (In some instances, "total births," including stillbirths, are used as a base, rather than "live births." However, because of variations in definitions of stillbirths and incompleteness with which they are reported, the number of live births is the commonly accepted base.)

Infant Mortality Rate. The number of deaths of infants under 1 year of age per 1000 live births.

Neonatal Mortality Rate. The number of deaths of infants under 28 days of age per 1000 live births.

Morbidity Rate. The number of reported cases of a given disease (e.g., tuberculosis, cancer, etc.) per 100,000 population.

Case Fatality Ratio. The number of deaths ascribed to a specified disease or condition per 100 reported cases of the same disease or condition.

Birth-death Ratio. The number of live births per 100 deaths in a specified population.

The Crude or General Death Rate and Its Calculation. The general death rate portrays the total number of deaths from all causes and at all ages, both sexes and including all races, per 1000 population per year. Example: A county of 60,000 population had 720 deaths in 1950. To calculate the rate, one may conveniently fall back upon ratio and proportion, of arithmetic days, using the following formula:

$$720 : 60,000 = x : 1000$$

In such an equation the product of the means (the middle figures, 60,000 and x) is equal to the product of the extremes (the outside figures, 720 and 1000). Then $60,000x = 720,000$. Divide to find the value of x.

$$60,000 \overline{)\ 720,000\ (\ 12}$$
$$\underline{600\ 00}$$
$$120\ 000$$
$$\underline{120\ 000}$$
$$x = 12$$

The general death rate, therefore, would be 12 deaths per 1000 population.

A shorter way of calculating this rate, and others, is to multiply the number of deaths by 1000 or whatever population basis is used for the rate, and divide by the total population figure, somewhat as would be done in estimating per cent relationship between two numbers. Such a procedure, shown by the formula below, is the method conventionally followed:

$$\frac{\text{Number of deaths } (720)}{\text{Number in population } (60,000)} \times 1000 = 12 \text{ (rate per 1000)}$$

The general death rate (provisional) for the United States in 1950 was 9.6 deaths per 1000 population.

Caution as to Drawing Conclusions from General Rates. Earlier in this chapter, it was indicated that in comparing two groups of figures, one must be certain that they arise from truly similar groups. The observation of this precaution is so important that it is here restated. For instance, it may be found that in City A the mortality rate is 9 per 1000, and in City B, 14 per 1000. Before one would be justified in assuming that the conditions in B are much worse than A, many factors would have to be determined.

Assuming completeness of reporting in each city, some of the more important considerations would be these: Are the age constitutions of the populations of Cities A and B comparable, or does one contain a greater proportion of older persons than the other; is the white-nonwhite proportion similar in the two cities, or does the nonwhite reach a relatively high proportion in one of them; do the health authorities of both cities scrutinize death certificates to be sure that a death which occurred in the city is the death of a resident, and similarly does each receive, and charge against the city, deaths of residents which occurred away from home; is one a hospital center or a sanatorium town and the other not, etc.

The higher death rate of City B might well be due to one of the more important of these factors or to a combination of them, and the death rate there when properly adjusted may be, in fact, no greater than is the case in City A. Further, if one were contemplating a public health program it would be vitally important to determine the causes of death in each city, and the circumstances in which these individual causes are operating at a high or low rate; at what ages, in which sex, and by color, occupation, economic situation, residence, season, etc. A general or crude rate, then, is only the roughest sort of index. Such rates must be broken down if one is to obtain a true insight into the dynamics of health and disease.

The 10 more important causes of death in the United States, with death rates, 1956, are shown in Table 2.

TABLE 2

THE 10 DISEASES PRODUCING THE GREATEST NUMBER OF DEATHS,
UNITED STATES, 1956*

Cause of Death	Number of Deaths per 100,000 Population
Diseases of the heart (410–443)†	360.5
Malignant neoplasms (140–205)	147.9
Vascular lesions affecting central nervous system (330–334)	106.3
Accidents (E800–E962)	56.7
Certain diseases of early infancy (760–776)	38.6
Influenza and pneumonia (480–493)	28.2
General arteriosclerosis (450)	19.1
Diabetes mellitus (260)	15.7
Congenital malformations (750–759)	12.6
Cirrhosis of liver (581)	10.7

* National Office of Vital Statistics: *Vital Statistics of the United States*, 1956. Government Printing Office, Washington, D.C., 1958.

† The numbers in parentheses refer to the classification in the 1955 revision of the *Manual of the International Statistical Classification of Diseases, Injuries, and Causes of Death*. World Health Organization, Geneva, Switzerland, 1957.

Deaths by Age and Sex. Tables 3 and 4 give an idea of the distribution of deaths by age and sex. It is important to avoid confusion as to what these tables mean. Table 3 indicates that of 1000 deaths at all ages what proportion of such deaths occurred in a given age group. It is not a particularly significant table, inasmuch as it does not take into account the number of persons in each age group. When compared, however, with similar tables from past years, it shows that children fill a far less proportion of coffins than formerly.

TABLE 3

DEATHS FROM ALL CAUSES (EXCLUSIVE OF FETAL DEATHS)
BY AGE AND SEX IN THE UNITED STATES, 1956*

Age	Number of Deaths per 1000 Deaths of All Ages		
	Total	Male	Female
All ages	1000	1000	1000
Under 1 year	69	70	68
1–4 years	11	10	11
5–14 years	9	10	9
15–24 years	16	19	11
25–34 years	23	25	20
35–44 years	44	47	41
45–54 years	91	102	77
55–64 years	165	185	137
65–74 years	244	253	233
75–84 years	229	204	261
85–94 years	91	69	120
95 years and over	7	5	11
Unknown ages	1	1	1

* National Office of Vital Statistics: *Vital Statistics of the United States,* 1956. Government Printing Office, Washington, D.C., 1958.

Table 4 is more significant in that it relates the number of deaths in each age group to that part of the population contained in that age group: an age-specific mortality. Thus, the number of deaths under 1 year, per 1000 population, was 29.6 in 1956. In 1900 the same rate was 164. Here it should be noted that this is not the infant mortality rate. The latter is calculated in relation to the number of live births. The particular thing that Table 4 shows more clearly

TABLE 4

DEATH RATE, BY AGE AND SEX IN THE UNITED STATES, 1956.
RATES PER 1000 POPULATION (ESTIMATED) IN EACH GROUP*

Age	Both Sexes	Male	Female
All ages	9.4	10.8	7.9
Under 1 year	29.6	33.6	25.5
1–4 years	1.1	1.2	1.0
5–14 years	0.5	0.6	0.4
15–24 years	1.1	1.6	0.7
25–34 years	1.5	1.9	1.1
35–44 years	3.0	3.7	2.3
45–54 years	7.4	9.6	51.3
55–64 years	17.5	22.1	12.2
65–74 years	39.9	49.8	31.0
75–84 years	89.4	102.3	78.4
85 years and over	189.7	193.9	186.2

* National Office of Vital Statistics: *Vital Statistics of the United States,* 1956. Government Printing Office, Washington, D.C., 1958.

than Table 3 is that age-specific death rates, after 15 years of age increase with age. Differences in death rates, specific for age and sex, also invite study. On the average, women live longer than men.

Births and Birth Rates. In 1956 in the United States, 4,163,000 live births were reported, a birth rate of 24.9 per 1000 population. Viewed over a period of years, it is to be noted that in the United States there was a fall in birth rates from 29 live births per 1000 population in 1915 to about 17 in the early 1930's. In 1941 the rate began to rise, and reached a peak of 27 in 1947. Since then it has tended to level off and in 1956 was 25 per 1000 estimated population. As a rule, birth rates rise temporarily with wars.

The nonwhite birth rate is consistently higher than that of the white. The former in the United States in 1956 was 34 per 1000 population, the latter was 24. Rural birth rates generally are higher than urban, and the lowest birth rates are ordinarily to be found in the great metropolitan areas. Other things being equal, the birth rate is higher in the poor than in the very wealthy, and, on an international basis, the so-called more highly civilized countries tend toward low or moderate birth rates.

Statistical Analysis. Previous discussion has dealt mainly with the legal and administrative requirements in the collection and processing of vital statistics. Incident to this processing, simple methods of calculation of rates, ratios, and proportions are used, and these ratios are established in more or less routine categories; rates by causes of death, or illness by age, sex, race, or by place of residence, and by combinations of these specific factors.

Quite aside from statistical material of this sort, many other data arise in public health work, and there is the opportunity or necessity to determine just what they mean. As a rule, the point to be established is whether or not a factor, *known* to be operating, is responsible for a constantly occurring result. Occasionally the problem may be the reverse of this, that is, *what* factor or factors may be responsible for an observed result, such as illness, death, or immunity. One, therefore, may start with a known factor, and, as it were, work forward, or begin with a result and work backward. In analyses of this sort there are a number of snares for the unwary and the lazy-minded. One such pitfall is the observation of association of some factor with an observed result. For example, before typhoid fever came under control, in many communities a good case could be made on the basis of association for straw hats as a cause of that disease. The seasonal distribution of typhoid fever was such that it might have been observed that cases began to occur each year shortly after people began wearing straw hats; and when straw hats were put into storage for the winter, cases of typhoid fever became infrequent. Conclusions no less fantastic than this have been drawn in grave seriousness.

A second consideration arises in deciding whether or not some particular factor, force, or element is actually responsible for an observed result. The result might be a lowered infant mortality rate. Is the child health program responsible? Or is the result due to an unrelated decrease in the number of cases of some disease? Is a recently introduced vaccine to be credited? Are the results noted due to a new form of treatment of some disease? Is the treatment really responsible for the seemingly improved situation? In such problems the first necessity is to make certain that some other factor or combination of factors has not been at work; and the second point to determine is whether or not the result is likely to have occurred by mere chance.

To resolve such questions, it has become customary to select two groups (man, monkey, or mice) as nearly alike as possible. One group is given the treatment or vaccine or some particular protection or exposure, and the other is not. In this way, in a well-planned study, the only difference in the two groups is the factor introduced in the one but not in the other. An excellent example of this approach is the nationwide study of the effect of Salk vaccine against poliomyelitis undertaken a few years ago. Thousands were studied; one group received the vaccine, another group received a placebo, that is, an injection that contained no vaccine. Neither those who gave nor those who received the injections knew whether it was vaccine or not. Those who studied the resulting data (subsequent incidence of paralytic poliomyelitis) did not know whether a given case had received the vaccine or the injection containing no vaccine. Finally, when all the results were in, the "key" to the result was taken from under seal, and the effect of the vaccine could be interpreted.

Not infrequently, the difference of results in two groups may not be great, and it is here that consideration must be given to chance as a factor. By mathematical formulas one may calculate how likely a given result may occur as a result of chance. Thus, if there is a roulette-like wheel, with numbers one to ten, and it is spun a hundred times, it should stop ten times on each number. Actually, this probably will not be the case. It may stop more often than that on one number, and less often on another. But if the wheel were spun a thousand times, it would even out more completely; and if it were spun a million times, there would be even less variation between the number of times it stopped on each number.

It should be noted from the above that the greater the number of observations, the more the element of chance tends to be offset. Similarly, if there appears to be a favorable result (after vaccination or a particular treatment) in thousands of instances, this is far more suggestive of the efficacy of the drug or vaccine or public health program than if there had been comparatively few observations, and mathematical formulas as to the likelihood of an occurrence by chance bear this out. These mathematical formulas fall generally

under the heading of probability determination, and they are somewhat difficult of understanding by the nonmathematically inclined
student. With the exercise of proper precautions, however, they may
be used by any intelligent and interested person. Utilizing these tests
of probability in the evaluation of data that arise in public health,
one may say that a given result or an observed difference in two
groups is unlikely to have occurred by chance, and by the use of
tables one can estimate the degree of probability of the observed
result occurring solely by chance. One may then say that the results
are "significant," and here a warning must be given. When the data
studied indicate that there is a significant difference in the findings
in two groups, this does not necessarily mean that the vaccine or
treatment tested is the factor that has brought about the difference.
The term "statistical significance" merely means that *pure chance*
has played an *insignificant* role. It is then the duty and the opportunity of the analyst of the data to determine whether his test, vaccine,
or treatment is the *sole* factor responsible. Parenthetically it should
be noted that such studies are not limited to testing vaccines or treatment. Well-planned research, with its controls and subsequent data,
may be directed to the determination of the cause of disease, such
as in the early studies of yellow fever and in the more current studies
of the epidemiology of cancer and heart disease. Studies such as the
recent investigation of the relationship of cigarette smoking to cancer of the lung illustrate clearly the need for careful statistical analysis of observed data.

It should be pointed out that not all discoveries of the relationship
of various factors to disease must wait upon formal statistical analysis. There were only crude and somewhat uncontrolled data available in the early days of evaluation of small pox vaccination. William
Budd in his classic on typhoid fever and John Snow in his studies
of cholera relied mainly upon inductive reasoning, and made valuable contributions to our knowledge of these diseases long before
adequate statistical confirmation of their observations was available.

It must be emphasized that the above discussion of statistical
analyses is necessarily superficial and oversimplified. Those interested
are referred to texts and studies particularly devoted to this subject.

Some Precautions to Be Observed in the Interpretation of Statistics. In a simple or complex manner, for this purpose or for that, almost every person draws on statistics in daily life, for statistics are essentially the summation of experience, or what the user thinks is a correct summation of experience. He may be wrong. No infallible rules can be given for avoidance of pitfalls in the interpretation of statistics, but the following considerations may help in avoiding trouble:

1. For figures to represent true happenings, the initial observation of each item or event, on which the figures are based, must have been accurately made and recorded.

2. The smaller the number in the group under observation, the less likely are the observations to be representative; and where time is an element, short-period observations are less likely to be significant than are observations over a long period of time.

3. Even though one event appears to follow another, this alone is not necessarily proof that the one caused the other.

4. Sheer chance plays a definite part in the *frequency* and *sequence* of events, and must be eliminated or given due weight as a factor.

5. Before assuming that events in a sample group (as shown by statistics) are truly representative of what happens in the whole group, in similar circumstances, one must take every precaution to ensure that the group studied is a true sample of the whole. Stated in another way, one must be sure that the group or situation studied is not a peculiar and unrepresentative one.

6. In comparing the number, sequence, and character of events that occurred in one group with similar events in another group, one must be certain that the two groups are truly comparable: Figures representing births, marriages, and deaths in 1000 persons over 60 years of age and similar figures from 1000 young adults do not arise from comparable groups.

7. One must be exceedingly careful in drawing conclusions from averages: The average figure obtained from a series of divergent numbers is not so likely to be representative of each figure in the series as would the average from a series of nearly uniform figures; and, as a

rule, the smaller the number of items on which an average is based, the less likely is the average to be truly representative.

8. In interpreting statistics, one must never allow a wish or a preformed opinion or a prejudice to lead to a conclusion—which is an easy and human thing to do.

REFERENCES

Bernstein, L., and Weatherall, M.: *Statistics for Medical and Other Biological Students.* The Williams and Wilkins Co., Baltimore, 1952.

Hill, A. Bradford: *Principles of Medical Statistics,* 6th ed. Oxford University Press, New York, 1955.

International Statistical Classification of Diseases, Injuries, and Causes of Death. World Health Organization, Geneva, Switzerland.

Mainland, D.: *Elementary Medical Statistics.* W. B. Saunders Co., Philadelphia, 1952.

Periodicals published by the U.S. Public Health Service, Children's Bureau, etc.

Publications of the Bureau of the Census.

Puffer, R. R.: *Practical Statistics in Health and Medical Work.* Blakiston Division of McGraw-Hill Book Co., Inc., New York, 1950.

Vital Statistics of the United States. Prepared annually by the National Office of Vital Statistics, U.S. Public Health Service; published by the Government Printing Office, Washington, D.C.

chapter 3

Organization and Administration of Public Health Work

WHETHER IN THE field of health or education or commerce or any other, government or stockholders must work through an organized group to which has been given definite authority, responsibility, and money for carrying on its work. The health department of a community, therefore, is nothing more nor less than government's designated instrument for performing inherent and assumed responsibility.

The amount and kind of authority vested in a health agency, and the character and extent of its undertakings, quite obviously depend upon whether or not the agency springs from a governmental or nongovernmental group. If from the former, the organization and work of the health service will reflect its national, state, or local background; if from a nongovernmental agency, the operating unit will, likewise, proceed in conformity with the policies of its parent organization.

The operating health agency must coordinate the highly specialized activities within itself, must give an accounting to citizens and the appropriating body which provides its funds, and must study needs of the health situation on the one hand and resources in authority, knowledge, and facilities on the other. Guiding each health organization is a chief administrative officer who is responsible for the organization as a whole. He or she is responsible for employment and discharge of personnel and for general procedures and relationships.

The kinds of agencies carrying on public health work may be divided into two principal categories: (1) official, (2) voluntary. In addition, no small contributions to the public health are made by agencies whose major interest is in another field: welfare, education, etc.

Official agencies are those supported and operated by the federal, state, or local government.

Voluntary agencies are those not operated or supported by the government, but which obtain funds from endowments, donations, patients' fees, campaign subscriptions, or contracts.

The way in which an official health agency approaches public health problems depends to some extent upon the agency and the problem. In ordinary circumstances the health department's work has been confined to measures designed to maintain health in the population as a mass and to prevent disease. In the past, it has generally been considered that any service rendered by a health department to an individual was only because he might spread disease to others. Thus, an individual with syphilis was treated at a health department clinic only because he might otherwise serve as a danger to his associates. A newer concept is that the individual, as a citizen, has a right to expect the government to furnish treatment if he is otherwise unable to obtain it, regardless of the character of his illness.

The official agencies are responsible for carrying out the public health laws; for enforcing quarantine; for various types of inspection, such as food, ventilation, sewage disposal; for vital statistics collection and preservation.

The United States Government in Health Matters. The authority and responsibility of the federal government in matters pertaining to the public health rest upon those parts of the Constitution which provide authority to regulate commerce with foreign nations and among the several states; authority to make treaties; unusual powers in relation to military safety; in federal districts, parks, reservations, etc.; and, finally, responsibility for the general welfare. As social, economic, and governmental problems and relationships within the

United States become more complex, there is a correspondingly increased tendency to utilize the "welfare clause" of the Constitution. Much of this country's more recent social legislation, including health provisions, rests upon this concept of national responsibility for the welfare of its citizens, regardless of the fact that an individual is the citizen of a given state.

It must be remembered, however, that the fact that a constitution indicates authority along a given line does not mean that an executive department may carry out what it considers to be the intent of the Constitution. Congress must pass laws based on authority in the Constitution, and these laws must direct that a given department shall be responsible for carrying out certain functions.

There is quite a difference in the authority and responsibility of the federal government and of state governments in health matters. The former is concerned with (1) the prevention of the importation of disease from abroad, (2) the prevention of interstate spread of disease, and (3) the maintenance of the health of the nation as a whole, in general but not in detail. A state has as its duty the prevention of diseases only within its borders and with maintenance of the health of its own citizens.

There is no national ministry or department of health in the United States government as there is in most countries. In 1879 Congress authorized the formation of a national board of health, but its functions and relationships were ill defined and, consequently, in 1893 the act creating the board was repealed. Public health activities did, however, develop in various departments of government. The Marine Hospital Service, later the U.S. Public Health Service, was established in 1798 and was for many years in the Department of the Treasury. The Children's Bureau was first organized in the Department of Labor in 1912. Less important public health activities were developed in various departments and agencies of the federal government. In 1939 there began a series of executive reorganizations which brought together in a newly created Federal Security Agency many of the health activities of the federal government together with programs for education, welfare, and social security. In 1953 there was created by an act of Congress a Department of Health,

Education, and Welfare, giving departmental status to these somewhat related activities. The Department of Health, Education, and Welfare is headed by a secretary who is a member of the President's Cabinet. He is assisted by a special assistant secretary for health matters. Within the department the principal health agency is the U.S. Public Health Service. The Public Health Service is divided into four major parts: the Office of the Surgeon General, the National Institutes of Health, the Bureau of Medical Services, and the Bureau of State Services. Each of these major administrative units is divided into subunits necessary for the performance of functions.

Quarantine stations operated by the U.S. Public Health Service are located at all the seaports and airports which have foreign commerce. Every ship, either American or foreign, coming from a foreign port must obtain health clearance from the quarantine station of the first United States port entered, as must airplanes, and the passengers of both.

While the ship lies anchored at "quarantine," passengers and crew are rapidly inspected for signs of the more dangerous diseases. As yellow fever mosquitoes and plague fleas constitute a potential menace, ships in foreign trades are fumigated at quarantine stations, from time to time as the need arises. Spraying with insecticide the interior of airplanes from tropical countries is now a regular procedure as a safeguard against infected mosquitoes.

The purpose of these stations is to prevent the importation of diseases from abroad. On the basis of past experiences there were especially stringent regulations as to (1) plague, (2) typhus fever, (3) cholera, (4) leprosy, (5) smallpox, (6) yellow fever, (7) anthrax. In recent years, the U.S. Public Health Service has effected an arrangement whereby radio reports from inbound ships, as to the state of health of passengers and crew, may be sent to the quarantine station before arrival. If the condition is found to be satisfactory, permission may be granted to come directly to dock, without waiting at the quarantine station.

Coastwise ships going from one American port to another are not ordinarily required to clear at quarantine stations.

The U.S. Public Health Service further attempts to prevent the importation of disease from abroad by maintaining officers in various foreign ports, and these physicians examine emigrants bound for this country, before embarkation at their home ports. Immigrants are again examined on landing in American ports.

The contribution of the U.S. Public Health Service in preventing the interstate spread of disease in this country is along the following lines:

1. By scientific research and the development of new knowledge in health and sanitary matters. Research is carried on directly by the service and through grants-in-aid to university workers, etc.

2. By lending specially trained personnel to states and cities, to assist them in developing and operating competent health departments.

3. By assigning experts to assist local authorities in study and control of epidemics: poliomyelitis, epidemic encephalitis, Rocky Mountain spotted fever, tularemia, psittacosis, brucellosis, malaria, etc.

4. By grants-in-aid from Congressional appropriation. These are designed to improve state and local health services.

It should be realized that, in providing this financial assistance to states or in lending officers, the U.S. Public Health Service does not in any way assume responsibility or authority which rightly belongs to the state. In obtaining grants the state health department submits a budget and plans to the Public Health Service or the Children's Bureau, and the federal agency approves, disapproves, or confers with the state health officer concerned. Once a grant is made the state health department is entirely free to proceed under its own policies so long as it operates within the limits of the plan agreed upon. When a federal public health officer is detailed to a state to assist, his authority does not supersede that of either state or local health officers as long as the problem involved is an intrastate one. In a serious interstate health situation, the U.S. Public Health Service could assume control, but generally it would act in liaison capacity between the authorities of the states involved.

The National Health Institutes. As indicated above, these research institutes are part of the U.S. Public Health Service. They grew from small beginnings, under highly competent scientists. There are now seven national health institutes: Allergy and Infectious Diseases, Arthritis and Metabolic Diseases, Cancer, Dental Research, Heart Disease, Mental Health, Neurological Diseases and Blindness. Allied to these institutes, which are located at Bethesda, Maryland, near Washington, is the Clinical Center, which is a research hospital, and a Communicable Disease Center, in Atlanta, Georgia. The Surgeon General has authority to establish other highly specialized institutes should the necessity arise.

Children's Bureau. Another important health agency of the federal government is the Children's Bureau. Formerly in the Department of Labor, this unit is now a part of the Department of Health, Education, and Welfare, but not under the direction of the Public Health Service. This bureau is interested broadly in the welfare of women and children. It focuses its activity on these specialized phases of public health work, including in its program the care of crippled children. It has done and is continuing to do valuable work in bringing to the attention of the public and of health officers, hospitals, and physicians the potentialities for maintenance of health, prevention of disease and disability, and saving of life in mothers and children.

Other Agencies of the Federal Government Which, Directly or Indirectly, Engage in Health Work. The more important are:

1. The Bureau of the Census.
2. The Department of Agriculture.
3. The Veterans Administration.
4. Medical Corps of Army, Navy, and Air Force.
5. A number of other agencies in highly specialized or minor matters.

The State in Health Matters. Each state, as a sovereign power, has the responsibility for and authority to guard the health of its citizens. Through their respective constitutions, which set forth this responsibility and authority as general principles, through acts of their respective legislatures, which provide specific health laws, and through board of health regulations, which restate the laws, but in more detail, every state is more or less adequately provided with the necessary authority for engaging in public health work.

In connection with this legal aspect of public health work, one should have clearly in mind the difference between a law and a regulation. A state law is an act of the legislature, based upon constitutional authority; a state health regulation emanates from the board of health or commissioner of health, and is based upon some specific law passed by the legislature. The regulation is more detailed, converting the general phraseology of the law into specific statements. Its requirements must remain within the limits of the particular law on which it is based. Properly drawn and reasonable, health regulations have the same authority as laws.

The Organization and Operation of a State Health Department. There is usually:

1. A board of health.
2. A state health officer.
3. A number of administrative divisions or bureaus: *communicable disease control* (sometimes including tuberculosis and venereal diseases, and if not, these are provided as separate divisions), *sanitation, laboratories, maternal and child hygiene, local health work, public health nursing, health education, food sanitation, vital statistics.* Many departments now include a division of *industrial hygiene.* Others have divisions or bureaus that relate to special problems or interests: *malaria, cancer control, nutrition, dental hygiene, chronic disease, mental hygiene, and medical care.*

The practice in the past was to create an additional administrative division for every new activity. At present, the tendency is to consolidate administrative divisions on the basis of function, regardless of age groups served or of professional personnel involved.

The state board of health usually consists of from five to seven members, appointed by the governor in most states. Occasionally membership is incident to some other major office in the state medical association or in the state government, such as the attorney general. The state health officer is usually an ex officio member of the board.

Boards may be all medical or partly medical and partly lay. The latter type is more frequently seen than formerly. The board serves the health officer in an advisory capacity, promulgates regulations, holds hearings, and acts in a liaison capacity between the operating health department and the public. Ordinarily it has no administrative functions. Some states have no board of health, but a public health council. It is unusual for members of the board of health to receive a salary. State boards of health usually meet once a month and in emergencies.

As a rule the state health officer is appointed by the governor, for the term of the governor's administration. The governor's choice may be limited by nominations from the state board of health. Most states have divorced health work rather completely from politics, and competent state health officers may remain in office indefinitely. In some states, however, the health officer changes as frequently as the governor.

The manner of appointment of subordinate personnel in a state health department differs in the various states. In most there is civil service; appointment must be made from a list of eligibles. Under civil service, favoritism is decreased to a minimum but many mediocre persons get permanent appointments. The old direct appointment system had much to commend it as long as the state health officer based his appointments on efficiency. If the state health officer is political-minded, he makes a sorry mess of things regardless of the system under which he works. The worst situation of all is where the governor sends over one of his political creditors with a request, practically an order, that a place be found for "my good friend." Fortunately, this gubernatorial practice is disappearing. No good health department can remain good under such a regime.

In the main, the state health department obtains its funds from taxes. Some states receive grants, for special purposes, from philanthropies, and varying amounts from the federal government. The amounts received from the latter source have increased greatly since 1935.

The Cost of State Health Activities. It is not easy for one to make an unqualified statement as to how much money is spent in the average state for public health work. This difficulty arises because of a number of factors. First, all health activities in a state are not carried on by health departments. There may be special independent commissions, such as a tuberculosis commission or a committee for the blind, or the department of welfare or labor may expend funds for health activities. Again, all funds expended in public health activities in a state may not be state funds. They may be derived from the federal government or a philanthropic organization or from other sources.

It is estimated that the total annual expenditure of official state agencies for state health activities in 1956 was in excess of $3.00 per capita, or more than $500,000,000 for these services. These estimates include funds made available to the states as state grants by the U.S. Public Health Service, the Children's Bureau, and other federal agencies as well as funds appropriated by local governments and state governments. In 1954 federal grants for general health services to the states amounted to approximately $24,000,000. Certain of the states have markedly increased the scope of public health work within the state and, accordingly, have increased expenditures for these services. For example, the state budget for public health in New York was approximately $7,000,000 in 1940 and was $55,000,000 in 1957. In Maryland the budget of the state health department increased during the same period from approximately $1,000,000 to $21,000,000 as a result of expansion of services in the fields of chronic disease and medical care, and as a result of the transfer of the tuberculosis hospitals from an independent agency to the health department. There is an increasing tendency for state governments to provide state aid for the development of local health services, with an increasing share of the responsibility for these services being placed upon the state.

The Types of Service Which a State Health Department Ordinarily Renders. These services are in connection with (1) maternal hygiene, (2) the hygiene of infancy and young childhood, (3) school hygiene, (4) control of acute communicable disease, (5) tuberculosis, (6) venereal diseases, (7) sanitation—pure water supplies, sewage disposal, (8) industrial hygiene, (9) milk and food sanitation, (10) nuisance abatement, (11) public health education, (12) collection of vital statistics, (13) special problems and programs. In recent years many state health departments have added services in dental hygiene, heart disease, cancer, and mental health.

The state health department is concerned with the whole state and in most instances renders its service to the people indirectly, through city, county, district, or township health agencies. In ordinary circumstances the responsibility is that of the local government concerned. In the event a locality fails or refuses, or is otherwise unable to cope with its health problems, the state may either lend assistance or assume control.

Note the difference in this relationship and that between federal and state governments, in health matters: The federal government may assist and advise the state on its internal health affairs, but not supersede it, as the authority of each is distinct. The local government, however, has only that authority which the state delegates to it. Although the state may assume control in health matters, it seldom does. To do so would be somewhat comparable to the situation where the state militia supersedes the local sheriff or police, under martial law.

The Organization and Operation of a Local Health Department. Each local health department has, as its head, a health officer, appointed by the mayor or county commissioners or board of health. Usually there is a board of health which acts in an advisory capacity. The administrative divisions of the larger local health department are similar to those in a state health department. Subordinate personnel may be appointed directly by the health officer or may be drawn from a civil service list, or may be foisted on the health officer by a strong politician. Fortunately, there is an increasing tendency for local politicians to acquiesce in the removal of the local health department from politics.

The functions of local health departments vary from place to place and depend to some extent upon the size of the department, its policies, and whether urban or rural. In general, activities may be listed as follows:

1. It investigates communicable diseases, including tuberculosis and venereal diseases, and institutes precautions designed to prevent spread of these diseases.

2. It investigates and supervises general sanitary conditions, especially as they relate to the safety of water and the disposal of human excreta.

3. It inspects and supervises the production, pasteurization, and distribution of milk.

4. It supervises the quality and safety of food and meat for public consumption, and attempts to exclude carriers of disease organisms from among the workers in food establishments.

5. It carries on regular inspection to obviate dangers to workers in industrial plants of various sorts.

6. It examines school children for the discovery of communicable diseases or physical defects, notifying parents and school authorities of findings, and urges that the family physician or a clinic be consulted for treatment. In some places school health work is a responsibility of the department of education.

7. It maintains health conferences for expectant mothers, infants, and young children not otherwise under medical supervision.

8. It conducts free clinics for the early diagnosis of tuberculosis, and may conduct mass surveys for discovery of cases.

9. It conducts free clinics for the diagnosis and treatment of venereal diseases in those not able to pay for this care.

10. It conducts clinics for the administration of protective agents against: diphtheria, smallpox, typhoid fever, and sometimes other inoculations.

11. It conducts special clinics: in relation to vision, heart, cancer, mental hygiene, etc., for selected groups.

12. It maintains a public health nursing service, which participates in many activities—in clinics, in schools, in health education—and makes instructive visits in certain cases, thus assisting the family in

carrying out the physician's orders or the regulations of the health department.

13. It provides a laboratory service for assistance to any physician in diagnosis of communicable diseases, including tuberculosis and syphilis.

14. It acts as one part in the vital statistics collection system, and keeps an orderly record of births and deaths.

15. It usually provides, to physicians, free smallpox and typhoid vaccine, diphtheria toxoid, and certain antitoxins, such as diphtheria and tetanus antitoxin.

16. It conducts, continuingly, a program of public health education.

17. It occasionally has as responsibilities the conduct of hospitals (particularly isolation hospitals) and the operation of the garbage collection system and inspection of tenements and housing.

18. It investigates complaints and takes action as to health and sanitary conditions.

19. It may have other miscellaneous duties, not necessarily of importance from a public health standpoint, but which have become responsibilities through local custom.

The Cost of Local Health Service. The generally recognized minimal standards of one medical health officer per 50,000 of the population, one public health nurse per 5000 of the population, and one sanitarian per 15,000 of the population plus the necessary supporting budget result in a per capita cost of $2.00 to $3.00 at prevailing salary scales. Thus a city of 100,000 population should provide between $200,000 and $300,000 per annum for the work of its health department. If unusual responsibilities are placed on the department, such as the operation of a communicable disease hospital, provision of medical care service, and the collection of garbage, or if intensive work is done in some particular activity, as in tuberculosis, then the budget must be increased accordingly. As a matter of fact, a large proportion of local health services operate on a budget much less than that recommended. As a result of these limiting budgets many public health services are inadequately provided or not provided at all.

It should not be assumed from the foregoing discussion of federal, state, and local health work that everything is as it should be. Much remains to be accomplished. Governments at all levels emphasize and reiterate the importance of the public health, but remain tight-fisted as to appropriations. There are still many places in the United States where the kind and amount of public health service available is as of the nineteenth century.

Public Health Personnel. In carrying out their programs, health agencies must have able, interested, and competent workers. They employ physicians, dentists, nurses, sanitary engineers, statisticians, bacteriologists, chemists, veterinarians, inspectors, experts in public health education, and technicians of various sorts. Public health work is a specialty and requires careful and extensive study and experience. Some of the larger universities have well-organized and well-equipped schools of public health.

Not infrequently there arises this question: Is the person with a basic professional education—as a physician, nurse, dentist, engineer —equipped, by this knowledge and training alone, to engage in public health work? If one answers "no," it would tend to place beyond the pale many of the present leaders in public health work. On the other hand, to answer "yes" would be unfair to those just entering and hoping to advance, in this specialty.

One can do satisfactory work in public health without special post-graduate study, but not be prepared so well as the individual who has had it. The worker who brings only some basic professional training must be more involved in trial and error than one who has been taught and guided. Further, the latter is more likely to have a broader perspective, a more objective and systematic approach, and a better understanding of procedures, purposes, and relative values. It is therefore desirable that those entering the public health field have special training. Of just what this postgraduate work should consist, no one person—or group—is at present qualified to delineate with finality. The demands in the various services are undergoing change. New prob-

lems arise, old ones are partially solved. New methods, new techniques, and new standards tend to replace those previously accepted.
Responsibilities of health departments increase and decrease. For
these reasons, it would be exceedingly unfortunate should there develop a fixity of ideas as to the content of postgraduate study in the
field of public health, and, as a general principle, an imposed cur-
riculum is detrimental to education.

With these cautions in mind, it may be said that the physician entering this field needs to be a man with a good cultural background.
Merely to be a college graduate is not enough; he must be also an
educated man. He must be broad-minded and emotionally balanced.
He should be able to see the health problems of the mass as well as of
the individual, and he must see health and disease in their biological
and social relationships. He must be conscious of his own work as but
one cog in society's machine for human betterment. If this work is
going to place him in contact with the public, then he cannot succeed
unless he is a good practical psychologist—one who knows and senses
human reactions; who can inhibit the unsatisfactory and stimulate
the satisfactory responses in others, at the same time deserving and
gaining the respect and liking of those with whom he comes in contact. He must understand local politics, not for the purpose of practice, but to avoid entanglements and pitfalls. And he must possess
imagination, mental keenness, and honesty of mind. With driving
energy he must drive himself as well as others.

Compensation in public health work varies within rather wide
limits. There has been a noticeable tendency for all public health
workers' salaries to increase in recent years. There has also been a
tendency to permit supplementation of salaries, particularly for
teaching responsibilities, in order to attract more competent professional health workers in the more important posts. A study carried
out by the U.S. Public Health Service in 1956 gave the range for state
health officers' salaries as $7500 to $18,500 per annum. In certain instances the health officers' salaries in the larger cities exceed those
paid in state health departments. The range in salaries for major
bureau directors in the same study was $6210 to $15,000 per annum.
The salaries of county health officers show an even greater variation in

different parts of the country. The most recent figures available indicate a range of $8000 to $20,000 for county health officers. Full-time health officers, such as those mentioned above, are not permitted to engage in private practice.

Public Health Nursing. Because public health nursing constitutes an important part of community health programs, it seems advantageous here to present certain generalities relating to the public health nurse and her work. Her part in various activities is mentioned more specifically in subsequent chapters.

The second edition of the *Manual of Public Health Nursing* defines this activity as: *

An organized community service, rendered by graduate nurses to the individual, family and community. This service includes the interpretation of medical, sanitary and social procedures for the correction of defects, prevention of disease and the promotion of health and may include skilled care of the sick in their homes.

The third edition of the same publication carries this statement: †

Public health nursing includes all nursing services organized by a community or agency to assist in carrying out any or all phases of the public health program. Services may be rendered on an individual, family, or community basis in home, school, clinic, business establishment, or office of the agency.

Among other things, the public health nurse:

1. Helps to secure early medical diagnosis and treatment.
2. Renders or secures nursing care of the sick.
3. Teaches by demonstration and interpretation, and supervises care given by relatives or attendants.
4. Assists the family to carry out medical, sanitary, and social procedures for the prevention of disease and the promotion of health.
5. Helps to secure adjustment, as possible, of social conditions which affect health.

* The National Organization for Public Health Nursing: *Manual of Public Health Nursing,* 2nd ed. The Macmillan Company, New York, 1932, p. 3.
† The National Organization for Public Health Nursing: *Manual of Public Health Nursing,* 3rd ed. The Macmillan Company, New York, 1939, pp. xi, xiii–xiv.

6. Influences the community to develop public health facilities for the promotion of a sound, adequate community health program, and shares in action leading to betterment of health conditions.

In their daily work public health nurses have contact with many and various sorts of people, who may be catalogued in this way:

1. The public: rich and poor, intelligent and stupid, ignorant and educated, broad-minded and prejudiced.
2. Private physicians, most of whom are cordial, some of whom are antagonistic, to the public health nurse.
3. School principals, teachers, and other officials.
4. Representatives of social agencies.
5. Medical social workers from hospitals.
6. Other nurses from other agencies.
7. Parent-teacher association officers.
8. Representatives of churches and religious organizations.
9. Politicians and persons with special axes to grind.

The major requirements for a successful public health nurse are a pleasant personality, judgment, tact, energy, and intellectual honesty; ability to present technical matters in a simple, understandable, and interesting manner; a willingness to teach by demonstration (with the sleeves rolled up). She needs a good preliminary education, at least high school, preferably college, and a well-rounded nursing education. She should have postgraduate work, preferably a full academic year, in public health.

Salaries paid to public health nurses vary from time to time and from place to place. The average is about as follows: staff nurses, from $3000 to $4000; supervising public health nurses, $3800 to $8000. Voluntary agencies and departments of education tend to pay public health nurses more than do health departments.

The Voluntary or Nonofficial Health Agencies. These agencies occupy a most important place in public health work. They differ considerably in their make-up, purposes, policies, etc., but the one factor they have in common is that they are not tax-supported and, correspondingly, not subject to the somewhat rigid pattern of performance that tends to become established in governmental undertakings.

A voluntary health agency usually comes into existence because some citizen, or a group of citizens, feels that there is an unmet need or a necessity for new knowledge in a particular field. Those interested then band together on a local, state, or national basis and form an organization whose activities are directed toward the end in view. Thus the National Tuberculosis Association arose in 1904. Other national organizations, with an interest in a particular field of health, have subsequently developed: the American Social Hygiene Association (1914), the National Foundation for Infantile Paralysis* (1938), the American Society for the Control of Cancer (1913), the American Heart Association (1933), the National Association for Mental Health (1950), and others.

Some of these national groups have well-organized state associations into which focus the local units. This is perhaps more clearly evident in the National Tuberculosis Association than in any of the others, insofar as concerns day-by-day programs of local work.

The more centralized voluntary agencies, such as the National Foundation and the American Cancer Society, carry on an extensive program of support for research in the cause and prevention of these diseases. In addition, they carry on an extensive public education program and a program of professional education through fellowships and scholarships. All of the voluntary agencies have as one of their major purposes public health education. The National Foundation differs from most other voluntary agencies in that it carries out an extensive program of patient care. This program provides not only funds for the care of the acutely ill patient but also extensive support for his rehabilitation and long-term care.

Financial Support of Voluntary Health Agencies. In general such organizations as these are supported by thousands of small contributions, annually, from the public. Actually, there are now so many voluntary health agencies, with diverse purposes and separate appeals

* In July, 1958, this organization announced a broad, new program, concerned not only with poliomyelitis and virus research but also with disorders of the central nervous system, arthritis, and congenital malformations. Accordingly, the name of the organization was shortened to the National Foundation.

for funds, that the public is becoming annoyed by the multiplicity of requests for money. Because of this situation, it has been suggested that there be one coordinated over-all fund-raising drive for health, and that from the proceeds of this each agency share.

There can be no question but that fewer appeals for funds would be welcomed by the public, would be less confusing than at present, and would seem to be a logical approach. Practically, however, there are two great difficulties:

1. The public does not give as readily or in as large amounts to general appeals as it does to specific; response is better when one is asked to help fight tuberculosis or poliomyelitis than when urged to give money for "good health" or the "conquest of disease."

2. Voluntary public health groups that have already established successful fund-raising procedures are not likely to give them up for a vague and untried method, based on theory and logic. People do not make donations for health and charitable causes on the basis of logic, but rather because of emotions.

The move for federated fund raising, nevertheless, is a very live issue. Among its proponents are numbered many of those who are viewing the matter logically but not necessarily practically, plus representatives of those health agencies which need funds from the public but have no device for obtaining them. Opposing the idea of one over-all campaign are generally to be found those who represent organizations with a tried and true and sure-fire method of getting public financial support, plus others who believe that a number of separate appeals is desirable in order that the public may preserve its right of free choice as to what it supports.

The voluntary health agencies, particularly those representing a disease which has a particular appeal to the emotions, have constantly increased their goals and have been remarkably successful in attaining these goals. In 1957 the four largest voluntary health agencies, representing interests in infantile paralysis, cancer, tuberculosis, and heart disease, raised a total in excess of $100,000,000.

Funds for support of voluntary health efforts are, in the main, raised by local committees as part of a national drive, at some designated time of the year. Perhaps the three best known of these campaigns are the Red Cross (not limited to health), the National Tuberculosis Association (the Christmas Seal), and the National Foundation (the March of Dimes).

Some of the newer health groups in their appeal for funds have adopted freshly modern methods, on a national basis: radio series, television "marathons," etc. Such methods have raised millions and, under the aegis of stage personalities, who are continuingly on the air waves, bring to the public repeated reminders as to the problems and opportunities and necessities for support in this or that special field of health. An encouraging aspect of this newer approach is that there has been a strong emphasis on the support of research. On the other hand, the participation of thousands of local citizens in fund-raising efforts for health, in their own communities, is of the utmost benefit.

The distribution of funds, between the national associations, the state associations (or societies), and the local associations, varies with the organization concerned. Some of the national associations receive as much as 50 per cent of the total funds raised in drives; others get much less: the National Tuberculosis Association receives only 6 per cent.

The Organization of National Voluntary Health Agencies. The national voluntary health agency usually has a board of directors or some similar governing body. There is a tendency in some to have a prestige board: one in which there are outstanding leaders in industry, business, the arts, the professions. Others have a mixture of persons outstanding in the profession concerned in the undertaking, plus representative directors chosen by the constituent or affiliated state and local associations. The officers, generally, are president, vice-presidents, treasurer, secretary, etc.

Under a constitution, which generally is more verbose and detailed than is necessary, the authority and responsibility for the affairs of the voluntary health organization rest in the board of directors. However, as such a group is usually quite large (from 50 to 100 members) and its members live in various parts of the country, it is not practicable for them to meet very often—perhaps only once a year at the annual convention. In the circumstances, a smaller executive committee conducts most of the business, meeting every two or three months.

In addition to the executive committee, most national health organizations have various special committees, concerned with one aspect or another of the program. These committees are not, however, operating or administrative, but are concerned rather with findings and deliberations as a basis for decisions and policies by the executive committee or board of directors.

Boards and committees cannot administer a program, whether in government, or citizen groups, and all national health organizations therefore have a secretariat or administrative staff. The principal officer is usually designated by a title comparable to executive director. In addition there are others who are deemed particularly competent in the several subunits of the organization's undertaking: a business manager, comptroller, public information (public relations) officer, technical directors, with necessary clerical services.

Voluntary health associations, on a state basis, are organized somewhat as indicated above, in the case of national groups: a board of directors with officers and committees, and some operating staff.

Local voluntary groups, concerned with some particular aspect of health, may be formally or loosely organized. They may carry on a continuing program of health education, demonstration, stimulation of communities to provide obviously needed services and facilities, and fund raising. In the past, many of them provided direct services in the community, such as public health nursing, clinic services, even hospitalization. At present, the trend in activities of voluntary agencies is toward popular education in health, community organization, the promotion of governmental health services when appropriate, better health service by hospitals, schools, industries, etc.

The Interrelations between National, State, and Local Voluntary Health Associations. In a given association, the national group establishes general policies, provides leadership, produces educational and publicity material, guides the program in a general way, and may conduct or support research. The state groups, in their respective organizations, give broad leadership, stimulation, and guidance to the local affiliates, rendering expert service in program planning and execution, in budgets and fund raising; conduct surveys; etc.

The local health associations, in their respective fields and communities, attempt to further a public understanding of the problems faced, and seek support of programs designed to improve this aspect of health locally.

There is a National Health Council, designed to coordinate the activities of all the separate and specialized nongovernmental groups which are in the health field nationally. Efforts have also been made to establish similar coordination on a state basis and in local areas.

The Value and Disabilities of Voluntary Health Agencies. One of the greatest values of voluntary health agencies is perhaps a by-product: experience and understanding gained by hundreds of thousands of private citizens who participate in work for the benefit of their communities. Such participation increases the civic stature of each person concerned and, by example, shows to others an opportunity and duty of active citizenship.

More direct values are produced as the result of work done, with new knowledge gained by research, by better definition of problems and the institution of measures to correct them, by public information as to the situation involved. Further, as previously mentioned, the voluntary health agency has the opportunity for great elasticity in its program. It does not have to follow a conventional path beaten down by precedent. It may explore new fields, going into the frontiers of public health with the vigor and vision of pioneers. Thus the great opportunity of the voluntary health agency is to blaze a trail which the more routine-bound may later follow.

The greatest potential deterrent to sound and progressive programs in voluntary health agencies is that they may lose the pioneer spirit; that having engaged in a given phase of activity, they may exhibit an unwillingness to move forward, in spite of the fact that a health department is able, willing, and might properly now take over.

Visiting Nurse Associations. These are voluntary agencies, local in character, designed primarily to render nursing aid to the sick in their homes. Each organization usually has a board of directors, an executive, and a staff of nurses. They attempt to work in close cooperation with the local health department, and, except for a first visit of investigation, all cases served by the visiting nurse must be under the care of a physician, to whom the nurse reports. The service is essentially a free one, although patients may pay a small fee if able to do so. A visiting nurse does not spend all of her time with one patient but visits a number of homes each day.

Visiting nurse associations are usually supported from two or more of the following sources:

1. Moderate fees collected.
2. Fees received from insurance companies for care of their policyholders.
3. The community fund.
4. Income from endowments.
5. Private subscriptions.

Public Health Associations. Those engaged in the public health field have somewhat dual affiliations with professional organizations: one with the professional group to which they primarily belong, and the other with associations having public health as a special interest. Physicians engaged in public health work have their membership in their local societies, state medical associations, and the American Medical Association. The basic affiliation for nurses is similar, their national body being the American Nurses' Association. The basic national organization for sanitary engineers is the American Society of Civil Engineers; for bacteriologists, the Society of American Bacteriologists; and for statisticians, the American Statistical Association. Within the field of public health, workers in these diverse specialties come together by membership in the American Public Health Association. In addition, there are a number of special-interest organizations: the American Epidemiological Society, the National League for Nursing (a national group particularly concerned with public health nursing), the American Society of Tropical Medicine, and others. Most of these basic and special organizations publish monthly journals or, from time to time, reports of their meetings.

International Health Organization. The aims of the presently existing World Health Organization are far more comprehensive than those of any international health organization that has existed in the past. Its resources, too, are greater than those in movements that preceded it. But the World Health Organization did not suddenly spring into existence as a by-product of the efforts for the United Nations. In effect, the present interest, facilities, and coordination of effort for better health in all nations arose long ago, with small sporadic and intermittent manifestations here and there.

Recognition of International Health Problems. From very early times, association of a well individual with a leper had been regarded as dangerous or at least unaesthetic, and from this there developed in tribes religious and secular practices of setting lepers aside: in effect, a sort of quarantine. Again, it had been observed that the ingress of goods and persons from one city into another was not infrequently followed by the occurrence in the visited city of an epidemic which was prevalent in the city from which the visitors had come. Going from the particular of quarantining lepers as individuals, cities began to set up quarantine periods for groups of people, usually in ships, coming from other parts when it was known that an epidemic existed in the area from which the ship had come. From records available, this procedure seems to have begun in the Middle Ages. But it was on a city-by-city basis for a very long time, and except in those instances where a city-state (as Venice) took the action, there was the anomalous situation of individual cities, through quarantine regulations, dealing with parts or all of foreign governments. This was the case for a long time in the United States. New York City, for instance, operated its own foreign quarantine until 1923.

First International Agreements. As would be expected, maritime quarantine developed first in those ports where visiting ships or travelers came in large numbers from various parts of the world and, in particular, from those areas in which epidemic diseases prevailed. Thus one of the very early international agreements in relation to health came about in 1831 in connection with commerce in Egypt. Cholera was at that time almost world-wide, and plague offered a serious threat from India. There was then established, at Alexandria, the Egyptian Quarantine Board. This board, however, and a similar one established in Turkey in 1838, arose from pressure rather than mutual agreement. In both instances, the various foreign powers concerned in commerce with Egypt and Turkey demanded such boards and were strongly represented upon them. But there was recognition that health conditions in one country could affect those in others, and the action taken was international in character. The first of these boards lasted only a short time. The second carried on, with intermittent activities, until 1923.

More Modern International Health Agencies. A short-lived international health agreement came out of a conference of some 12 nations, held in Paris in 1851. The conferees reached agreement on certain basic international quarantine procedures but, generally, the nations which they represented did not confirm the arrangements, and the movement made no more lasting contribution than to indicate the necessity for further consideration and action.

Subsequent conferences led to the establishment of an International Office of Health with headquarters in Paris in 1907 (*L'Office Internationale d'Hygiene Publique*). This organization had a Permanent Committee to which 55 governments sent delegates, and there was a paid worker; a sort of world-wide epidemiological service was set up. This international office continued in operation until it became a part of the World Health Organization in 1947.

In the Western Hemisphere, it was the problem of yellow fever that gave rise to the first international health conference. In 1887, Paraguay, Argentina, and Brazil entered into agreements as to regulations designed to prevent the spread of this disease between their respective countries. Out of this, or at least subsequent to and in association with it, grew the Pan-American Sanitary Bureau. The latter became a formal entity (as the International Sanitary Bureau) in 1902, adopting its later name in 1924, and continued a vigorous program in epidemiology, training of professional personnel, development of sound organization, encouragement of research, etc. It became a regional office of the World Health Organization in 1949.

League of Nations: Health Section. This health organization, with headquarters in Geneva, was established in 1923. It provided a Health Commission of 12 members, with four meetings a year. Some coordination with the International Office of Health was arranged through having the Permanent Committee of the latter organization serve as the General Advisory Committee of the League's Health Section.

The Health Section provided a secretariat: a director and small staff. Its broad objectives were to strengthen national health services, and maintain epidemiological intelligence on a world-wide basis. Considering the limitations under which the Health Section operated and the early evidence of dissolution in the League, of which it was a part, good and constructive work was done.

World Health Organization. Previous to establishment of the Health Section of the League of Nations, efforts to develop international cooperation in health were directed mainly to finding an international sanitary code strict enough to prevent importation of disease from one nation to another but not so strict as to interfere with commerce. The World Health Organization, in intent, goes much further, and evidences an interest in all health of all people in all nations, regardless of whether the problems are social, economic, infectious, mental, nutritional, acute or chronic, etc.

Groundwork for the World Health Organization was laid at the Conference of Nations on International Organization held in San Francisco in the spring of 1945. A representative from Brazil had the word "health," as an interest of the proposed United Nations, introduced into the document under consideration, and the Conference approved, as a declared purpose, the establishment of an international health organization. Subsequently there were international conferences directed toward making this intent a reality. An interim committee served, pending formal organization, and the World Health Organization, through ratification by the respective governments concerned, came into existence April 7, 1948. It occupies the status of a specialized agency in the framework of the United Nations. A nation may be a member of WHO without membership in the United Nations.

The charter adopted is broad, perhaps somewhat verbose. There are 19 chapters with 82 articles. In the preamble, five principles are set forth, and these to some extent are repeated in objectives. In essence the latter are: ". . . the attainment by all people of the highest level of health." And health is defined as "a state of complete physical, mental and social well being and not merely the absence of disease or infirmity." Organizationally, there is provision for a World Health Assembly, an Executive Board, and a Secretariat.

The World Health Assembly is made up of delegates from member nations. There may be as many as three delegates from each nation, but only one vote. There must be at least one meeting a year.

The Executive Board. This has 18 members, designated by the Assembly, with due consideration to geographic (and national) arrangement. This body must meet at least twice a year, and its responsibility, relationships, and functions are set out in detail.

The Secretariat. The principal officer is the Director-General, appointed by the Assembly on nomination of the Executive Board. In addition, there is a technical staff and a complement of clerical personnel.

As adjuncts to the organization, there are various panels of experts who are called upon from time to time for advice or service in special problems.

Headquarters for WHO is in Geneva, Switzerland.

Regional Offices. There are six regional offices located as follows:

1. Washington, D.C., U.S.A.: Office for the Americas.
2. Copenhagen, Denmark: Office for Europe.
3. Alexandria, Egypt: Office for Eastern Mediterranean area.
4. New Delhi, India: Office for South East Asia.
5. Brazzaville, French Equatorial Africa: Office for Africa.
6. Manila, Philippines: Office for Western Pacific.

The breadth of WHO's approach to the problems of international health is seen in its functions, as set forth in the constitution: *

(a) to act as the directing and coordinating authority on international health work;

(b) to establish and maintain effective collaboration with the United Nations, specialized agencies, governmental health administrations, pro-

* Hyde, H. van Zile: *World Health Organization—Progress and Plans.* (Department of State, Publication #3126). Government Printing Office, Washington, D.C., 1958.

fessional groups, and such other organizations as may be deemed appropriate;

(c) to assist governments, upon request, in strengthening health services;

(d) to furnish appropriate technical assistance and, in emergencies, necessary aid upon the request or acceptance of governments;

(e) to provide or assist in providing, upon the request of the United Nations, health services and facilities to special groups, such as the peoples of trust territories;

(f) to establish and maintain such administrative and technical services as may be required, including epidemiological and statistical services;

(g) to stimulate and advance work to eradicate epidemic, endemic, and other diseases;

(h) to promote, in cooperation with other specialized agencies where necessary, the prevention of accidental injuries;

(i) to promote, in cooperation with other specialized agencies where necessary, the improvement of nutrition, housing, sanitation, recreation, economic or working conditions, and other aspects of environmental hygiene;

(j) to promote cooperation among scientific and professional groups which contribute to the advancement of health;

(k) to propose conventions, agreements, and regulations, and make recommendations with respect to international health matters and to perform such duties as may be assigned thereby to the organization and are consistent with its objective;

(l) to promote maternal and child health and welfare and to foster the ability to live harmoniously in a changing total environment;

(m) to foster activities in the field of mental health, especially those affecting the harmony of human relations;

(n) to promote and conduct research in the field of health;

(o) to promote improved standards of teaching and training in the health, medical, and related professions;

(p) to study and report on, in cooperation with other specialized agencies where necessary, administrative and social techniques affecting public health and medical care from preventive and curative points of view, including hospital services and social security;

(q) to provide information, counsel, and assistance in the field of health;

(r) to assist in developing an informed public opinion among all peoples on matters of health;

(s) to establish and revise as necessary international nomenclatures of diseases, of causes of death, and of public health practices;

(t) to standardize diagnostic procedures as necessary;

(u) to develop, establish, and promote international standards with respect to food, biological, pharmaceutical, and similar products;

(v) generally to take all necessary action to attain the objective of the organization.

The inside cover page of the *Chronicle of World Health Organization* (published monthly in several languages) contains this succinct statement:

The scope of WHO's interests and activities exceeds that of any previous international health organization and includes, in addition to major projects relating to malaria, tuberculosis, venereal diseases, maternal and child health, nutrition, and environmental sanitation, special programmes on public-health administration, epidemic diseases, mental health, professional and technical training, and other public-health subjects. It is also continuing work begun by earlier organizations on biological standardization, unification of pharmacopoeias, addiction-producing drugs, health statistics, international sanitary regulations, and the collection and dissemination of technical information, including epidemiological statistics.

REFERENCES

Annual Report of the Department of Health, Education, and Welfare. Government Printing Office, Washington, D.C.

Annual Report, Surgeon General, United States Public Health Service. Government Printing Office, Washington, D.C.

Mountin, J. W., and Flook, Evelyn: "Distribution of Health Services in the Structure of State Government. I. Composite Pattern of State Health Service," *Pub. Health Rep.*, **56** (No. 34): 1673–98, 1941.

chapter 4

Health Education and
Related Activities

IT IS ESSENTIAL that the public be informed on matters pertaining to health. These matters may vary from personal hygiene to bond issues for a new water supply. The activity of health agencies designed to furnish such information is designated as "health education." Perhaps this term is not completely accurate, but it has general understanding and acceptance.

The amounts and kinds of work done as health education are quite broad, and there are many related activities which might be considered to be health education by one user of the term or by a health agency, but not by others. Viewed from one standpoint, practically every activity of a health agency has within it some element of health education—even the prosecution of a violator of a sanitary code would be informative to the community, if not educational.

Perhaps the two activities most closely related to health education, from a practical and operating standpoint, are public relations and community organization. These will be dealt with more specifically, below.

The Purpose and Methods of Health Education. The activities that are carried on as health education are designed to supply the public, or occasionally some particular part of the public, with information as to health matters and with stimulus to do something about their personal or community health. Obviously, what the individual might do could vary within rather wide limits.

The process of health education is a continuing, vigorous process, adopting psychological techniques as regards individuals and crowds, adapting (cautiously) scientific information to terms understandable by the public, bringing to bear the experience of education, advertising, and propaganda, and utilizing all available media for mass communication.

The Growth of Health Education. This activity has grown tremendously in the last half century, as has the public's knowledge of health matters. The necessity of informing and guiding the public along these lines has long been realized, but only comparatively recently have there been well-organized and continuing programs directed to these ends. In times of great epidemics, boards of health issued brochures and handbills, advising citizens what to do personally to avoid infection, and laid down rules of hygiene and sanitation. But health agencies did not act unless there was an epidemic and, having acted, then remained quiescent until another dramatic threat to health became imminent.

Perhaps the first sustained effort in health education in relation to a nonepidemic but still a communicable disease was that of the National (U.S.) Tuberculosis Association, which undertook to carry information on this disease to the public early in the present century. Out of this, antispitting campaigns arose, and the danger of the common drinking cup was pounded into the public consciousness. Later came the "swat the fly" programs in connection with intestinal diseases.

Over the years, programs of health education have broadened and changed in character. Particularly significant has been the inclusion of what might be called a positive aspect: a change from advice on how to avoid sickness to advice on how to maintain health. One of the best illustrations of the latter approach is to be found in health education in relation to nutrition and diet.

It should be noted that there is a place for both the positive and negative approach. It would be just as great a mistake to outlaw health education that deals with the prevention of disease as it would be to rely entirely upon scaring people to death in an effort to keep them healthy. At the moment, in modernly trained health educators, the reaction against the negative approach is rather strong, possibly too strong in view of the fact that the border line between health and disease is vague. People generally work harder against something specific which they can visualize than for something which is vague and not dramatic.

Other factors that account for the increase in health education activities, and for greater public information and the results attained in health, are these: the availability of a greater fund of scientific knowledge; a population in which illiteracy has been reduced; the incorporation of health teaching in schools; the provision of sanitary facilities in homes, schools, etc.; the wide reading of newspapers, magazines, etc.; radio, television, and advertising. The latter groups do not always portray accurately or without a commercial interest, but they are of great importance.

Essentials in a Health Education Program. In undertaking health education there are certain essentials. First, and of extreme importance, is the necessity that there be a scientific basis for the material presented. This need for accuracy is sometimes overlooked because of enthusiasm, paraphrasing, and the urge for slogans. Further, not only must the information given be sound, but it must be constructive and applicable. There would be but little benefit in presenting the cold fact that rabies is a fatal disease in man; nor would a recommendation, even though substantiated scientifically, be of much value in a health education program if the measures advocated were quite beyond the limits of practical application.

A second essential in a health education program is that the information presented be in understandable terms. It is in this area that the physician, with no graduate training or experience, is likely to be inadequate. But regardless of the means or methods of presenting health education material, technical terms in medicine, psychology, the social sciences, education, economics, etc., must be avoided. This is not always easy, because not only is it convenient to use these terms, but many workers appear to feel that such usage is a badge of erudition.

Closely allied to the necessities for simplicity is the requirement that not too much of one thing or too many different things be presented to one group at the same time. There is a definite limit to the absorptive qualities of audiences. A great gush of words, spoken or written, urging them to refrain from a lot of things and to embrace in their everyday lives many and diverse chores, is certainly not productive.

A fourth necessity in a health education program is communication of information and stimulus to the public or to the particular group to which the program is directed. Means of communication are various: as simple as a mimeograph machine, as complex as a television show. Included in means of communication, too, would be the entree to strategic persons or organizations: entree to a superintendent of education in a matter having to do with schools; entree to reporters or editors, to the key man at a radio station, etc.

Finally, a fifth essential in a health education program is concerned with the staff workers and resources. The latter relate to funds available, etc., and are of great importance. But it is of even greater importance to have at the head of the program a competent person, with imagination and vigor. Such a person can overcome most difficulties, and without him or her, the finest resources and theories remain static. The trained health educator, with good personality, sound general knowledge, and fine perspective, has the qualities of leadership, an ability to obtain the understanding and participation of other workers in allied fields. The latter are qualities that a guild-conscious, overaggressive, or shrinking health educator does not possess and cannot accomplish.

Sciences and Disciplines Contributing to Health Education. The above discussion of essentials in a health education program is far from complete. Space limits discussion. Further light, however, is shed upon health education programs, their inclusiveness and requirements, by a consideration of the sciences and disciplines from which procedures in health education draw. The influence of some of them is quite specific, others are vague. The more important are the following:

Medicine. The basic facts as to health and disease naturally derive from this source, and its collateral sciences: physiology, nutrition, microbiology, diagnosis, therapy, etc.

Education. The art and science of pedagogy contribute to health education both in knowledge of how people learn and in methods.

Psychology. Both in theory and practice, it is essential that programs of health education pay due attention to what makes people, individually and in the mass, act and react in the ways that they do. Basic principles, in these connections, are drawn from the field of psychology, and are utilized more or less by workers in health education. Some workers, though well trained, find it difficult to apply these principles directly and practically; others, trained or untrained, demonstrate a grasp of psychological principles almost intuitively.

Arts and Letters. Because health education utilizes the written word to a great extent, the art of clear expression is an essential. One seldom needs to present material in the leisurely style of an essay; in fact only rarely is such a presentation justified. But the clarity, conciseness, simplicity, and interest, similar to that seen in a good news article or magazine, are essential.

Advertising and Propaganda. Although health education would not wish to emulate all the pressures, exaggerations, and ruthlessness sometimes exhibited by advertising and propaganda, much of practical value has been drawn from these fields.

There are other areas of human endeavor from which the practice of health education has drawn substance and inspiration from time to time, but the above listing seems sufficient for present purposes.

Agencies That Conduct Health Education Programs. Practically all health departments and voluntary health associations now have well-defined programs in health education. To the voluntary agencies must go the credit for being the first to embark upon long-range continuing activities designed to inform and guide the public in the maintenance of health and the prevention of disease. Elementary and secondary schools attempt to inculcate the principles of healthful living in their pupils; teachers colleges include courses for those who will in turn give instruction in health and hygiene. A number of insurance companies have found it to be good business, as well as an opportunity for public service, to prepare and distribute health education material. They are naturally concerned with prolonging the lives of their policyholders, but vast public benefits come from the well-written, restrained, and sound advice they give incident to national advertising campaigns.

As regards health education in official and nonofficial health agencies, it may be said that excellent contributions are made available by the U.S. Public Health Service and the U.S. Children's Bureau. A list of their publications and the publications themselves may be obtained, at small cost, from the Government Printing Office. The various state, city, and county health departments are engaged in health education to an extent depending upon their respective resources and predilections.

In the voluntary agencies a similar situation exists. National agencies, in one special field or another, set the pace for their state and local groups. The cumulative effect of these endeavors is telling, although there is some danger that the groups with the cleverer appeals and inherently dramatic subject matter may attract more attention and make a greater impression upon the public than is deserved, comparatively, by the problem which they are attempting to solve.

Many social agencies find it desirable and productive to carry on programs of health education incident to their major functions. They are naturally concerned most with the health of those who come under the care of social services or the welfare department, but the effect of their activities reaches the community as a whole.

Kinds of Health Education Programs. As indicated in previous discussions, many different kinds of agencies with varying purposes are engaged in health education. Although these programs are broadly similar, they are healthily different in detail. They vary in scope, as between national, state, and local. They vary in content, as between the inclusive program of a large health department and the specialized interest of a small local voluntary health agency.

Some health education programs are concerned with one selected population group, as in maternity hygiene or schools; another, as in heart disease, would be particularly concerned with health education as it relates to prevention, early diagnosis, care, rehabilitation, and occupational adjustment of those affected. Such an agency, however, would also be interested in health education for all the public in an effort to prevent heart disease where practicable. Somewhat similarly, health education programs in nutrition would be concerned with wide public dissemination of information as a mass undertaking, and also with the focusing of the program on those who need information most: mothers of young children, perhaps the overweight.

Health education programs vary, too, in the degree to which they use the different media and methods for dissemination of information. These media are discussed below in more detail.

Methods in Health Education. Methods in health education partake of and are shaped by the dignity of conservative educational processes on the one hand and the techniques of advertising and propaganda on the other. Obviously, methods are but means to attaining an end. The end, in the case of health education, is to have individuals take those actions that will be beneficial to their own and the community's health. Behind the methods adopted must be a shrewd determination of what has made people act favorably in similar circumstances in the past or is likely to attain favorable results in the given situation.

Will they act because of a profit motive? Will they act through fear? Will they act to inflate or gratify the ego? Will they act through pure reason? Or because it is the decent thing to do? Or the popular thing? Will women diet because of vanity, rather than for health? Will people be more likely to read this poster (and act favorably) if it carries a flavor of ham or cheesecake?

The above are only some of the questions that may be considered in adopting methods. A decision must face the old problem of how far one is justified in using means to attain ends. Health educators and psychologists generally deprecate the use of fear as a motive for action, although no inconsiderable portion of the public behaves itself or pays its taxes because of fear. Most persons in health education would eschew, and quite properly, the blatant and crude in posters and publications, but they must at the same time avoid stuffiness.

The final decisions that have determined methods and policies have depended upon a nice discrimination and balance between all the elements involved, with due consideration of the materials to be used, the audiences to be reached, the media of communication, and in accordance with good taste and practicalities.

Materials Used in Health Education. These vary from a mimeographed information sheet to the more complex scripts: stage, moving picture, radio, and television. Brochures, newsletters, magazines, etc., are adapted to various methods and audiences. Posters and exhibits play an important part. The preparation of such material, if it is to be effective, requires skill and experience. Most brochures, and in fact much of the written material used in health education, are profligate of words. It requires much more talent to write simply and briefly than wordily in polysyllabics.

In general, commercial agencies interested in health education produce more attractive, interesting, and effective material than do health agencies. Because of strict budgets and inability to engage consulting art talent, the health material of official agencies is likely to be colorless if not drab.

In the distribution of materials, lists by categories of interest are kept alive. Where the agency is specialized this is comparatively easy. Where diverse activities are engaged in, as by a health department, more discrimination is necessary in distribution of material—and of services: brochures dealing with problems limited to one sex or one age group would not profitably be sent to another.

Means of Communications in Health Education. It will be apparent that there is here a close relationship to methods and materials. Thus, written words may constitute material and serve as a means of communication. Generally speaking, the means of communicating health education to others are as follows. Some comment is made in each case.

Word of Mouth. This may be from one individual to another, as given by a doctor to his patient, a nurse to a parent, etc. The spoken word, however, may be from one informed person to an audience: the talk or speech.

Because one must so often, or does so often, make speeches in health education, it may be helpful to consider certain guides:

1. One cannot speak with conviction or arouse enthusiasm unless he is himself (or herself) well informed on the subject. Effective speeches, to a great extent, depend upon the speaker's information.

2. A speech from notes is usually more effective than the reading of a prepared paper. The latter is desirable if accuracy cannot otherwise be assured, as in reports of research, but reading, except by a master, is usually stiff and impersonal.

3. The speech should always be organized beforehand, either by writing in full, by notes, or clearly in the speaker's mind. Extemporaneous speeches are seldom orderly, and frequently are superficial and irrelevant. Most of the effective, yet apparently extemporaneous speeches, are not in fact extemporaneous. They come from individuals who are well informed and who, on the basis of previous speeches on the subject at issue, have the material already organized, mentally, for presentation.

4. If one finds himself in danger of being called upon for an extemporaneous speech—and usually one can tell from the category of persons upon whom the chairman is calling—a little quick thinking along two lines may help to make the speech less futile than it would have been: first, mentally formulate the opening remarks, and the closing remarks. Even though the material in the middle is a bit jumbled, a good start and a vigorous finish may offset such deficiencies.

5. It is much better to make a speech shorter than was permitted or expected, than longer. Very few speakers can hold an audience for more than half an hour, at the most. The continuing sound of the speaker's voice does not entrance hearers to the same degree that it does the speaker.

6. It is unwise in a speech to attempt to cover a number of subjects or to go into great detail on any one subject. This is not so much a question of the audience's intelligence but rather of its subconscious resistance. Statistical data are not well received by lay audiences. If figures must be used, they should be kept, at the least, on the left-hand side of the decimal point.

7. There are various speaking techniques that improve the talks that those in health education must make, and certain obvious habits and mannerisms that may well be avoided.

On the positive side, it is necessary to speak loudly enough to be heard: it is good practice to speak to those in the next-to-back row of the room or hall. Where there is wiring for sound, nice judgment is necessary.

A change of rapidity of words or in loudness of voice breaks the monotony, gives emphasis, and may waken the interest of one on the verge of somnolence.

An anecdote or story not only eases audience tension or lack of attention, but may emphasize a point that otherwise would have gone unnoticed.

Among the things a speaker should avoid are: um-ming and ah-ing, too much physical motion, such as putting hands into pockets and out, toe rocking, table leaning, etc.; an oratory where ringing phrases are uncalled for; a breathless spate of words; playing with chalk or a paper clip or rubber band, or twirling a Phi Beta Kappa key.

A speaker needs to remember, too, that his hold on the audience's attention is a narrow, marginal thing. They will escape from the sound of his voice and his demand for continuing attention at the slightest opportunity. They turn to view a latecomer not because of avid interest in who comes, but as an escape; for the same reason they become fascinated with the movie operator who is adjusting his machine in the back of the room.

The above suggestions as to the art and science of public speaking are, of course, incomplete and spotty. There can be no assurance that those who observe these tacit do's and don't's will immediately thereafter receive applause and commendation for what they have had to say.

The spoken word is also used in circumstances more complicated than in speech, as in radio, television, specially prepared sketches for short plays, etc. These are effective when the aspect of health concerned lends itself to such presentation and when there is a selected audience. Institutes and workshops, where the audience participates actively, are also much in vogue, and special class sessions provide a means of conveying information to groups.

The Written Word. This method of communication naturally occupies an important place in health education. Information is thus presented in newspapers, as news articles, feature stories, questions and answers, special stories or articles, etc.

Pamphlets, brochures, and periodic publications are used extensively. National magazines, particularly those addressed to women, carry regular or occasional articles on one aspect of health or another. Considering the circumstances in which the latter are prepared, they are remarkably good and reach and influence vast numbers of people. Occasionally such publications do some harm through prematurity or incompleteness, and arouse unjustified hopes in those who read them; but on the whole, in the United States, they contribute to a better informed and more alert public in matters of health.

Some of the deficiencies in pamphlets and brochures have already been referred to. Although they suffer some from drabness and verbosity, they are productive of much good.

Audiences in Health Education. Some reference to selected audiences has been made above. The points that must be borne in mind are that the methods of presentation, the materials used, and the subject matter must be suitable to the audience to which the information and stimulus of health education are directed at a given time. There would be but little use in distributing brochures to those who cannot read, or to present something in English to those who know only French.

But the matching of presentation and audience must go much further than this. There must be consideration of the audience's stake in the problem and measures. Does the problem come home to them in terms of age, sex, family, community, etc.? Are the measures advocated practicable for this audience, and will they be interested and benefited, or gratified if the measures are carried out? These considerations and many others are necessary in the approach to audiences within the public.

The kinds and varieties of audiences are almost unlimited. Many come to attention only as some specialized undertaking gets under way. Thus audiences in tuberculosis would be different from those one might wish to reach in control of the venereal diseases, as would the group concerned in restaurant sanitation differ from those concerned with an early cancer diagnosis program.

Schools, churches, civic organizations, unions, chambers of commerce, the ministerial groups, physicians, lawyers, parents of children of various ages, sufferers from particular diseases (tuberculosis, heart disease, diabetes, rheumatic disease), the aged—all these have their particular interests, motives, and potentialities for health education.

Participants in Health Education. Everybody should take a part. More particularly, however, it needs to be emphasized that from the health agency standpoint, the entire burden and prerogative of the health education program should not rest on or with those persons labeled as health educators. In a generalized health service, health education should permeate practically every service. There is some danger, however, that with the development of health education specialists, others who are not specialists may tend to withdraw from this aspect.

The health educator himself or herself is relatively a new specialist. One may stand too much, or not enough, in awe of those in the more established professions: teachers, engineers, nurses, physicians. It is from these and other fields that the health educator must draw his basic information and content. His is largely a matter of methodology, with nice discrimination as to approach and pursuit in given circumstances. Nearly all health educators become addicted to the use of jargon and clichés. As they become more seasoned, they slough this off and return to normal diction.

Public Relations. This important aspect of public health work is closely related to health education. It has only recently been recognized as a necessary element in health unit practice, and its place organizationally is not clearly cut. In some health departments or voluntary agencies, the same service operates both: public relations becomes a part of health education or vice versa. There is no objection to this, provided the basic difference between the two undertakings is clearly recognized. Health education is designed to provide information and stimulation that will benefit individual and community health. Public relations work is designed to gain among individuals, groups, and the community a favorable and supporting attitude toward the health agency itself.

Here, again, public relations is a job in which all persons in the health agency must participate. Thus the voice answering the telephone is an important factor in public relations. Treatment of reporters plays no small part. The wisdom and style of letters, the personality of those who represent the health department or agency contribute for good or ill. One's attitude and expressions on matters of public interest, and the way he says or does things, may tell a harmful or helpful story.

The Effectiveness of Health Education. It is difficult to measure the result of educational or informative processes. One can, of course, examine groups in colleges as to what information was gleaned from a given course, but obviously education is concerned with more than information, and the results of examinations are not completely satisfying. In health education one cannot examine the public, and even if this were practicable, there is no assurance that, because one knows, for instance, that his food should contain certain essential elements, he will necessarily be sure he eats a balanced diet. Most educated men know that overweight carries with it a shorter than average life expectancy, but comparatively few fat men attain leanness.

In spite of the fact that the results of health education cannot be measured as could the incidence of smallpox in the vaccinated against the unvaccinated, there are reasons for believing that gradually the information and stimulus which the public gets through health education is producing beneficial results. People, as a whole, do eat more balanced meals; women, at least, and some men, consider weight. The public will support measures designed for community health; hospitals are now recognized as places where one is most likely to regain health, not as places to die. Extraneous, variable, and uncontrolled factors enter into all the situations to which the above examples relate, but the American public on the whole is better informed as to health and more interested in it than formerly. Some of this is due to health education.

But because there is so much not specifically or immediately measurable in health education, it is essential that its personnel look at their work objectively from time to time. They must not assume that because a given means or practice is the conventional approach, it will necessarily and assuredly reach the end originally in view, or that it may not be improved upon or replaced by another approach.

Efforts are being made to study the logic and effectiveness of various practices in health education, and such studies should be supported and furthered. At best, however, the procedures must remain largely empirical.

REFERENCE

Kleinschmidt, Harry E., and Zimand, Savel: *Public Health Education—Its Tools and Procedures.* The Macmillan Company, New York, 1953.

chapter 5

The Acute Communicable Diseases

A COMMUNICABLE disease is one which may be communicated directly or indirectly from one host to another. The "host" may be either human, lower animal, or insect, but most often human. The term "communicable disease" to a great extent replaces the older designations "infectious disease" and "contagious disease," formerly used in this connection.

There are one or two other definitions which should be borne in mind in relation to the communicable diseases. "Sporadic" means that the disease occurs fitfully or intermittently. "Endemic" indicates that a disease is constantly present in a given locality but affects only a very small proportion of the population. "Epidemic" means that an unusually large number of persons in a given area are affected by a disease. "Pandemic" indicates that the epidemic is nationwide or world-wide. Thus rabies occurs *sporadically;* measles is *endemic* in all large cities, and tends periodically to become *epidemic;* a *pandemic* of influenza occurred in 1957.

"Epidemiology," as applied to the communicable diseases, may be defined as the science concerned with the mass interactions between man on the one hand and his parasites on the other; and with those factors which influence these interactions. The word *incidence* refers to the occurrence of the disease on a given date, whereas *prevalence*

89

refers to the existing number of cases on a given date. Thus, in an epidemic of typhoid fever, the incidence as of January 14 would include only those cases which occurred on that date. The prevalence on January 14 would be the incidence of that day, plus the incidence of previous days, minus those that have recovered or died. A *contact* is one whose history indicates probable exposure to the infectious material of a communicable disease.

It was not so long ago that the major part of health departments' time was given to efforts for the control of communicable diseases. Great reliance was placed upon quarantine, not infrequently enforced by guards, and upon the assumed efficacy of fumigation for the destruction of bacteria. Gradually, procedures have evolved along more or less scientific lines. Fumigation is no longer practiced for the destruction of infectious material, and quarantine requirements are not nearly so strict as formerly. With the application of measures for community sanitation, and with an increasing proportion of the population protected by vaccination against smallpox, typhoid fever, and diphtheria, and, perhaps, with the operation of certain natural forces not at present understood, the acute communicable diseases are not so much of a problem as they once were. They are still important, however, and, in some, such as the common cold, control measures are no more effective than they were a thousand years ago.

Every case of a communicable disease is an instance of *parasitism*, where one organism lives in (endoparasites) or upon (ectoparasites), and at the expense of, another. The invaded organism is the *host*, the invading organism is the *parasite*. If the parasite has more than one species as host, and reproduces sexually and asexually, the one in which its sexual phase occurs is known as the definitive host; the other is the intermediate host. Parasitic relationship is seen in an endless variety of instances in both the plant and animal kingdom, e.g., plant lice and viruses; any infection in animals, infestation with ticks, intestinal worms, etc. It is the latter which one is more likely to think of as parasites, but cases of scarlet fever or poliomyelitis are just as definitely manifestations of parasitism.

The Essential Causes of Communicable Diseases. Every communicable disease is due to some living organism, usually microscopic, although not necessarily so. There is no consensus as to the finer separations of these causative organisms, but the following is a reasonably conventional classification.

1. *Bacteria,* as in diphtheria and typhoid fever. Bacteria are minute living organisims, belonging to the lower order of the plant kingdom. Relatively few of the existing bacteria produce disease in man. Indirectly, some are highly beneficial.

2. *Protozoa,* as in malaria and amebic dysentery. Protozoa belong to the simplest, unicellular order of the animal kingdom.

3. *Spirochetes,* as in syphilis. Spirochetes appear to occupy a position between bacteria and protozoa, though usually classed with the former.

4. *Viruses,* as in yellow fever and measles. Typically, viruses are substances so small as to pass through the finest filters. An entirely acceptable system of classification has not yet been achieved.

5. *Rickettsiae,* as in typhus fever. Rickettsiae are bacteria-like bodies. Although at present there is no agreement as to their precise place in any scheme of classification, they are now recognized as a special group of microorganisms.

6. *Molds,* as in ringworm. Molds are low forms of plant life (fungi), characterized morphologically by filamentous, weblike structures and abundant spores.

7. *Yeasts,* as in thrush and coccidioidal granuloma. Yeasts are closely related to molds, being fungi of much simpler form.

8. *Trematodes* (flukes).

9. *Cestodes* (tapeworm).

10. *Nematodes* (hookworm, ascaris).

Factors Concerned in the Prevalence of a Communicable Disease. For a communicable disease to occur in a community, there are three essential elements: a focus, from which may come the causative organism; an individual who is susceptible to the disease; and an avenue, a way, for the causative organism to get from the focus to the susceptible. Lacking any of these three, the disease will not occur unless imported. Thus, at present in the United States, the yellow fever mosquito is relatively abundant in certain localities, and practically the whole population is susceptible to that disease—but there is no focus.

There are, of course, conditions which modify the operation of these factors and which, in the presence of focus, susceptibles, and means of transmission, determine whether or not a given disease will be sporadic, endemic, or epidemic. For instance, temperature and associated factors have considerable effect upon the seasonal occurrence and distribution of many diseases. Travel enters strongly into the situation in certain diseases, as do the customs, dietary habits, and personal hygiene of the people concerned.

The kind, the number, and the virulence of the organism, as well as the resistance of the individual, play important parts in determining whether or not a disease will occur when the specific living agent gains access to the body. Thus A, vaccinated against typhoid fever, might without harm swallow a glass of water containing some typhoid bacilli, the same number of which would produce the disease in unvaccinated B. But if the number of bacilli which A swallowed were large, or if the organisms were unusually virulent, he would develop typhoid fever, as his immunity is only relative.

The Ways in Which Infectious Material Leaves the Body. This depends largely upon the character of the disease. Generally the natural orifices of the body are the means of exit of material containing the specific causative agent of the disease. Of course, there can be no discharge of such causative organisms from an individual unless they have previously been introduced into that individual: No possible combination or interaction of secretions or of excretions or of tissues can produce the protozoa of malaria or the typhoid bacillus, since these are living organisms and must have ancestors. The summary which follows indicates the principal means of exit:

1. Through the intestinal tract: in the stools, as in typhoid fever, cholera, dysentery.

2. Through the urinary tract: the bacillus of typhoid fever.

3. From and about the genital organs: the causative organisms of gonorrhea and other venereal diseases.

4. Through the mouth and nose: secretions and excretions of the

mouth, nose and throat, bronchi, as in diphtheria, scarlet fever, tuberculosis, secondary stage of syphilis.

5. Through the eye: not so important as most of the others, but a factor to be considered.

6. From the blood: when the skin is punctured and the blood drawn by some insect, as by the mosquito in malaria.

7. Through milk: particularly important in connection with dairy cattle and the spread of brucellosis and bovine tuberculosis.

The Ways in Which Infectious Material Gains Access to the Body. Broadly speaking, although there are exceptions, the portal of entry of any given microorganism is into the same general system as that through which the infectious material is discharged from the body. Those which are discharged through the intestinal and urinary tracts are swallowed; those in the excretions of the nose and throat enter through the mucous membranes of these orifices; those leaving via the blood only through a biting insect gain entrance through the bite of the same kind of insect. Pneumonic type of plague exhibits a sharp exception to this. Examples of atypical portals of entry for diseases which usually infect by some other route are wound diphtheria, diphtheria of the vagina, gonorrhea of the eye.

The Ways in Which Communicable Diseases Are Transmitted. That communicable diseases cannot just spring up, but can arise only from a pre-existing organism of the same sort, is not only a fact, but the bedrock of epidemiology. As simple as this principle now appears, it is the dividing line between the ancient and modern conceptions of communicable diseases.

Transmission may be *direct* from the case or carrier to a susceptible, through immediate contact such as transfer of secretions from mouth to mouth, as in kissing; contamination of hands of one person by excretions of another, with subsequent transfer of this contamination to nose or mouth; a dog bite, as in rabies; an infected cut, as from cleaning a rabbit, in tularemia.

Transmission may be *indirect*, where some intermediate agent carries infectious material from case or carrier to a susceptible: (1) Air acts as the agent in "droplet infection," where coughed or sneezed moisture remains suspended for a short time; (2) water or food, including milk, may be an intermediate agent, as in typhoid fever, diphtheria, scarlet fever, bovine tuberculosis, brucellosis; (3) soils may serve as an intermediate agent, as in hookworm infestation or tetanus; (4) insects may act as agents, either by mechanically carrying infectious material, such as flies contaminated with dysentery bacilli, or because the organism goes through a stage of development in the insect, as malarial parasites do in mosquitoes; (5) contaminated articles (fomites) if freshly soiled may occasionally act as agents in certain diseases, but their importance has been greatly overrated.

Knowledge of this sort is necessary in public health work in order that prompt disinfection may be practiced on infective discharges, during the course of a given disease, and also in order that household and community measures may be taken to erect barriers in the avenues along which infection travels.

Measures Taken to Prevent the Communicable Diseases. These are of considerable number and of many different sorts. They vary from vaccination to the building of sewer systems; from the destruction of mosquito breeding to the pasteurization of milk. Classified as to approach, such measures may be separated as follows:

1. Measures relating to a focus or the foci of a disease. They are designed to prevent the individual case or carrier from causing spread: isolation, disinfection, procedures which change cases from infectious to noninfectious stage, as in the early treatment of syphilis.

2. Measures designed to make immune to a given disease those now susceptible to that disease, before the disease occurs: vaccination against smallpox, or diphtheria. See page 105 in regard to immunity.

3. Measures designed to interpose a barrier between foci of infection and susceptibles: filtration and disinfection of water supplies, pasteurization of milk, destruction of insects, personal hygiene.

Isolation and Quarantine. The word "isolation," as used in public health work, has the following meaning: the separation of a case or

carrier of a communicable disease from other persons in such a way
and for such a length of time as may be necessary to prevent spread.
"Quarantine" refers to restrictions on the movements of those exposed to a communicable disease. Thus the child exposed to diphtheria may be quarantined at home until there is reasonable assurance
that he will not develop the disease. Within the home the person
who actually has diphtheria is isolated.

Some years ago far more reliance was placed upon isolation and
quarantine than is now believed justified. In those days guards were
quite often posted at entrances to prevent ingress and egress; the
householders were required to display red or yellow flags, and occasionally a cross was painted on the door with a lettered supplication.
Today, the rights and comforts of those quarantined are given consideration, and such persons are allowed freedom within the limits of
safety. Quarantine and isolation do some good, in that they separate
known sources of infection from contact with susceptibles and avenues of infection, but the control of communicable diseases cannot
be brought about by isolation and quarantine alone.

Some of the Problems Incident to Isolation and Quarantine

1. Some cases are not reported to the health department until
the disease is well advanced. In such circumstances the patient was
not in isolation during the early part of the period of communicability.
He may have infected many others during this time.

2. Carriers are seldom discovered and reported, and are difficult
to manage.

3. In many communities it is difficult to get persons with a communicable disease admitted to a general hospital, and the case must
remain at home.

4. In many homes, living quarters are so congested that it is not
practicable to effect complete separation of the case from other
members of the family.

5. Not infrequently, the mother of the sick child must act in the
capacity of nurse and also as cook and nurse for other children in
the family.

6. Not infrequently the intelligence or interest of the mother is

not such as to grasp the general principles and procedures in hygiene and disinfection.

7. Poverty may be such that it is impossible for the family to obtain the simplest essentials for disinfection: vessels in which to boil clothes, separate dishes, disinfectants.

8. In many instances the period of communicability is longer than the illness, and it is difficult for the health authorities to make the family understand that recovery of the patient does not mean cessation of danger to others.

9. To quarantine the breadwinner means no income for the family.

10. It is difficult for mothers to keep the well, but quarantined, children off the street. They may spread infection.

11. The quarantined family is impatient of restrictions and uses various means in trying to get the health department to "release" them before the danger of spread is past.

12. It is not always practicable to find contacts of cases; it is difficult at best to get contacts not in the family to observe restrictions during the period of incubation of the disease.

Disinfectants and Their Use. A disinfectant is an agent used to destroy pathogenic organisms. It will be noted that disinfection is less complete than sterilization, which destroys all organisms.

Concurrent disinfection is the immediate and continuing disinfection of infectious material as it arises during the course of a disease. It includes similar prompt action with articles freshly soiled by infectious material.

Terminal disinfection is the final disinfecting bath of patient, disinfection of clothes, bedclothes, and room or rooms which were occupied by the patient.

Contrary to what was formerly thought by the medical profession and at present thought by the public, terminal disinfection is of little importance compared with concurrent disinfection. If the latter has been properly carried out, there is but little infectious material left for terminal disinfection at the end of the period of communicability.

The principal kinds of disinfectants are:

1. Mechanical: removal of infectious material and its contained pathogenic organisms by scrubbing or washing.

2. Thermal: heat, cold.

3. Chemical: carbolic acid, chlorine gas or solution.

4. Light rays: natural sunlight or artificially generated rays.

5. Drying: probably effective in nature over periods of time.

6. Pressure: usually used in connection with heat, especially steam, as in the autoclave.

The strength of a chemical disinfectant is expressed in terms of phenol, which, under certain standard conditions, is given a disinfectant value of 1.0. Thus a disinfectant may be of an effectiveness of 1.5, 0.3, etc., in comparison with phenol. This comparative strength is known as the "phenol coefficient" of the disinfectant. The phenol coefficient is not an entirely satisfactory index of the general value of a disinfectant.

Certain Important Factors to Be Borne in Mind in the Use of Disinfectants. It should be remembered:

1. That except where there is actual destruction, as by fire, no disinfectant acts immediately. Therefore, sufficient time must be provided.

2. That the *mass* or *amount* of material to be disinfected must be taken into consideration: One quart of a 5 per cent phenol solution added to a quart of feces, has its disinfectant content reduced to 2.5 per cent.

3. That the disinfectant must come into contact with all parts of the material to be disinfected; thorough mixing is necessary.

Measures Usually Carried Out When There Is a Communicable Disease in a Home. The most worth-while instruction, so far as the home is concerned, is to advise sending the case to a hospital where isolation is practicable. Where this is not possible, the patient should be put in a well-ventilated room, preferably with a private bath adjoining. Convention prescribes that rugs and draperies be removed, although this is largely a gesture. The attendant is provided with two or three protective aprons and cap for hair, and there should be a supply of paper napkins or old cloths for mouth and nose secretions. On use, napkins are deposited in a paper bag within easy reach of patient and attendant. The bag and its contents are burned as soon as the bag is full.

There is maintained a stock of disinfectant solutions for hands, woodwork, sputum (if there is more than can be caught in handkerchiefs), stools, and urine. A nailbrush is needed for the attendant. It is very essential that there be covered receptacles (1) containing disinfectant solutions for bedclothes, pending boiling; (2) for boiling dishes; (3) for holding disinfectant solution in contact with stools, urine, sputum; also a basin for hand disinfectant solution. There should be separate dishes, boiled after each use, and milk receptacles, etc., for patient and attendant.

In concurrent and terminal disinfection, material listed below may be disinfected as indicated:

Mattresses and Heavy Bedclothes. By exposure to sun and air for at least 48 hours.

Soiled Linen. By immediate immersion in 2 per cent cresol solution, followed by boiling.

Floors and Woodwork. By thorough scrubbing with strong soap and water.

Sputum and Nasal Discharges. By catching in paper or rag handkerchiefs, and burning.

Stools and Urine. By 5 per cent fresh solution of chloride of lime for one hour. Amount of disinfectant equal at least to amount of material to be disinfected, and thoroughly mixed.

Dishes. By ordinary washing, followed by boiling.

Hands of Attendant. By scrubbing and immersion in bichloride solution, alcohol, or cresol solution.

Fumigation and Fumigants. As understood, at present, the word "fumigation" indicates the liberation, in a closed space, of chemicals in gaseous form, destructive to insect and rodent life.

Fumigation is used in destroying rats, mosquitoes, and fleas in ships. It is no longer relied upon by health departments for destruction of germ life, although not infrequently the public expects it. Because of an old faith in its efficacy, the householder will sometimes burn a few sulfur candles instead of using soap and water and sunshine in terminal disinfection.

Hydrocyanic Gas. This is used under pressure or through use of substances (cyanogen chloride) which will release the gas. It is highly efficacious, *but exceedingly dangerous.* Its use is mainly limited to ship fumigation, in the hands of experts, equipped with gas masks. It should not be used except by experts.

None of these cyanogen preparations should ever be used in home fumigation.

DDT. A residual spraying of DDT or related substances has largely replaced fumigation for the destruction of insects. DDT, used as a powder, is particularly effective for the destruction of lice in the control of typhus fever. Residual spraying of DDT or similar products has become a standard method for the prevention of malaria in a large part of the world.

The "Period of Incubation" of a Disease. The period of incubation is the lapse of time between the introduction of infectious material into the body and the development of the first symptoms of the disease. The length of time included in the period varies with the different diseases and also varies from case to case in the same disease. One should, therefore, know the minimum and maximum and average period of incubation for each disease.

The respective periods of incubation in the more common communicable diseases are:

Chickenpox. From 2 to 3 weeks.

Common Cold. About 1 to 2 days.

Diphtheria. From 2 to 7 days, usually 3 to 5.

Gonorrhea. Usually 3 to 5 days, may be a little longer or shorter.

Influenza. From 1 to 3 days.

Measles. Approximately 10 days to onset of fever, 14 to onset of rash.

Meningococcal Meningitis. From 2 to 14 days, usually only a few days.

Mumps. From 12 to 26 days, usually a little under 3 weeks.

Pneumonia, Lobar. As a rule, only 1 to 2 days.

Poliomyelitis. From 1 to 2 weeks.

Rabies. Quite variable. From 2 weeks to 6 months, usually a little over a month.

Scarlet Fever and Streptococcal Sore Throat. From 2 to 7 days, usually 3 to 5.

Smallpox. From 1 to 3 weeks, usually 14 days from exposure to rash.

Syphilis. Usually about 3 weeks, may be shorter or longer.

Typhoid Fever. From 1 week to a little over 3 weeks. Usually between 10 and 14 days.

Whooping Cough. From 1 week to 16 days, usually under 10 days.

Importance of Knowledge as to Incubation Period. Practical application of this knowledge is evident in the following instances:

1. A health officer, in placing restrictions upon the movements of a person known to have been intimately exposed to a given disease, keeps these restrictions in force in accordance with the maximum limits of the period of incubation. Sometimes the restriction period is only as long as the average incubation period of the disease concerned.

2. An epidemiologist searching for the source of an outbreak of disease, where most of the cases became sick about the same time, makes use of the known period of incubation of the disease in question in an effort to discover a past experience, or exposure, common to the group concerned. The same process may be gone through in search for source of disease in one individual: a search for some record of possible infection within the minimum and maximum limits of the incubation period.

3. A practicing physician, knowing a patient to have been exposed to a given disease at approximately a given time, can guide himself accordingly in administering prophylaxis or in observation.

The "Period of Communicability" of a Disease. The period of communicability of a disease is that time during which a person affected with a given disease is capable of transmitting it to others, either directly or indirectly. Communicability not infrequently begins in the latter part of the period of incubation. When, as sometimes happens, an individual continues to be a danger to others, after the usual period of communicability is passed, he is known as a "convalescent carrier." Convalescent carriers may become chronic carriers. The period of communicability varies with the different diseases. The end of the period, in any given disease, may be decided:

1. Bacteriologically, when this is possible, as in diphtheria, or
2. By a regulation of the health department, setting forth what shall officially be regarded as the minimum period of communicability for the disease in question, where there are no complications, or
3. By clinical judgment, as in mumps.

The respective periods of communicability in the more common communicable diseases are:

Chickenpox. From just before the eruption to somewhat less than 10 days after its appearance.

Common Cold. Mainly during acute stage.

Diphtheria. From 2 to 3 days before illness, and until the nose and throat are free of diphtheria organisms. This freedom from organisms is based upon two consecutive negative nose and throat cultures, taken not less than 24 hours apart. It is unusual for a case of diphtheria to remain in the communicable stage for more than 4 weeks, although this occasionally happens.

Dysentery, Amebic. Varies with length of illness and infection.

Dysentery, Bacillary. Until causative organisms are absent from stools.

Gonorrhea. As long as causative organism is present. Once this was for months, but modern treatment shortens period of communicability of most cases to a few days.

Influenza. Probably just before and for a day or two after acute illness ends.

Measles. From 3 to 4 days before and for about 5 days after appearance of rash.

Meningococcal Meningitis. Possibly communicable before onset, and for about 2 weeks after.

Mumps. From a day or two before onset and until glandular enlargement disappears. Usually from 1 to 2 weeks.

Pneumonia. Probably just before and during acute stage of disease. Knowledge not exact.

Poliomyelitis. Probably during latter part of the period of incubation and for 1 or 2 weeks thereafter.

Rabies. The period of communicability in animals (dogs) is the point of practical importance. This is believed to be from about 2 weeks before the onset of symptoms and throughout the time the animal lives thereafter.

Scarlet Fever and Streptococcal Sore Throat. Probably a day or two before onset of symptoms, and for a period of 2 or 3 weeks after onset if case is untreated; but only for a day or two after effective antibiotic treatment is begun. It is prolonged by discharging ears, infected sinuses, etc.

Smallpox. From 3 to 6 days before appearance of rash and until all scabs have disappeared, usually some 3 weeks after appearance of rash.

Syphilis. While there are open lesions of skin or mucous membranes. Few untreated cases of syphilis are communicable after the second year. Prompt and effective treatment greatly shortens the period of communicability.

Typhoid Fever. From latter part of incubation period and until stools and urine are free of organisms: Usually determined by two negative stool and urine cultures, taken about 1 month after fever disappears. Modern treatment shortens period of communicability.

Whooping Cough. From catarrhal stage, before whoop, and for about 3 weeks after onset of whoop. Modern treatment shortens period of communicability.

Practical Use of Knowledge of the Period of Communicability. Health departments, in placing restrictions upon a case of one of the communicable diseases, continue isolation of the patient until the period of communicability is believed to be ended. Also, in searching for the probable source of a new case, the investigator needs to know whether or not the person suspected as having been the source was, at the time of exposure to him, in a stage of communicability.

Although knowledge of the period of communicability may be applied along fairly definite, reasonable, and effective lines in connection with most diseases, it fails in connection with carriers. This is for two reasons:

1. Seldom does anyone know who the carrier is, in any given circumstances, and the period of communicability of carriers varies not only with the disease but with the individual carrier.

2. The discharge of organisms may be intermittent: communicable today but not tomorrow, not this month but next month.

Some of the Difficulties in Discovering the Source of a Disease. These are many and complex. The principal ones may be listed as follows:

1. The inability of most persons to give a clear and trustworthy account of their affairs for a week or two in the past: what and when and where they ate, or drank water or milk; when and with whom they came in contact.

2. Lack of knowledge on the part of both investigator and patient as to what or whom in the patient's immediate past might have carried infectious material. He may have been in contact with carriers, subclinical cases, missed cases unknowingly, or similarly may have partaken of contaminated food or drink.

3. The difficulty in determining the real significance of a suspected food or contact. Something might appear to be of importance, but it may be an appearance tending only to mask the true operative factor or person.

The fewer and more scattered the cases, the less likely is one to discover some factor common to all; and the less one knows of the subject, the more likely is he to be dogmatic in saying that the source of a given case was this or that. Thus most city people consider the visit to the country, if there was one in the past few weeks, as the place of infection with typhoid fever; and people living in the country are quite likely to blame a visit to the city or town.

Carriers, Subclinical Cases, and Missed Cases. A carrier is one who harbors and discharges infectious material of a communicable disease, but who does not show symptoms of the disease. The carriers about which most is known are the typhoid and diphtheria carriers. It is believed that there are carriers of meningococcal meningitis, polio-myelitis, streptococcal and other diseases. Present knowledge of carriers is quite limited, but they are exceedingly important sources of spread.

Carriers are grouped into various classifications, some of which include individuals who are not truly carriers, inasmuch as their carrier stage is either incident to an oncoming disease or to recent recovery from a disease. The former are sometimes called "incubationary" or "precocious" carriers, and the latter "convalescent" carriers.

Aside from the above types, a true carrier may be either a:

1. *Temporary carrier:* One who carries and discharges the organisms or virus of the disease for a relatively short time, as in contacts of diphtheria cases, or a,

2. *Chronic carrier:* One who carries and discharges organisms or virus for an indefinite time.

Carriers may be further subdivided in terms of organs affected. Thus the carrier in typhoid fever may be an intestinal carrier, where the organism is located in the gallbladder, ducts, and duodenum, and discharged in the feces; or a urinary carrier, with organisms in the pelvis of the kidney and the bladder, discharging bacilli into the urine.

The *subclinical* case of a communicable disease is one where true infection exists but which presents symptoms so mild as to escape recognition in most instances. Thus a person with a communicable disease might have only headache, or a little fever for a day or two; the manifestations of a true poliomyelitis in a child might be considered as only an upper respiratory infection.

The dividing line between the carrier, in whom absence of symptoms is assumed, and the subclinical case, in which symptoms are slight, is not clearly drawn.

A "missed" case is one which is not known to the health authorities. It might be:

1. A subclinical case, either with or without a physician in attendance, and not reported.

2. A typical case, but with no physician in attendance and hence not reported.

3. A typical case in which a physician failed to make a correct diagnosis.

4. A typical case in which a physician made a correct diagnosis, but failed to report it to the health department.

Immunity as It Relates to Public Health. As indicated above, the establishment of immunity to a given disease in one or a number of individuals is a highly important method of protection. Even the casual student of public health needs to know some of the elements of this subject.

By "immunity," as the term is usually used, is meant resistance to a particular communicable disease. Immunity to one disease does not mean that there is immunity to another. The apparent robustness of an individual is not an index of his resistance to infection by the organisms of an acute communicable disease: An invalid, successfully vaccinated against smallpox, would be far less likely to develop that disease on exposure than would the unvaccinated wrestling champion in similar circumstances.

Resistance to diseases may be classified either as natural immunity or as acquired immunity. *Natural* or *inherited immunity* is a condition wherein the individual, human or lower orders, is immune, usually completely immune, to some particular disease because all members of the species to which he belongs are immune. Animals have an immunity to syphilis,* typhoid fever, and most of the acute communicable diseases; man has an immunity to chicken cholera, Texas fever of cattle, and many virus diseases affecting the lower animals.

Animal experimentation in the diseases of man is limited to those animals that are susceptible to the infectious agent responsible for a particular disease. For example, experimental work in poliomyelitis was limited markedly because only primates are naturally susceptible to the disease, and then only in limited degree and under special circumstances. In some instances it has been possible to adapt the

* Except the rabbit.

causative organism of certain diseases to animals not naturally susceptible to these infections. For example, certain strains of the poliomyelitis virus have been adapted to animals not naturally susceptible to the infection.

The temporary, passive immunity to certain diseases, transmitted by immune mothers to their infants, is sometimes included in the heading "natural" immunity. This is really an immunity which the child acquires in utero, but it is acquired only if the mother herself possesses the particular immunity. It is not a common heritage of the species, but may be called a congenital immunity.

Some races appear to have a higher resistance than others to certain diseases, but there is not complete assurance that this is not an acquired immunity.

Acquired immunity is a resistance which the individual develops, other than through a commonly held species immunity, as follows:

1. In many communicable diseases, by having had the disease, although there are exceptions.

2. In a number of diseases, by receiving from others doses of infectious material sufficiently large to cause the tissues to produce antibodies, but neither large enough nor strong enough to produce clinical symptoms of the disease.

3. In certain diseases, through artificial immunization (see below).

4. By passage of antibodies of certain diseases through the placenta to the developing infant. Obviously, as stated above, if the mother does not possess these antibodies, she cannot transmit them.

Acquired immunity is seldom absolute. An individual might successfully resist infection from an ordinary "dose" of typhoid bacteria of average virulence, but would develop the disease if he swallowed large amounts of milk or water containing a great number of highly virulent typhoid organisms.

Two kinds of immunity may be produced by artificial immunization against certain diseases.

1. *Passive Immunity.* Immunity received when material already containing antibodies is injected, as diphtheria antitoxin, or con-

valescent serum. In such procedures the resistance to newly formed toxin produced by the infecting agents is rapid, from 12 to 48 hours. However, passive immunity is of short duration, passing off in 3 to 4 weeks.

2. *Active Immunity.* Immunity developed when material ("antigens," see below) introduced into the body causes the tissues to form their own antibodies. This is the type of immunity developed as the result of a case of whooping cough or measles or as the result of vaccination against smallpox or diphtheria. Active immunity usually develops much more slowly than passive, but is more lasting.

A person possessing passive immunity is like a warehouse: a temporary storage place for a product manufactured elsewhere. One with active immunity is comparable to the manufacturing plant itself.

Vaccines are used to produce active immunity; sera to confer passive immunity.

The substances in the blood stream and tissues upon which immunity is believed to depend are of two kinds, both known by the general term "antibodies."

1. Those which tend to destroy the invading organism, and
2. Those which tend to destroy or neutralize the toxins of the invading organisms.

Included in the first group are substances which the tissues produce, each one specific for a particular organism. These are called lysins, precipitins, agglutinins, opsonins. In addition to these antibodies, which are not really "bodies," but chemicals, are the leukocytes, or white blood cells, which are nonspecific and tend to destroy any invading organisms through engulfing them (phagocytosis).

In the second group, those which tend to destroy or neutralize toxins are the antitoxins. These are produced only in response to a definite toxin ("exotoxins," see below) manufactured by the invading organisms.

The term *virulence,* to which reference has been previously made, indicates two factors in an organism: (1) its relative capacity to overcome tissue resistance, thus establishing itself parasitically; and

(2) its ability to produce or otherwise yield toxin. Because the former function cannot at present be definitely measured, there is a tendency to consider that toxin production is an index of virulence and to designate as virulent those organisms which produce toxin under laboratory conditions. In this connection, two factors should be borne in mind. The first is that laboratory procedures in testing virulence are not necessarily the same as, and frequently are sharply at variance with, those conditions which obtain in nature; the second, that an organism's ability to produce a powerful or abundant toxin does not necessarily indicate a corresponding ability to overcome tissue resistance.

The subject of virulence is quite complex. Variations in virulence of the same kinds of organisms must be recognized but cannot be predicted. The question of strains, varying qualitatively as well as quantitatively in their virulence, adds to an already confused situation and encourages assumption.

Somewhat related to the matter of virulence is the problem of "resistant" strains or forms of organisms. These have become the object of much attention since the introduction of the sulfonamides and the antibiotics. In effect, certain organisms, such as the gonococcus or the tubercle bacillus, tend to become resistant to the drug used. There is a justifiable but sometimes overemphasized fear that if and when these resistant organisms are passed on to others they will remain impervious to what is, in general, successful therapy; and that these hardy survivors may establish a new and widespread strain causing disease more intractable than ever before.

Research suggests that combination of the antibiotic with some other drug may lessen the rise of resistant organisms: thus the combination of aminosalicylic acid (PAS) with streptomycin.

Exotoxins and Endotoxins. An *exotoxin* is the chemical product resulting from metabolism in the organism, and thrown off during the life of the organism. The best-known exotoxins are those of the tetanus and diphtheria bacilli.

An *endotoxin* is the chemical product resulting from the death and subsequent degeneration of the organism. The toxin of the typhoid organism, and from a number of others, appears to be an endotoxin.

It is probable that many organisms, at present thought to produce only the one type of toxin, will later be found to release both.

Tissue reaction to an exotoxin is to produce a specific antitoxin. The reaction to an endotoxin is to produce specific bacterial antibodies such as lysins, agglutinins, precipitins.

Factors Which Largely Determine Whether or Not an Individual Will Develop an Acute Communicable Disease upon the Introduction of Infectious Material

1. The character of the infective agent; some organisms have an affinity for human tissues, others have not, in ordinary circumstances.

2. The virulence of the organism or virus.

3. The numbers of the organism or the amount of virus.

4. The specific immunity of the individual concerned.

5. To a limited extent, in certain conditions, the general health of the individual; perhaps certain specific elements in nutrition play a part.

6. Probably, in certain instances, local tissue resistance.

7. The route through which the infectious material is introduced; if the portal of entry is not suitable there is no tissue damage.

Susceptibles. A susceptible, to some particular disease, is one who, because of no immunity, or lack of reasonably effective immunity to that disease, is likely to develop the disease on exposure. As in immunity, susceptibility is a relative term. An individual vaccinated against smallpox 20 years ago might be an immune, so far as infection with a mild virus is concerned, but a susceptible as regards a virulent strain of smallpox virus.

Antigens. The word "antigen" is the scientific designation given to any material capable of stimulating the tissues to the production of antibodies: diphtheria toxoid, virus of smallpox vaccine, typhoid vaccine. Antigens are not necessarily associated with microorganisms or viruses. Such commonplace substances as egg albumen, or beef soup, fulfill the requirements for antigens.

Correct Usage of the Word "Serum." One may use this term if the material in question comes from the blood serum of an animal, as diphtheria antitoxin, tetanus antitoxin, antistreptococcus serum. One may not designate, as sera, agents used to develop active immunity, for they are usually bacteria, viruses, or their immediate products. It is painfully bad usage to speak of diphtheria toxoid, or typhoid vaccine, or rabies vaccine, as a "serum." Incidentally, although the word "vaccine" comes from the Latin, *vacca*, meaning "cow," and although only smallpox vaccine comes from the cow, custom has made acceptable the use of the word "vaccine" to indicate any agent used to produce active immunity.

Anaphylaxis, Allergy, Protein Reaction, Serum Sickness. The phenomena manifested in these conditions are exceedingly complex and not clearly understood. It is probable that they are all closely related, and incident to quite similar physiological processes. They appear to be due to some toxic product formed by the action of previously sensitized tissues on certain substances, mainly proteins, when these are taken into the body. Persons who have had one injection of a particular protein, such as the protein in a horse serum antitoxin, are to some extent sensitized to future injections and may react by "anaphylaxis" or by "serum sickness." A similar sensitivity may be brought about by previous inhalations or ingestions of other materials such as horse dandruff, pollens, foods. One who has had a previous injection containing horse serum, or who suffers from asthma or hay fever, should never be given horse serum injections without first testing for sensitivity by injecting a drop of the serum into the skin and noting whether or not an urticarial wheal forms. If there is such a wheal, serum may be given safely only in small divided doses, frequently repeated. Some individuals, with no history of previous serum injections and no other indications of sensitivity, react sharply to the first injection of a serum. The following, as commonly used terms, probably overlap each other either quantitatively or qualitatively, or both.

Anaphylaxis is the term employed to describe symptoms of shock which, in these sensitized individuals, appear immediately upon the injection of the substance to which they are sensitive. The use of the term is largely limited to reactions seen after the introduction of a serum.

Allergy is a term used to describe such groups of symptoms as are seen in (1) hay fever, (2) asthma, (3) sudden illnesses and rashes incident to eating certain foods, and (4) local reactions manifested after certain skin tests: pollen, foods, dusts, and protein skin tests.

Protein Reaction. This is the term commonly used to describe disturbances, local and general, sometimes seen after injections of killed cultures of bacteria or their filtrates: after typhoid vaccine or diphtheria toxoid.

Serum Sickness. This is the term employed to describe late and relatively mild reactions, with urticaria, possibly arthritis, seen from the second to twelfth day after injection of a serum.

The Usual Legal Requirements in Regard to Communicable Dis. eases. Requirements vary from city to city and from state to state, but in general these may be listed as follows:

1. Communicable diseases shall be promptly reported, by the physician in attendance, to the local health officer. In absence of a physician, the head of the house is responsible for reporting.

2. They shall be promptly investigated by the health department, in order to determine source and prevent spread.

3. Such restrictions (isolation and quarantine) as are imposed by the health department must be observed, on penalty of a fine. It is also unlawful to interfere with or obstruct an agent of the health department in pursuit of his or her duty.

4. Quarantine placards, if used, may not be removed by any person other than a member of the health department.

5. School children, teachers, or persons engaged in food handling, who have recently had one of the more serious communicable diseases or who have been exposed to one of them, may not return to school or work until passed upon by the health department.

Physicians are rarely prosecuted for failure to report communicable diseases. If the doctor merely forgets to report a disease, the health department is ordinarily quite willing to assume good intentions on his part. He is courteously requested to be just a little more careful. On the other hand, if the physician point-blank refuses to make reports, and if discussion and attempts at persuasion are ineffective, there is but little for the health department to do except enforce the requirements by prosecution. Health officers, unless they are unusually unpleasant types, undertake this legal action only as a last resort. Quite often they attempt to have some mutual friends persuade the physician to observe requirements.

The health officer is inclined, too, to be sympathetic with families under restrictions because of communicable diseases. Even though regulations are violated, the authorities are willing to consider it as due to ignorance of the requirements, and a warning is issued. When the violations are deliberate, flagrant, and repeated, the health department has no satisfactory alternative to prosecution.

Important Public Health Points to Be Remembered in Connection with the Common Communicable Diseases. The physician, attending the patient, is concerned with etiology, pathology, symptomatology, prognosis, treatment, and to some extent prevention, as these subjects relate to the particular individual under observation. The public health perspective, although it is also concerned with the individual, sees the problem more as it relates to the community: the biological conflict between the human group and the causative organism; what circumstances are likely to give ascendancy to the one or the other. For these reasons, the practicing physician on the one hand and the epidemiologist on the other are interested in a different set of data. Actually the interests of these two are interdependent rather than mutually exclusive, but there is a strong tendency for each to lose interest in the field of the other.

The kind of communicable disease information in which the public health worker is particularly concerned, as it relates to any given disease, may be outlined as follows:

1. The causative agent of the disease, and its important characteristics. The likelihood of its survival or death in natural and artificially created environments; whether the organism is found only in human beings or also in animals, birds, insects, etc.; whether or not it exists for any length of time independent of a host.

2. Avenues of infection: the usual and occasional ways in which the disease is transmitted.

3. Through what portal of entry infection gains access to the body.

4. In what tissue and in what excretions the infectious material is found or is discharged from the body.

5. The period of incubation of the disease in question.

6. The period of communicability and how its end is determined.

7. Whether or not atypical or subclinical cases are likely to play a part as unrecognized and difficultly discoverable foci of infection; and the role of carriers, if any.

8. What aid the laboratory can give in arriving at a diagnosis of the disease or carrier state.

9. The morbidity rate: the annual number of cases of the disease per 100,000 population.

10. The mortality rate: the annual number of deaths from the disease, per 100,000 population.

11. The case fatality ratio: the per cent of cases of the disease which result in death.

12. The age group which the disease particularly affects, if in the various age groups there is a difference in the morbidity rate, the mortality rate, or the case fatality ratio.

13. The character of prevalence: whether sporadic, endemic, epidemic; and the frequency, extent, and peculiarities of the epidemics.

14. Immunity, as it relates to the disease: whether one acquires immunity as the result of an attack; whether any age groups tend to be immune; whether there are agents for the production of active and passive immunity.

15. The general measures taken to prevent and control the disease: isolation, quarantine, disinfection, community sanitation, personal hygiene.

Although it is considered unnecessary to discuss, in this presentation, each of the communicable diseases in the above terms, there are certain aspects of some that justify more specific mention, as follows.

Diphtheria. This was for long a highly fatal disease of childhood. It has to some extent been brought under control, but vigorous programs must be continued. Antitoxin and toxoid are the material most relied upon.

Diphtheria Toxin. Diphtheria toxin is the material, probably an excretion, possibly a secretion, which active living diphtheria organisms produce. This toxin is released into the tissues and blood stream during infection. It may also be generated in artificial culture. When filtered from laboratory cultures it is the basis of toxoid.

The Preparation and Use of Diphtheria Antitoxin

1. Active immunity is produced in the horse by injecting diphtheria toxin in increasing doses, over a period of months.

2. The horse is bled from jugular vein, under aseptic conditions.

3. Serum is separated from clot, concentrated, tested for sterility, tested for potency (number of antitoxin units* per milliliter), and put up in syringes for use.

4. Antitoxin is used to confer a passive immunity, mainly for the cure of diphtheria, dose from 20,000 to 80,000 units. It is sometimes used for immediate prophylaxis in children exposed to the disease, dose 10,000 units.

Immunity so conferred is *passive*. As the antibodies injected are contained in a foreign protein (globulin in horses' serum), the protection thus obtained will last only for so long as it takes the tissues to get rid of their foreign protein—about 1 month.

Although prophylactic use of antitoxin gives practically an immediate resistance (in 12 to 48 hours) to diphtheria, *there is no permanent immunity as a result of this process*. It should not be confused with the active and more lasting immunity conferred by toxoid.

The Preparation and Use of Diphtheria Toxoid

1. Diphtheria toxin is obtained by filtering laboratory cultures of diphtheria bacilli. The fluid portion passing through the filter contains the toxin. Diphtheria toxin has two very distinct elements: (1) the toxic, which causes tissue damage, and (2) the antigenic, which stimulates the tissues to produce antitoxin. It is desirable to reduce the former and conserve the latter. Formalin has this unique ability.

---

* A unit of antitoxin is the amount of antitoxin necessary to protect a 250-gm guinea pig against 100 times the minimal lethal dose of diphtheria toxin. The minimal lethal dose (frequently written MLD) is the least amount of toxin which, when injected into a 250-gm guinea pig, will cause death on the fourth or fifth day.

2. The toxin is treated with a solution containing 0.3 or 0.4 per cent of formalin, and thus is converted into toxoid.

3. It is allowed to "ripen" for a number of months, and then placed in bottles for use.

4. It is used to produce active immunity against diphtheria.

Alum-precipitated toxoid consists of toxoid prepared in the usual manner, to which is added alum (alum potassium sulfate) to precipitate out the antigenic elements. The precipitate is suspended in normal salt solution. The presence of alum prolongs absorption in the tissues, and, as this absorption goes on for 2 or 3 weeks, the effect of the dose is more continuing than with ordinary toxoid.

The Administration of Toxoid. The procedure is as follows:

1. An area on the upper, outer surface of the arm, just posterior to and above the insertion of the deltoid muscle, is cleaned with alcohol or acetone.

2. One milliliter of toxoid is injected deeply subcutaneously or into the muscle.

3. Sterile, nonrust needles, ½ in. long, 25 or 26 gauge, are used.

4. All-glass syringes (1-, 2-, 5-, or 10-ml capacity, in accordance with the physician's choice) are used.

5. With ordinary toxoid, the dose is repeated at monthly intervals until three doses have been given.

6. With alum-precipitated toxoid, one dose was, in the past, considered sufficient. The tendency at present is to give two doses, one to two months apart or preferably three doses of combined diphtheria pertussis and tetanus toxoid at monthly intervals.

Reaction Encountered in the Use of Toxoid. The reaction consists usually in a very slight redness, in 12 to 24 hours, in the area where the injection was given. Occasionally, there is malaise, with a slight fever. Older persons, and persons with "combined" Schick reactions (see below) usually have considerable discomfort, fever, headache. The dose for them should be smaller, or toxin-antitoxin may be used.

The Age at Which Toxoid Should Be Administered. When the infant is between 2 to 6 months of age he should be given toxoid.

If it was not given at this time, it should be administered as soon thereafter as possible. The reasons for this are as follows:

1. During this period infants lose the passive immunity usually transmitted by the mother.

2. Having lost this passive immunity, and not yet having acquired any active immunity, infants are particularly susceptible to diphtheria. Both case fatality and mortality rates are relatively high in these young children.

3. Infants give the minimum reaction to toxoid.

Approximately 85 to 95 per cent of those given toxoid will probably become immune to diphtheria in 6 weeks to 3 to 4 months. *Toxoid should not be relied upon to give immediate protection to a child already exposed to diphtheria.* The immunity stimulated by toxoid is fairly long lasting. How long it will last depends upon a number of factors, one of the most important of which is subsequent receipt of diphtheria organisms through association with carriers. If, or as, carriers in the population decrease, this means of stimulating immunity would tend to disappear, and toxoid injections would have to be repeated every few years.

The Schick Reaction. This is a skin test, for the determination of the amount of diphtheria antitoxin an individual possesses. It is usually interpreted as indicating the diphtheria immunity status of the individual.

A solution of diphtheria toxin, so made that 0.1 ml contains $\frac{1}{50}$ of a minimal lethal dose of toxin (see page 114, fn.), is the material used. One tenth of a milliliter is injected *into* the skin (between the layers of the skin, not subcutaneously) on the anterior surface of the forearm.

If the person's blood contains as much as $\frac{1}{30}$ or even $\frac{1}{40}$ of a unit of antitoxin, per milliliter, this will neutralize the toxin injected and no reaction occurs—a negative. If there is less than the above amount of antitoxin in the blood, the injected toxin causes redness around the site of the injection—a positive.

A "control" is used on the other arm. The control material is the same as the Schick test solution, except that it has been heated to

75° C (167° F) for a few minutes in order to destroy the toxin. It therefore contains all the elements of the Schick test material except toxin. Because the use of toxoid has become so common in the United States, the Schick test is rarely employed except in "spot checking" of immunity in population groups.

Measles. There is no drug that has a direct effect upon the virus of measles—a serious disease in infants and young children. The antibiotics do, however, act to prevent the development of pneumonia, which causes most of the measles fatalities.

Reasonably satisfactory protection can be assured young and delicate children by injecting gamma globulin a short time after known exposure. This material is derived from pooled human blood. As most adults are immune to measles, this pooled blood contains measles antibodies and gives recipients a protection against measles similar to that provided against diphtheria by diphtheria antitoxin.

Vaccination against Smallpox. Vaccination, as it should be done today, is a simple, rapid technique, not painful. The technique described below is known as the multiple-pressure method. The procedure is essentially as follows:

1. An area about the insertion of the deltoid muscle, usually left, is cleaned with acetone.

2. The small, sealed glass capillary, in which the virus is contained, is cleaned with alcohol or acetone, its ends broken off, a bulb, supplied in package, is applied to one end, and the virus expelled on the cleaned area of the arm.

3. The arm is supported with the left hand; in the right is held a sterile needle (supplied in package), *parallel* to the plane in which the vaccination is to be done.

4. The side of the needle point is *pressed*, with a rapid up-and-down motion, about 20 to 30 times through the virus, against the skin. This causes a minute fold of the epidermis to lap over the needle point. Pressure should be limited to an area of not more than ⅛ in.

5. The vaccine is immediately blotted off, with a piece of sterile gauze. No dressing is applied.

Reaction to Smallpox Vaccine. When an attempt is made to vaccinate an individual against smallpox, one of three things must happen, providing the virus is potent and is properly inserted: *

1. Vaccinia, or primary reaction.
2. Vaccinoid, or a modified reaction.
3. Reaction of immunity.

In the *primary reaction* or "take," the following is the usual sequence of events:

1. For the first 3 or 4 days, nothing seems to be happening.
2. About the fifth or sixth day the vaccinated area becomes reddened, and in another day or two a disk-like pustule is formed.
3. The vaccination is at its height from the tenth to twelfth day; there is a flat, umbilicated pustule, surrounded by a reddened area; the axillary glands may be enlarged; there may be a degree or two of fever, and malaise, lasting for about 24 hours.
4. The pustule hardens, becomes a thick dark-brown scab. In 1 to 2 weeks after the vaccination reaches its height, the scab drops off.

Should the vaccinated arm become unusually sore, the child is kept quiet. If the vesicle has broken, a dressing, greased lightly with boric acid ointment, is attached to the inside of the sleeve over the vaccination. It is best not to put a dressing directly on the arm. Vaccination shields are dangerous and are mentioned only for condemnation. Painting the arm with iodine is *contraindicated.* Local inflammatory reactions arise sometimes because of secondary infection. They are not usually severe, but if serious may be treated with an appropriate sulfonamide or antibiotic.

Vaccinoid is a reaction grading somewhere between the reaction of immunity and a true take or primary reaction. Redness and a superficial vesicle appear in 2 or 3 days after vaccination. A flake-like scab is formed, this being thrown off in about a week or 10 days.

The *reaction of immunity* consists of slight reddening and edema,

---

* It is possible that, even when the virus is impotent or not properly introduced, the initial wound may be infected, thus producing a local reaction, usually mild and of pimple-like appearance.

with itching, around the vaccinated area. It makes its appearance in 12 to 36 hours after vaccination and remains only for 24 to 48 hours. It indicates that the person concerned is relatively immune to smallpox. It is seen in persons who have had smallpox or who have been vaccinated comparatively recently.

Postvaccination Encephalitis. A condition rarely seen, but occasionally reported, is postvaccination encephalitis. The condition seems not dependent upon any infection carried in the vaccine virus. It may be due to some virus previously latent in the person's tissues, which becomes active at the height of the "take" of a primary vaccination. It appears to be similar to the encephalitis sometimes seen after influenza, measles, and other acute infections, and is probably due to a similar chain of events.

The Best Time to Vaccinate against Smallpox. The best time to vaccinate against smallpox is within the first few months after birth. Very young infants stand vaccination excellently, and develop a high degree of immunity. It is doubtful that one is ever justified in vaccinating on the leg. Certainly it should not be done in adults or children old enough to walk.

Unfortunately, relatively few infants are vaccinated, physicians generally not insisting upon it. Only the more intelligent mothers are willing to have it done even when its desirability is called to their attention. They fear it may hurt the baby. Further, because smallpox is becoming more rare, and generally is seen only in a mild form, few people believe it necessary to be vaccinated. Antivaccination and antivivisection societies wage a continuing fight against the procedure. They have little influence with the intelligent but occasionally meet success with the uninformed. Sometimes they succeed in having vaccination laws repealed.

Vaccination against Smallpox after Exposure to the Disease. Whether or not a person, vaccinated after the process of infection has begun, receives protection depends to a great extent upon how early in the period of incubation the vaccination is done. If vaccinated within the first 4 or 5 days after exposure, the immunity resulting from vaccination will probably protect against the developing infection. It is always better to vaccinate exposed persons and hope for the best, regardless of how late in the assumed incubation stage the vaccination is done.

General Requirements of Laws Regarding Smallpox Vaccination. Vaccination laws vary with the different states. Some require, but seldom enforce, vaccination in the first year of life. Most cities and many states require vaccination for school attendance. Cities generally enforce the latter requirements. Unless there are competent rural health departments in a state, rural school children are likely to remain unvaccinated. Most state laws provide that if smallpox is epidemic, vaccination may be made compulsory, at the discretion of the health officer or board of health.

Vaccinations against Other Diseases. Typhoid vaccine has long been used successfully. With markedly decreased incidence of this disease, relatively a small proportion of persons, living under modern urban conditions, now receive this immunization. It is still important, however, in areas where there remains a heavy seeding of carriers and occasional cases, especially where protected water and milk supplies are lacking and where excreta disposal is primitive. It is effective in the protection of troops, and should be given to those who expect to travel or live in an environment not of the highest sanitary quality.

Whooping cough (pertussis) vaccine is reasonably effective and is attaining wide usage by pediatricians. Inasmuch as most fatalities from this disease occur in infancy, vaccination should be done between the second and sixth months of life. Antibody development against whooping cough by infants under 2 months appears to be weak.

Tetanus vaccine (toxoid) is extremely important, because the disease itself, once developed, is highly fatal. Formerly, when one received a wound in which there seemed a chance that tetanus might develop, tetanus antitoxin was given. This was a passive and therefore transient immunity and had to be repeated when there was a second nail in the foot, scalp wound, etc. Unfortunately, many of those who received tetanus antitoxin experienced sharp allergic reactions because of the accompanying horse serum.

Tetanus toxoid, usually two or three doses, establishes a protective immunity. For safety sake, a recall or "booster" dose of tetanus toxoid is usually given if or when new wounds are received. The initial doses are given before there is any wound, frequently in combination with whooping cough vaccine and/or diphtheria toxoid.

In pediatric practice as well as in public health clinics there is a growing tendency to give a combined antigen containing diphtheria toxoid, pertussis vaccine, and tetanus toxoid, the so-called DPT injections. To be most effective this combined immunization should be started between 2 and 6 months of age and should consist of three injections at approximately 1-month intervals. A recall or "booster" dose should be given during the preschool period (at 2 to 3 years of age) and upon entrance to school. For continuing maximum protection, small recall or "booster" doses may be given during childhood and adolescence at intervals of 3 to 5 years. If protection has been neglected in infancy the full program should be carried through as soon as the opportunity arises.

Vaccination against Poliomyelitis. In 1953 Dr. Jonas E. Salk introduced a poliomyelitis vaccine prepared by (1) growing, in separate monkey kidney tissue cultures, a strain of each of the three types of poliomyelitis virus, (2) inactivating the viruses with formalin, and (3) mixing the three inactivated virus types. This vaccine gave promise of producing immunity, at least for a period of time, to all three types of poliomyelitis virus—and without the potential undesirable effects of the Howe vaccine, which was prepared from virus grown in the central nervous system tissues of the monkey. In 1954 the Salk vaccine was subjected to extensive field trial by an evaluation team headed by Dr. Thomas Francis, Jr. Since the field trial seemed to prove beyond reasonable doubt that the vaccine was safe and effective in preventing paralytic poliomyelitis, a nationwide campaign for immunization against this crippling disease was undertaken in 1955. Unfortunately, when the vaccine was adapted to mass production, the specified methods for virus inactivation were not entirely adequate; and several early lots of vaccine apparently contained some live virus, thereby producing a limited number of cases of the disease. More stringent specifications for the inactivation of the virus have prevented any subsequent accidents of this kind. The Salk vaccine has been used widely throughout the United States as well as in other countries, and preliminary evidence would indicate a marked reduction in the incidence of paralytic poliomyelitis.

It is recommended that the Salk vaccine be given in three doses, the first dose being administred preferably in the early fall, the second dose following after an interval of 1 to 2 months, and the third dose being given in the spring, well in advance of the poliomyelitis season. Vaccination is recommended particularly for infants and young children and for adults up to the age of 40 years.

The duration of immunity produced by the inactivated or killed virus is as yet unknown. However, there is some reason to believe that the killed-virus (Salk) vaccine will produce immunity of a shorter duration than might be expected from an attack of the disease or by vaccination with a live virus. Attenuated strains of types 1, 2, and 3 virus have been shown capable of producing antibodies for all three types, and it is possible that an attenuated live-virus vaccine may produce immunity of greater duration than the inactivated or killed virus. Nevertheless, the live-virus vaccine is still in the experimental stage, and adequate evidence of its safety and efficacy must await extensive field trials.

Influenza Vaccine. Active immunization with available influenza vaccines has been shown to reduce substantially the incidence of the disease provided the prevailing strain of virus corresponds to those strains used in the production of the vaccine. At least three major types of influenza virus have been recognized as occurring in epidemic form in the United States prior to 1957. These major types contain several serologically distinct strains, and the vaccine to be effective must be prepared from viruses corresponding to the prevailing strain in the community to be protected. The duration of immunity is probably short, and revaccination is recommended at yearly intervals for maximum protection. The vaccine must be prepared from a number of different strains in order to provide protection of broad valency. Under these circumstances general vaccination of a population is not usually recommended.

Early in 1957 a previously unrecognized strain of influenza virus was isolated from cases associated with extensive epidemics of influenza in the Orient. It was early recognized that this strain of influenza virus has been introduced into the United States by travelers from the Orient. Preliminary studies indicated that immunity to this strain of virus in all probability did not exist in the population of the United States, and that vaccine produced from known domestic strains would be ineffective. The possibility of a widespread epidemic was, therefore, clearly recognized. Heroic efforts were made to develop a suitable vaccine, and, in a matter of weeks after the isolation of the strain, what appeared to be a satisfactory antigen was produced, and in a matter of months vaccine was produced in sufficient quantity to make a vaccination control program feasible. General vaccination of the population with this Asian strain vaccine was recommended by the United States Public Health Service, and millions of Americans received the vaccine prior to the height of the expected influenza epidemic period. It is difficult to evaluate the effectiveness of this vaccine and of the program of vaccination. It seems probable that there was some reduction in the extent of the epidemic, and it is clear that the vaccine was safe and free from serious reactions. It is doubtful if generalized vaccination against influenza will be justified, but a multivalent influenza vaccine may be very useful under special conditions of exposure, particularly in the case of a special hazard as in institutional populations or in the military forces.

Antibiotics as a Factor in the Control of Communicable Diseases. Reference has already been made to the fact that the length of illness, complications, and fatalities in many communicable diseases have been decreased through use of the antibiotics. The agents act effectively in many of the diseases due to bacteria and in some caused by rickettsiae. Their ability to control virus diseases, however, is limited, sometimes nil.

Aside from the beneficial effect of the antibiotics as regards life-saving and their contribution to early recovery in the individual, they play an important role in the mass control of disease. This is effected through shortening the period of communicability, thus neutralizing a focus of spread that might have remained operative for weeks instead of days. As an offset to this, however, it must be remembered that some of the antibiotics in certain diseases (as streptomycin in tuberculosis) may precipitate the development of resistant strains. (See p. 147.)

REFERENCES

American Public Health Association: *Control of Communicable Diseases in Man*. The Association, New York, 1955.

Anderson, Gaylord, W., and Arnstein, Margaret G.: *Communicable Disease Control*, 3rd ed. The Macmillan Company, New York, 1953.

Maxcy, Kenneth F.: *Rosenau's Preventive Medicine and Hygiene*, 8th ed. Appleton-Century-Crofts, Inc., New York, 1956.

chapter 6

Tuberculosis as a
Public Health Problem

AS A PUBLIC health problem, tuberculosis presents a maximum of interests and responsibilities: (1) it is a communicable disease; (2) within certain limitations, it is preventable; (3) it affects relatively large numbers of people; (4) in most states and cities there are laws and ordinances requiring that the health department institute measures to prevent spread of the disease; (5) although public opinion is not sufficiently crystallized to provide adequate facilities and measures for maximum obtainable control of the disease, each individual in the public is prepared to demand that the health department do something when he believes that he or his family is endangered by tuberculosis in some other individual or family.

Public health interests and responsibilities arise also because of problems peculiar to this disease. The interrelation of tuberculosis and poverty; the chronicity of the disease; the necessity for hospitalization in most cases; the need for family adjustments incident to loss of income for a number of months; the carrier role played by cases of tuberculosis; the comparative lack of symptoms in the early stages in many cases: all of these factors add to the complexity of the problem. Public health measures for the control of tuberculosis can never produce their fullest results unless supplemented with generous and intelligent social relief by government.

125

Important Public Health Points to Be Remembered. These, briefly, are as follows:

The disease affects fish, flesh, and fowl. Birds may suffer with the disease (avian form); it spreads rapidly in cattle (bovine tuberculosis); and certain fish harbor organism with some of the characteristics of bovine tubercle bacillus. The bovine type appears to be the only one of these forms transmissible to man.

The disease is due to the tubercle bacillus, the human type of which has a high power of resistance to drying and will remain alive in dark, dry places for many months. Tuberculosis is not an inheritable disease. Theories, difficult either to prove or disprove, have been advanced to the effect that one might inherit either a susceptibility or a resistance to the disease. Tuberculosis has *appeared* to be inheritable because it so often manifests itself in a number of members of the same family. This, it is now believed, is incident to continuing exposure to infectious material.

Age is a matter of great importance in tuberculosis. Youth and early adult life are the periods when *infection* is most likely to occur; adult life is the age at which the more common forms of the *disease* manifest themselves; and old age is the period in which the *death rate* is highest. Sex, as it relates to age, is important and complex. These factors are discussed below more fully.

It is generally believed that in certain racial stocks pulmonary tuberculosis runs a more virulent course than in others, both as to spread in the group and extension in the individual. This also appears to be the case with groups only recently exposed to the tuberculosis hazards of civilization. In considering situations where race susceptibility appears to play an important role, one must, however, be cautious in drawing conclusions. The real factors may be in the mode of living, such as congested tenements, poor food, insanitary conditions, and exhausting work, rather than in racial susceptibility.

The length of the period of incubation in tuberculosis is not clearly defined. Lodgment of the organism and protective tissue-response are not immediately accompanied by symptoms at present recognizable nor by incapacity, as in the acute communicable diseases. Nor does the end of the period of incubation mean that the disease, in the sense in which this term is ordinarily employed, is in progress. The infected person may never give any outward evidence of the infection; or, in a short time, may develop a tuberculosis meningitis or disseminated tuberculosis; or may give clinical evidence of the disease some 10 to 20 years after this first infection with tubercle bacilli.

Whether or not a case of tuberculosis acts as a focus of spread depends upon the discharge of tubercle bacilli. Persons discharging tubercle bacilli are not isolated (as they would be in acute communicable diseases), and many of them are not incapacitated. These people act in the capacity of carriers, and few localities have laws authorizing forcible hospitalization of sputum-positive cases.

The laboratory can give definite aid in establishing a diagnosis when tubercle bacilli are being discharged. When bacilli are found it means that the individual concerned has tuberculosis. Failure to find the organisms does not mean that the individual does not have tuberculosis since he might have discharged bacilli in some other specimen of sputum. Gastric washings, as well as sputum, are examined, and, in addition to the usual smear or slide examination, cultures and even animal inoculation are becoming routine before it is concluded that the person is not discharging bacilli.

In pulmonary tuberculosis, the infectious agent is essentially the sputum. Some sputum is swallowed and excreted in the feces. Excreta in such cases is dangerous, but not in a degree comparable with sputum. In other forms of tuberculosis, excretions, secretions, and discharges from the area affected may carry the bacilli but, after all, the material which is essentially responsible for the spread of the disease is sputum. Milk from tuberculous cattle is the vehicle of the bovine form in transmission to human beings.

Infectious material gains access to the body most commonly through the gastrointestinal system, the respiratory system, or the tonsils. When tubercle bacilli are swallowed they get into the general circulation through the intestinal lymphatics. Their place of final lodgment is usually in a pulmonary capillary but may be elsewhere. Bovine bacilli swallowed in milk also follow this route. Infected dust and spray from tuberculous coughing are probably the more important avenues through which the organisms gain access to nose and mouth. Here they may lodge in the tonsils or be carried into the bronchi and lungs by respiration. Kissing may transfer infectious material from one person to another.

An individual with pulmonary tuberculosis remains in the period of communicability as long as he is discharging tubercle bacilli. From a public health standpoint, the case of tuberculosis discharging bacilli is in an entirely different category from the one who is not discharging them, and is far more dangerous. To prevent spread, therefore, it is highly important to hospitalize, and keep hospitalized, sputum-positive cases, regardless of the chances of the patient's recovery. Many sanatoria, with the patient's recovery as the principal objective, feel they ought to reserve their beds for cases which they can help. This attitude, however, means lack of hospitalization for far-advanced cases, and is therefore in conflict with the sound public health policy of removing the focus from contact with others. *No sputum-positive case of tuberculosis should ever be discharged from a sanatorium.*

Tuberculosis does not flare or flash into epidemics as do the acute communicable diseases, but is endemic in all parts of the world.

There is conflicting evidence as to the immunity conferred by an attack of tuberculosis, but there can be no question of the existence of natural resistance to infection. Many individuals withstand the primary infection and successfully resist subsequent infections. It is also clear that immunity conferred by the initial infection is not a solid immunity because active tuberculosis can develop at a later date in such a person. Comparisons between the occurrence of tuberculosis in those who have a positive tuberculin reaction and those who are negative are difficult to interpret for several reasons. The person who has suffered a primary infection in early life has in all probability been exposed to tuberculosis to a greater extent than has the person with the negative tuberculin reaction. The two groups also usually differ with respect to socioeconomic level, crowding, and other factors of hygiene. The endogenous and exogenous sources of the reinfection are obviously of importance but not clearly understood. A greater ability to resist the disease appears to exist in populations that have for generations been exposed to the disease. The evidence of a reduced incidence of active tuberculosis in persons receiving BCG vaccine suggests that the vaccine has given partial protection possibly similar to the immunity produced by a primary infection.

Calculation of the Death Rate from Tuberculosis. The death rate from tuberculosis is expressed as the number of deaths per 100,000 population, during a given time and in a given place, as in 1950 in the city of Baltimore, or the state of Michigan, or the United States.

Assume that in a city of 180,000 there were 45 deaths from tuberculosis. The rate would be calculated as follows:

1. Multiply the number of deaths by 100,000
$$45 \times 100,000 = 4,500,000$$
2. Divide by population figure
$$4,500,000 \div 180,000 = 25$$

or, by ratio and proportion:

$$x : 100,000 = 45 : 180,000$$
$$180,000x = 4,500,000$$
$$x = \frac{4,500,000}{180,000}$$
$$x = 25$$

The tuberculosis death rate then, in this hypothetical case, is 25 deaths per 100,000 population.

The Trend in Tuberculosis Mortality. The decline in the death rates of tuberculosis has been continuous since the beginning of the twentieth century, but has been greatly accelerated in recent years. In 1900 the death rate from tuberculosis in all forms in the U.S. registration area was 194.4 per 100,000 population. In 1910 the mortality rate had decreased to 154 per 100,000. In 1920 it had gone further down to 113 per 100,000. In 1930 it had decreased to 71, and in 1940 to 46. In the decade from 1940 to 1950 the decline became even sharper, so that by 1950 the rate for the United States as a whole was 22 per 100,000, a percentage drop of over 50 per cent. Preliminary figures for 1957 show a mortality rate in the United States, as a whole, of 8 per 100,000, an even more rapid rate of decline.

It is of interest that mortality from tuberculosis in the United States declined quite consistently at a rate of between 2 and 3 per cent per year until the advent of chemotherapy at which time there began a precipitous decline in mortality for the country as a whole, at an approximate rate of 9 per cent per year. A similar experience has been observed in many other countries in which chemotherapy has been used extensively.

Probable Causes of the Decline in Death Rate from Tuberculosis. There can be little doubt that many factors have contributed to the decline in mortality from tuberculosis, particularly in the early part of the twentieth century. During the first half of the century it seems probable that the following factors have all played a part, acting and interacting with each other:

1. Higher standards of living.
   a. Improved housing and household cleanliness.
   b. Better nutrition.
   c. Shorter working hours and less exhaustion.
2. Social legislation and social service resulting in less neglect of the unfortunate.
3. Improvement in community sanitation and personal hygiene.
4. Raising of general educational levels, and a public better informed as to tuberculosis.
5. Increased medical knowledge and facilities for the treatment of the disease, including earlier diagnosis, bed rest, and sanatorium treatment, providing for a larger proportion of those suffering from the disease.

The markedly accelerated decline in tuberculosis mortality in the past ten years can only be explained on the basis of newly developed drug therapy. In 1947 streptomycin for the first time became generally available for the treatment of tuberculosis, and in 1949 aminosalicylic acid (PAS) was developed and was promptly demonstrated to be effective particularly in conjunction with streptomycin. In 1951 isoniazid was dramatically demonstrated to be effective in the prevention of death from tuberculosis and came into general use in 1952. These three antimicrobial agents in various combinations have become almost standard therapy for tuberculosis. During this same period there has also been considerable improvement in the surgical treatment of tuberculosis, particularly in conjunction with the drug

therapy. It should be pointed out that these encouraging developments have had their most marked influence on mortality. Morbidity
from tuberculosis has not by any means declined at the same rate as
has the mortality. Only time will tell whether the recent and presently
encouraging results from modern therapy will eventually result in the
relegation of tuberculosis, as a disease, to a minor position among the
public health hazards of the country.

Age and Sex as Factors in Tuberculosis Mortality. If one compares
the number of deaths from tuberculosis, in a given age group, with
the number of people in that age group, thus obtaining an *age-specific
death rate,* it will be seen in the United States in 1956 (1) that the
lowest death rate from tuberculosis, all forms, was in the group 5 to
14 years of age (0.2 deaths per 100,000 persons in that age group);
(2) that the death rate gradually increases with age so that, in the age
group 75 to 84, the rate was about 31.6 deaths per 100,000 persons in
that age group. A similar trend is found in previous years.

The age at which the mortality from tuberculosis is greatest, when
expressed as age-specific rates, has undergone a marked change in the
last 50 years.

In 1900, the highest rate was in children under one year of age:
311 deaths per 100,000 infants in this age group. Then, quite early in
the century, the death rate in this group began to drop more quickly
than in the group with the next highest rate (25–34 years), and the
latter became established as having the highest of all the age groups:
262 per 100,000 in 1902. The death rate in this group then began to fall
a little faster than in older groups so that by 1935, when the age-
specific death rate in the 25–34 group was 74, all older groups had
higher rates, with the exception of those 85 years of age and over,
for whom data are not always as precise as would be desired. As of
1956, the tuberculosis death rate in the older age groups remains
higher than in the younger.

The essential point in regard to age as a factor in tuberculosis mortality is this: death from this disease is being pushed back into the
older group. Whereas infants died of this disease at the rate of more
than 300 per 100,000 in 1900, now less than 3 infants per 100,000
die each year. Or, again, of those who died of tuberculosis in 1910,

67 per cent were under 40 years of age, whereas in 1956 the percentage of deaths in those under 40 was reduced to 17 per cent of the deaths that occurred at all ages from this cause.

Careful study has shown that the death rates from tuberculosis in older people tend to reflect those death rates which were in existence when these old people were young and does not, therefore, indicate any particular susceptibility of old people to this disease. The death rates are also falling in those past middle age, but not so rapidly as in younger persons. It is important, however, to bear in mind that tuberculosis is not uncommon in the old. If this is not remembered a grandmother or grandfather might pass unnoticed as a source of infection.

Mortality in tuberculosis is not the same in males and females. It would appear that some part of this may be due to differences in exposure, such as between the employed man and the housekeeping woman, but with the increasing proportion of women in business and industry, these differences in environment are less marked. Further, epidemiological studies suggest that the basic differences in male and female physiology play a role in the respective mortalities of the two sexes.

The male death rate as a whole has always been higher than the female, although at the beginning of the century the difference was not great. In 1956 the gap between these rates had widened to such an extent that in the white population (where decline in tuberculosis rates is first manifested) the tuberculosis death rate of females was less than 40 per cent that of males: 4 females to 10 males. A similar phenomenon, though not in the same degree, is evidenced in tuberculosis mortality in nonwhite males and females. However, mortality from pulmonary tuberculosis is greater in young adult females than in males. As a result, although females generally have lower mortality rates from tuberculosis, they die earlier: the average age at death from tuberculosis is around fifty in males, about forty in females. The death rate from tuberculosis in nonwhites is about three times that of white persons, but rates are declining.

The Prevalence and Incidence of Tuberculosis. There are no figures from which one may draw exact conclusions as to just how much tuberculosis exists. The main reasons for this are (1) difficulties in drawing a line between latent, active, and "cured" tuberculosis, and in keeping posted as to what happens in each case; (2) difficulties in discovering all tuberculosis in a given community; and (3) variability of prevalence from place to place. In these circumstances, estimates must be relied upon, but with understanding caution.

A recent estimate has been made of the prevalence of tuberculosis in the United States in 1956, and this estimate has been compared with a previous estimate made by the same group in 1952. The sources of information for such estimates are many and varied, but include the following:

1. The Public Health Service tuberculosis bed census of April 1, 1956, giving the number of tuberculosis beds occupied in all federal and nonfederal hospitals except mental and penal institutions.

2. The Tuberculosis Hospital and Sanatorium Directory, published by the National Tuberculosis Association, showing the number of tuberculosis beds in mental and penal institutions.

3. Annual tuberculosis reports prepared by state health departments.

4. Tuberculosis case register summary reports received by the Public Health Service from state and local health departments.

5. The nationwide nonhospitalized tuberculosis patient study conducted as part of the tuberculosis program of the U.S. Public Health Service in 1954 and 1955.

On the basis of information obtained from the above-mentioned sources, it is estimated that at the beginning of 1956 there were 250,000 active cases of tuberculosis in the continental United States. Of this number 150,000 or 60 per cent, were known to state and local health departments. The rest of the estimated number comprised unknown cases, that is, currently unreported cases and a small number of previously reported cases since lost from supervision. The estimates suggest that there were 550,000 inactive cases. Of these, 250,000 were known to health departments, and 300,000 were not known. In addition, it was estimated that 1,200,000 persons who once had tuberculosis do not now require supervision according to state and local health department standards. Although these persons do not require public health supervision, they constitute a reservoir of former cases susceptible to reactivation.

A comparison of the prevalence of tuberculosis in 1952 and 1956 was made on the basis of corresponding information for those years. It was estimated that the total number of active cases had decreased from 350,000 in 1952 to 250,000 in 1956 or a percentage change of approximately 30 per cent, and that the inactive cases had decreased from 600,000 in 1952 to 550,000 in 1956, or a percentage change of approximately 10 per cent. The conclusion is that, if these trends persist, the combined number of active and inactive tuberculosis cases will continue to decline. This decline will be the consequence of the continuing decrease in incidence and the increasing recovery rate.

It would seem that better case finding, mass x-ray programs, better diagnostic and hospital facilities, etc., are bringing to light cases that would otherwise have remained undiscovered. Doubtless this explains a part of the continuing high prevalence data, but not all of it. Actually, mass x-rays account for only a small proportion of new cases reported; and in connection with the assumption that there is more prompt and complete reporting of tuberculosis than heretofore, it must be borne in mind that in the United States from 15 to 50 per cent of patients who die of tuberculosis are not reported as having the disease before death. Expressed otherwise, it may be said that the death certificate, with tuberculosis as the cause of death, was the first notice received by the health department.

An encouraging and partial explanation of the relatively slow decrease in cases as compared with decrease in deaths is that many persons with tuberculosis continue to live under modern treatment and therefore tend to keep the number of cases large. A quarter of a century ago, they would have swelled the number of deaths and decreased the number of cases.

Tuberculous Infection. If an individual shows a positive tuberculin reaction (see below) he is considered to have been infected, at one time or another, with tubercle bacilli. The proportion of individuals who respond positively to this test appears to depend largely upon whether or not the conditions under which the group of persons lived were such as to make exposure to tubercle bacilli probable. Most adults who have lived under urban conditions give a positive tuberculin reaction. Practically all children exposed to active tuberculosis in the family show a positive reaction. The majority of young children, living in rural areas, respond negatively to the tuberculin test. Until comparatively recently, from 25 to 50 per cent of urban school children and 10 to 25 per cent of rural school children reacted positively to a tuberculin test. This condition is changing, however, and current findings are much lower.

Figures and findings in one section of the country are not necessarily correct for another section; and even findings in one group of school children may not be indicative of the situation existing in another group of school children in the same city. Other things being equal, the older the group tested, the greater will be the proportion of positive reactors.

A child with only a positive tuberculin reaction, or nothing more than x-ray evidence of old tuberculous involvement of glands in the chest, should not be considered as a case of tuberculosis. Children with such evidence of past infection, apparently well offset, do not need treatment or nursing care as in pulmonary tuberculosis. As in other children, physical defects should be corrected, nutrition kept at optimum, with normal rest, fresh air, and play, and they should be guarded from strain and exhaustion in the period of adolescence. If the focus from which they have received infection is known, it should be removed. They should be examined from time to time, but the mere tuberculin-positive reaction or evidence of an old childhood tuberculosis means only that they have gone through a human experience quite usual in the present civilization.

Classification of Cases of Pulmonary Tuberculosis. The National Tuberculosis Association has established certain diagnostic standards and classifications of tuberculosis which are generally accepted and utilized. In relation to pulmonary tuberculosis, the pathogenesis of the condition is divided into *primary* tuberculosis and *reinfection* tuberculosis. Formerly these were designated, respectively, as childhood type and adult type. It must be recognized that, as the one might merge into the other, a sharp line of demarcation is somewhat arbitrary. However, the primary phase represents the physiological and anatomical reaction of the pulmonary system to a first experience with the tubercle bacillus. Here there is a small focus of infection, or more than one in the lung tissue itself, with lymphangitis. As the lymph drains into the tracheobronchial lymph nodes, a lymphadenitis occurs in this area. In most cases there is the classical sequence of healing, with characteristic x-ray findings. The lesions may rarely go on immediately to further local tissue destruction and may be disseminated as a generalized tuberculosis. The *primary phase* is seen most often in infants and children, but is not necessarily limited to this group. The tuberculin reaction becomes positive.

The *reinfection phase* represents chronic tuberculosis of the lungs. It may arise either from the introduction of a new dose of bacilli (exogenous reinfection) or by the breakdown of some already existent but latent focus (endogenous reinfection). The *reinfection phase,* with its subsequent chain of events, is the source from which the disease spreads: a pulmonary lesion breaks through and into a bronchus and tubercle bacilli are present in the sputum.

The extent of pulmonary lesions is indicated in terms of *minimal, moderately advanced,* and *far-advanced* lesions, and symptoms that might accompany are indicated as *none, slight, moderate,* or *severe.*

Certain terms and definitions are adopted for purposes of classification of the status of the tuberculous lesion: *inactive, arrested, active condition of cases.* The latter usually, but not always, is discharging tubercle bacilli and has symptoms.

As a matter of convenience and practical importance, public health workers tend to make another differentiation between cases of tuberculosis. They speak of "open" cases of tuberculosis, indicating that the case is discharging tubercle bacilli. So far as concerns degree of danger to others the latter is the immediate and vitally important question in any given case of tuberculosis.

It is probably true that the well-trained tuberculous patient evidences great care in coughing and sneezing and in the disposition of sputum. Even when he is most careful, if his sputum contains tubercle bacilli, he is of some menace to those about him. Even experts sometimes are careless in handling dynamite, and only a relatively small number of the existing cases of tuberculosis are effectively careful. Therefore, regardless of how well the patient may seem, or how careful he may appear to be, the sputum-positive case of tuberculosis remains a potential danger to his associates, especially those in his family.

From such data as are available it would appear that a married person exposed to a tuberculous partner is about twice as likely to die of tuberculosis, though not necessarily immediately, as is one who is not so exposed; and that the child exposed to a tuberculous parent or tuberculous parents is two or three times more likely to die of that disease before reaching the age of 20 than is the child not exposed in this way. This increased hazard of the child is probably incident to intimate exposure, rather than to the mere blood relationship.

Tuberculin and the Tuberculin Test. Tuberculin is the concentrated filtrate of a killed culture of tubercle bacilli, mixed with glycerin. A somewhat more refined and stable product, also used in the tuberculin test, is a purified protein derivative, usually designated as PPD. This product has about one hundred times the concentration of tuberculin.

The *tuberculin test* is a procedure designed to show whether or not an individual has ever been infected with tuberculosis. Those who respond to the test in one way are said to be *positive;* in another way, *negative.* It is extremely important here to bear in mind a fact previously mentioned: a positive test means that the person concerned has once had the primary type of tuberculosis, but does not, necessarily, now have the disease. Practically all persons with the disease give a positive reaction.

It is believed that the tuberculin reaction is due to an allergic response. When tubercle bacilli are taken into the body, the tissues naturally respond in a protective manner; they acquire some ability, through antibodies, to destroy the tubercle bacillus and to break down its endotoxin, which is essentially protein in nature. These partly broken-down protein products are irritants, causing an inflammatory reaction. Thus when tuberculin is introduced into the skin of the arm, the antibodies, resulting from previous tissue experience, enter into combination with the tuberculin, producing inflammation in and around the area of irritation.

There are a number of methods of performing the tuberculin test. Those most used at present are the Mantoux, in which a measured amount of tuberculin is injected into the skin; and the "patch test" in which a small bit of material soaked in tuberculin is strapped to the arm. Though simple, the selectivity and reliability of the patch test compare favorably with others.

Utilization of the Tuberculin Test. The tuberculin test has been widely used in public health work and by physicians in private practice, especially those engaged in pediatrics and tuberculosis.

A negative tuberculin test is of more significance than a positive, except in very young children. The infection that gives rise to a positive tuberculin in an older person may have been acquired years before, and therefore does not necessarily bear any definite relation to the condition of the individual as of today.

At one time it was believed that because a positive tuberculin in a young child meant relatively recent infection from one of a limited number of associates, an investigation of that child's family offered an unusually good chance of finding cases of tuberculosis. Some cases may be found in this way, but it is relatively a time-consuming procedure and therefore expensive. It is likely too that a similar amount of work in unselected families in a slum area would lead to the finding of just as many, if not more, cases of tuberculosis.

Use of tuberculin testing has also been made in the schools. One can usually get good cooperation from parents and teachers and children in an undertaking of this sort, but unless it is practicable to follow through with ample x-ray examinations and with adequate provisions for those who need treatment, widespread tuberculin testing does little more than create ill-founded optimism on the one hand and undue apprehension on the other.

Another use of tuberculin testing is in connection with the administration of the BCG vaccine. In studies or in BCG programs, only those with negative tuberculin reactions are given the vaccine.

Chest X-ray Surveys. The x-ray has long been utilized in the diagnosis of tuberculosis, and in the study of the progress or regression of lesions in cases already diagnosed. Prior to the development of the small film photofluorograph, the use of the x-ray in diagnosis of tuberculosis was limited to a certain extent by the cost of the procedure. The cost of the large film x-ray was prohibitive for mass surveys for the detection of tuberculosis, but with the development of the low-cost, small-film screening technique, mass radiography for the detection of tuberculosis and other chest diseases came into great favor. Large sections of the population were screened for evidence of tuberculosis. This procedure was found to be a dependable tool in the selection of those individuals who should require more intensive study.

The mass survey approach rests upon the knowledge that in any large group there is a small proportion of individuals who have tuberculosis in one stage or another, many of whom do not have symptoms sufficient to make them seek medical advice. It was found that in certain groups as high as 1 per cent of those surveyed had evidence of tuberculosis not previously recognized. In addition, such conditions as lung cancer, nontuberculous pulmonary infections, intrathoracic tumors, and cardiovascular abnormalities could be detected with some accuracy by this method. The values of this procedure were promptly recognized, and extensive programs of mass photofluorography were developed in health departments and in voluntary agencies throughout the country. There can be little doubt that this technique was an important factor in early recognition and treatment of persons suffering from tuberculosis, and has been a valuable tool in the general tuberculosis detection and control program. But in recent years there has been increasing concern as to the possible harmful effects of radiation, whether from the newer developments in nuclear fission and thermonuclear reactions or from x-ray radiation. Both produce what physicists designate as ionizing radiation—a process which may be deleterious to the molecular structure of body cells. Studies carried out by the National Research Council of the National Academy of Sciences have pointed out the possibilities of a cumulative effect of background radiation plus various exposures to ionizing radiation including x-ray (see section on radiological health hazards, page 217).

In view of these considerations there is, at the present time, quite general agreement that exposure to ionizing radiation should be limited insofar as possible. There is some evidence that even low doses of ionizing radiation, if often repeated, may produce genetic effects that would be undesirable and even may produce direct harm to the individual subjected to the radiation. These findings have led to efforts to limit x-ray exposure to essential diagnostic and therapeutic uses. This has tended to inhibit the further development of mass x-ray surveys except for carefully selected groups. Mass x-ray surveys are now considered to be justified only if they can be expected to lead to the detection of a considerably significant number of previously unsuspected, clinically significant chest diseases that can be followed up with appropriate therapy. It is agreed that it is essential for those engaged in the detection of pulmonary disease to evaluate the yield from this procedure on a continuing basis. This does not preclude use of this valuable tool for the study of population groups in which there would be expected a high yield of tuberculosis. Furthermore, every effort should be made to reduce the exposure to ionizing radiation to a minimum in the process. Those procedures are not recommended which involve high dosage radiation, such as direct fluoroscopy, the taking of laminograms, or other prolonged exposure. In the use of the fluorographic unit great care should be exercised to limit the amount and duration of exposure, in order to reduce to a minimum the radiation dose for those being examined and to operators of the equipment. Proper safeguards, such as shielding, and exposure controls can do much to reduce the total body exposure of the patient and of the operator.

BCG Vaccine. The letters BCG stand respectively for Bacillus, Calmette, and Guerin. Calmette was a distinguished French authority on tuberculosis, Guerin an associate. BCG is a living culture of bovine tubercle bacilli. Calmette believed that through many years of artificial culture, the strain of bacilli which he used had lost its power to produce tuberculosis but possessed an ability to serve as an antigen: it would cause the tissues to produce antibodies against the tubercle bacillus. It was first fed to infants known to be exposed. At present, it is given hypodermically or by multiple minute punctures. In the former process it occasionally causes a small local abscess.

As would be expected, there was serious disagreement not only to the efficacy of BCG, but also to its safety. Its proponents believed that it was efficacious and safe. Its opponents believed neither. The American medical profession as a whole was skeptical for a long time.

At present, it is generally believed to be safe and to some extent effective in producing a resistance to tuberculous infection. Just how effective the vaccine is has not been determined, but from studies of relatively large groups, under conditions partially controlled, there seems less likelihood that children who have had BCG will develop tuberculosis than those, living under similar conditions, who have not had the vaccine.

It has been used more on a mass scale in Europe than in the United States. In this country its use is limited to studies and to those who are tuberculin negative but exposed to an unusual hazard of tuberculous infection: student nurses, medical students, hospital employees, etc.

BCG vaccine cannot be purchased through ordinary drug companies, as can diphtheria or whooping cough vaccines. Relatively few laboratories are licensed (by the U.S. Public Health Service) to manufacture BCG. These are essentially nonprofit organizations or state health department laboratories, and distribution of the material is for study and research purposes.

BCG is not yet established as comparable to the more conventional vaccines. More knowledge as to its efficacy is needed, and it would be unfortunate if it were used on a wholesale scale before this more complete knowledge is available.

The Purposes of the Public Health Program, As It Relates to Pulmonary Tuberculosis. The objectives in the anti-tuberculosis program may be listed briefly, as follows:

1. To prevent those not already infected, from becoming infected.

2. To prevent those already infected from developing active, clinical tuberculosis.

3. To prevent those with active clinical disease from dying, from spreading it to others, and, finally, to bring about the maximum recovery and rehabilitation.

While the above are the ultimate purposes of a tuberculosis program, they are goals rather than measures that one may apply immediately. In concrete terms, the latter may be set forth somewhat as follows:

1. To discover, by every means possible and at the earliest moment, all cases of tuberculosis that exist but are not suspected, and toward this end to conduct mass surveys and provide free x-ray, laboratory, clinics, and consultation services.

2. To aid in getting suspected cases and contacts into the hands of private physicians or clinics for examination; and where no other facilities are available, to supply such diagnostic clinics.

3. To teach the public the necessity for early diagnosis, regular medical observation, and continuing treatment.

4. To teach the person with tuberculosis and those of his immediate family the danger of exposure of others and the means of spread; and to instruct patient and family as to prophylaxis and disinfection.

5. As a supplementary diagnostic service, and for guidance in handling cases, to provide laboratory service for examination of sputum and other excretions or secretions.

6. To develop public consciousness of the need for sanatoria where there are inadequate facilities and to aid patients in getting sanatorium treatment; and to further economic betterment and good housing in the poorer elements of the population.

7. To carry on continuing study and research in an effort to increase knowledge of the disease and its control.

8. To carry on a continuing program of public health education.

What the General Public Should Be Taught about Tuberculosis. In a program for popular health instruction regarding tuberculosis, the public should be taught:

1. That tuberculosis in its early stages may exist, even in the apparently robust, without symptoms, and that a chronic, even though mild, state of ill health needs medical investigation.

2. That this is particularly necessary in (a) young adult life, (b) one who has been exposed to tuberculosis, (c) thin, delicate persons, (d) aged persons.

3. That loss of weight, a chronic cough, spitting of blood, and pleurisy are danger signals never to be disregarded even in a person who otherwise feels well or looks well.

4. That the first essential for recovery is early diagnosis.

5. That no physician may safely say a person does not have tuberculosis without a complete examination, *including x-ray,* and that failure to find tubercle bacilli in the sputum does not mean freedom from the disease.

6. That getting well of tuberculosis cannot be made secondary to or fitted into the ordinary schedule of existence. For the time being, getting well must be a full-time job.

7. That tuberculosis is a communicable disease; that persons living in the same home with a sputum-positive case of tuberculosis are subjected to a dangerous hazard.

8. That exposure, especially continuing familial exposure, is dangerous in any age, but particularly so in infants, adolescents, and young adults.

9. That the disease may appear in any family, regardless of wealth, social position, or assumed freedom from exposure.

10. That hospitalization of the tuberculous is as much for the community's protection (as in any communicable disease) as for the patient's benefit, and that such persons should not be required to stand a means test or take a pauper's oath as a preliminary to sanatorium admission.

11. That tuberculosis is a community problem, demanding organized and coordinated social action if better housing, economic conditions, and proper diagnostic and sanatoria facilities are to be made available for all those who need them.

Tuberculosis a Reportable Disease. Tuberculosis is a communicable disease and must be reported to the local health department by the physician in attendance. The usual report card used for this purpose gives name, age, race, sex, address, date of report, and the kind of tuberculosis—pulmonary, bone and joint, etc. In general, physicians are slow in reporting tuberculosis and report it rather incompletely. The reasons for this vary with the circumstances and with the physician. The following are the factors which appear to be of most importance in this connection.

1. Physician has difficulty in establishing diagnosis.

2. Assumption on physician's part that another physician who previously attended case had already reported it.

3. Urgent request of patient that case not be reported.

4. Physician fears that a health department investigator might alarm patient or otherwise irritate family.

5. Because of a real or fancied grievance in the past, physician wants no health department interference.

6. Physician intends to report, but forgets to do so.

7. Physician does not approve of health activities and, by principle, will not cooperate.

8. Other reasons having to do with personalities in the medical profession or in the health department, or with local custom.

Tuberculosis Cases Remaining at Home. It is obvious that the home is where most cases of tuberculosis first develop and, likewise, it is the place where the majority of cases are treated for the longest time, although this should not be so. They remain at home for a number of reasons: (1) because of failure on their part to present themselves to a physician or clinic, for examination, (2) because of failure of the physician or clinic to make a diagnosis, (3) because they are not advised by the physician to go to a sanatorium, (4) because the breadwinner feels that he cannot quit work lest his family starve, (5) because the mother fears that in her absence her children will not be cared for, (6) because of fear of a strange, possibly distant, sanatorium, or perhaps because of sheer stubbornness, (7) because of inadequacy of free sanatoria, (8) cost of sanatorium care.

In discussing the care of tuberculosis in the home, it must be emphasized that the home is a bad place for an active case and that the case is bad for the home. In not one home out of a hundred can conditions be made satisfactory. There is lacking in the best home that quietness, regularity, freedom from participation in little worries, close medical observation, instruction, etc., which are so essential to good care. Therefore, the home care of a case of tuberculosis is unsatisfactory as compared to hospital care. It is to be adopted only as a bad compromise.

Home treatment of tuberculosis means that a focus of the disease continues in contact with the patient's family. Special arrangements as to isolation, disinfection, and supervision of contacts are necessary in these circumstances. Sometimes screened porches are provided, and at least the patient should have a separate room, airy and easily sunned and scrubbed. His dishes should be boiled after each usage and they should be of a distinctive pattern, to distinguish them from those used by the rest of the family. Concurrent disinfection should be carried out as in one of the acute communicable diseases where nose and mouth secretions contain infectious material.

When, or if, the patient dies or moves, the following steps should be carried out in terminal disinfection:

1. At least two days of sunning and airing the rooms used by the patient.

2. Thorough scrubbing of floors and woodwork with particular care to cracks in the floor. This should be followed by sloshing the floor with some cresol disinfectant. Painting, or shellacking the floors, and repainting or papering the walls are desirable adjuncts in cleaning.

3. Sunning mattresses, etc., as in terminal disinfection after an acute communicable disease.

4. Underclothing, bed linen, dishes, knives, forks, etc., should be boiled for at least ½ hour.

5. Upholstered furniture should be scrubbed with a stiff brush soaked in cresol solution, and other furniture should be wiped with generous amounts of furniture polish.

The Nurse's Part in Home Care of the Tuberculous. Neither concurrent nor terminal disinfection will happen by chance. The family must be guided, and it is here that the public health nurse renders a most valuable service. She visits such cases with the following purposes:

1. To minimize chances of infection of others. This she does through isolation of the patient, concurrent disinfection, and personal hygiene in the family.

2. To teach some member of the family how to make the patient comfortable and how to carry out the physician's orders as to diet, rest, exercise, special treatment.

3. To bring about periodic physical examination of contacts, especially very young children, adults, and the aged.

4. To see that the patient, if ambulant, continues to report to the physician or clinic.

5. To guide the patient in getting into a sanatorium, if the physician orders this.

6. To guide the family in obtaining welfare relief if this is indicated.

7. To find the source of infection, if possible, instituting whatever measures appear to be indicated.

The Sanatorium and Tuberculosis. For the patient's recovery, to remove him from contact with his family, and to teach him how in future to maintain his own health and protect others, the sanatorium is a most important element in the program directed against the disease.

In the past, the basis for estimating hospital-bed needs for the tuberculous in a given community was one bed for each annual death from that disease. Even though some states failed even to meet this modest standard, the standard itself was raised to two beds. Since modern treatment, especially surgery, offers more to the patient than formerly, most authorities believe that, for many years to come, the recommended standard should be three beds per annual death.

The latest available figures indicate that, for the United States as a whole, the ratio of beds in 1950 to deaths from tuberculosis in 1948 was 2.86 beds per death from that disease: 125,398 beds, 43,833 deaths. This includes hospitals under federal control and also beds for tuberculosis available in mental and penal institutions. The ratio of beds for tuberculous patients, exclusive of beds in federal, mental, and penal institutions, in the United States was 1.96 beds in 1950 per death from tuberculosis in 1948.

In the individual states the ratio of beds to deaths varied markedly, from more than 7 in North Dakota and Colorado to 0.57 in Nevada.

The 125,398 beds for tuberculous patients are located in 870 institutions. Of these institutions, 87 are federal, 126 are general hospitals, 193 are state mental hospitals, and 38 are state penal institutions, and the remainder (426) are tuberculosis hospitals.

Of the beds themselves, 73,959 are in tuberculosis hospitals, 15,837 in federal hospitals, 12,095 in general hospitals, 22,139 in state mental hospitals, and 1368 in state penal institutions. It is interesting to note that state mental institutions have more than one fourth the number of beds available in all tuberculosis hospitals.

The Newer Treatment of Tuberculosis and Its Significance. The new drug therapy of tuberculosis in conjunction with approved surgical techniques have markedly altered mortality from this disease. Certainly hundreds of thousands of lives are being saved as a result of this improved treatment. It is still necessary, however, to recognize the need for hospitalization of a large proportion of active cases of tuberculosis. Ambulatory treatment may be found to be practical after a period of hospitalization, but for the vast majority of cases a period of careful study and treatment in a tuberculosis hospital will be necessary. The relatively small reduction in cases as compared with the marked reduction in deaths from tuberculosis calls attention to the urgent need for continuation of all possible control activity. Moreover, the evidence of the development of drug-resistant strains of the tubercule bacillus must temper optimism as to the eventual eradication of this disease. A tendency on the part of the public, legislators, and even health officers to assume that the fight against tuberculosis is won raises fears that the necessary provision of facilities and services for the continued attack upon the disease may be even more difficult in the future than in the past. It would be tragic if overoptimism and consequent failure to utilize to the fullest, available knowledge for the prevention and cure of tuberculosis should result from the great advances that have been made in recent years.

REFERENCES

Drolet, Godias J., and Lowell, Anthony M.: "Where to Tuberculosis?" *Am. Rev. of Tuberc. and Pul. Dis.*, **72**:419–52, 1955.

Glaser, Stanley; Trauger, Donald A.; and Wyman, Arthur H.: "Estimate of Tuberculosis Prevalence in the United States, 1952," *Pub. Health Rep.*, **72**:963–75, 1957.

National Tuberculosis Association: *Diagnostic Standards and Classification of Tuberculosis*. The Association, New York, 1950.

————: *Tuberculosis Hospital and Sanatorium Directory*. The Association, New York, 1951.

chapter 7

The Venereal Diseases

EFFECTIVE CONTROL OF the venereal diseases is one of the most important health problems that confront society. The stigma of having such a disease, the tendency to chronicity, the remote sequelae of some of them, and the cost and length of treatment complicate the problem for the individual. From the public health standpoint the venereal diseases are of significance: (1) because they are communicable, (2) because they are preventable, (3) because they affect relatively large numbers of people, (4) because systematized social action is necessary for their control, and (5) because, in most localities, it is required by law that the health department take action.

The diseases usually referred to when one uses the term "venereal diseases" are syphilis, gonorrhea, and chancroid. Two other venereal diseases of some importance are granuloma inguinale and lymphogranuloma venereum. The word "venereal" is an adjective qualifying the noun "diseases" to indicate conditions associated with or arising incident to sexual intercourse. Another term used to cover this group is *genitoinfectious diseases*. This is perhaps a better term, though "venereal diseases" has the strength of priority and common usage.

There is another term which may cause confusion: *social hygiene*. One finds social hygiene associations or a bureau of social hygiene. In many instances the term was chosen by health agencies, or in conversation, as a euphemistic retreat, it being less harsh than the expression "venereal disease." Actually, however, social hygiene as used in

149

this connection is the more inclusive term. It is concerned with all matters relating to the sexual problems of society: sex education, continence, morality and immorality, illegitimacy, perversions, prostitution, and diseases that arise because these problems are not controlled. Complete eradication of the venereal diseases would still leave social hygiene with a lot of problems on its hands. Social hygiene and venereal disease control, therefore, are related and overlapping, but not synonymous terms.

Syphilis. This is by far the most important of the venereal diseases. It is essentially a disease of human beings, there being no animal or insect reservoirs of the disease.

The causative organism is the *Treponema pallidum,* a form of life related to bacteria on the one hand and to protozoa on the other.

In the biological sense, syphilis is not inheritable, for it seems not possible that the *Treponema pallidum* can be carried by either the male or female germ cell. However, this must be remembered: the organism of syphilis has the ability to pass through the placenta, and thus to enter the fetal circulation. This results in syphilis in the fetus: congenital syphilis. By early and proper treatment of a pregnant syphilitic woman, congenital syphilis can be prevented. Hence the importance of routine serological tests, and of prompt and effective treatment in antepartum cases.

Infection with syphilis most often occurs in young adult life, with aftereffects manifesting themselves in middle or later life.

The period of incubation averages from 2 to 4 weeks, the first manifestation of the disease being in the nature of a small local sore at the site of infection. Here the laboratory renders important aid in the diagnosis. From the initial sore, slides are prepared and a search is made for the *Treponema pallidum.* This is usually spoken of as a "darkfield" examination, because of the light adjustment in the microscope. The other important laboratory aid is the serological test. This may be done on either blood serum or spinal fluid.

The *Treponema pallidum* may leave the infected individual (a) in the exudation from the venereal sore, (b) in the exudation from mucous patches in the mouth, throat, lips, (c) in the semen, (d) in milk.

Syphilis is transmitted essentially through sexual intercourse. Kissing must be recognized as a factor. In rare instances, syphilis may be contracted from using a glass recently contaminated by a person with mucous patches in the mouth. Though physicians have often to listen, sphinx-like, to tales of extravenereal contraction of syphilis, such stories must generally be considered as smoke screens. As indicated above, syphilis may be transmitted to the infant in utero; and a non-syphilitic baby suckling a syphilitic woman is quite likely to be infected. A person in a highly infectious stage may appear to be in good health and thus play the part of an unrecognized and difficultly discoverable focus of infection.

The period of communicability during which a person infected with syphilis may transmit it to others varies with cases. Every case is communicable as long as there is a venereal sore (primary stage), while there is a syphilitic rash and mucous patches in the mouth (secondary stage), and in certain circumstances in the later stages: though a syphilitic woman may eventually produce a nonsyphilitic infant, she usually continues if untreated to have stillbirths or syphilitic infants for a number of years after her primary and secondary manifestations of the disease. Even in a late stage, syphilitics may discharge treponemata in the seminal fluid. A syphilitic, then, may possibly transmit the disease even though open lesions disappeared years ago.

A decision as to when a syphilitic has recovered depends to a great extent upon how early the case received treatment: except in late cases, recovery from syphilis usually is considered to have occurred when, after a systematic course of treatment, the serological reaction is negative on a number of consecutive tests taken some months apart. Usually at least one negative spinal fluid reaction is required. Decision as to the recovery of any given case must rest upon the circumstances in that case, not upon any general rule.

There seems reason to believe that a fair proportion of cases of syphilis go on to what may be designated as spontaneous recovery. However, one should be cautious in the use of this term since no one knows exactly what it means, and evidence available as to spontaneous recovery is not completely satisfying. Further, it must be remembered that though some individuals may appear to withstand a syphilitic infection without development of chronic disability or death from that disease, they may, nevertheless, have served disastrously in spreading the disease during their period of infectiousness.

It is difficult to estimate what proportion of persons once infected with syphilis die of that disease for, in many instances, the role of syphilis in causing death is masked. It is suspected as a factor in a large proportion of deaths resulting from cardiovascular disease, and locomotor ataxia and general paralysis of the insane *are* syphilis. It has been estimated that about half the untreated syphilitics eventually die as a result of their infections—and a greater proportion would eventually die from this cause if they did not previously succumb to some other disease.

Syphilis must be regarded as an endemic disease. It has been estimated that from 3 to 4 persons per thousand contract the disease each year. Vonderlehr and Usilton studied the record of serologic tests in nearly 2,000,000 men, between the ages of 21 and 35, who were examined under Selective Service. They summarized their findings as follows:

The rate of prevalence based on positive and doubtful blood tests among the selectees examined is 45.3 per thousand. The rate of prevalence for the entire male population of the United States between the ages of 21 and 35 is estimated to be 47.7 per thousand.

The rate of prevalence among Negro selectees is 252.3 per thousand, among white selectees 17.4 per thousand. The estimated rate of prevalence for the entire male Negro population (aged 21 to 35) is 272 per thousand, for the entire male white population (aged 21 to 35) is 23.5 per thousand.

The rate of prevalence among selectees from rural areas is 43.8 per thousand, from urban areas 46.1 per thousand. The estimated rate of prevalence among the entire male population (aged 21 to 35) in rural areas is 49.4 per thousand, in urban areas 46.5 per thousand.

Highest prevalence rates (white and Negro) are found in the Southeastern states, the lowest in the New England, West North Central and Middle Atlantic States.*

In interpreting such data, one must be careful lest race and geography of themselves be considered too strongly. Consideration must

* Vonderlehr, Raymond A., and Usilton, Loda J.: "Syphilis among Men of Draft Age," *J.A.M.A.*, **120**:1369 (No. 17, Dec. 26), 1942.

be given to the influence of social, economic, educational, cultural, environmental, and perhaps other factors. Further, there is evidence that the situation has improved markedly since these data were gathered.

The number of persons reported as dying of syphilis may not be relied upon as reflecting completely the real death rate of the disease, but such data, nevertheless, are of value. Thus in 1940, the death rate in the United States was reported as 14.4 per 100,000 population. For 1956 the rate was 2.3. These rates include deaths from aneurysm of the aorta, locomotor ataxia, and general paralysis of the insane. If this marked decline truly represents the situation, it is encouraging. Closely related to the above data are the facts that, while in 1940 in the U.S., 6.6 per cent of all deaths from syphilis were in children under one year of age, in 1956 less than 1 per cent of syphilis deaths were in the under one group.

The Wassermann Test. The Wassermann test or some of its modifications is a procedure of tremendous value to the public health. The theory as to why a syphilitic gives a positive Wassermann reaction, the technique of the test itself, and the interpretation of results are highly complex. For a discussion of them the reader is referred to more specialized texts.

Recent Advances in the Treatment of Syphilis. Until the development of Salvarsan by Ehrlich in 1910, the treatment of syphilis was quite unsatisfactory. With the availability of this chemotherapeutic agent and it derivatives, and with the supplementary use of such heavy metals as bismuth, early control of the infectious stages became practicable and ultimate recovery more likely. One of the great difficulties, however, in applying this type of treatment was the length of time involved. At least 12 to 18 months were necessary, with subsequent periodic observation. The patient got tired, tended to skip treatments, and might stop altogether.

The demonstration in 1943 of the efficacy of penicillin in the treatment of syphilis revolutionized venereal disease control programs. It has been amply demonstrated that adequate treatment with penicillin will accomplish in days what previous methods of chemotherapy took weeks or months to accomplish. The simplicity of the treatment of this disease with this antibiotic has removed one of the greatest obstacles to the control of this serious problem, namely, holding of cases for sufficient length of time to be sure that the patient was rendered noninfectious and would continue the treatment necessary to produce a definite cure.

There is still some question as to the most desirable form of therapy but there is considerable evidence that a single injection of a slowly absorbed preparation of penicillin is effective in rendering the patient noninfectious, and producing a cure. Careful follow-up is, however, indicated in order to provide assurance that the disease has been completely cured.

Gonorrhea. Only such diseases as measles, whooping cough, and mild upper respiratory conditions exceed gonorrhea in prevalence. It is generally estimated that it is three or four times as prevalent as syphilis. It is difficult to obtain exact data as to its incidence, since the disease is poorly reported, and, perhaps of all serious diseases, it is the one which receives the greatest degree of self-medication and drugstore treatment.

This disease is responsible for much of the sterility found in both males and females, and is the underlying cause of no inconsiderable part of gynecological operations. Formerly, it contributed the majority of cases of blindness in babies and children, but this condition has been greatly improved since instillation of silver nitrate solution into eyes of the newborn has become routine practice and a legal requirement.

The infectious material of gonorrhea is contained in the discharges from the affected area: purulent urethral discharge in males, urethral and vaginal discharges in females, discharges from eyes in gonorrheal ophthalmia. While it is theoretically possible that gonorrhea of the genital tract in adults might be contracted otherwise than through sexual intercourse, this is an unusual happening; and if there were no genital tract gonorrhea in adults other than that contracted from toilet seats, the disease would be at the vanishing point. On the other hand, ophthalmia neonatorum arises from gonorrheal infection which the infant receives from the genital tract of the mother, and the vulvovaginitis of little girls is most frequently contracted from towels, clothing, etc., contaminated by an infected adult associate. Gonorrheal ophthalmia may also arise from the same kind of exposure.

In the diagnosis of gonorrhea, the laboratory can give definite aid. The most common procedure is by microscopic examination of a smear of the suspected pus. In males, the smear is made from urethral pus. In females, smears are made from the meatus of the urethra and from the cervix. Under the microscope these organisms may be confused with the meningococcus. Both are biscuit shaped, in pairs, tend to be within the cell, and are negative to the Gram stain. Because of this similarity, many laboratories report "Gram-negative, intracellular organisms" instead of "positive" for the gonococcus. A negative laboratory report does not mean that the case is not one of gonorrhea.

In recent years, laboratory culture of the gonococcus has been simplified and made more exact. This procedure has, therefore, come into more common usage and is the method of choice. It is of particular aid in reaching a conclusion as to whether or not a case has become noncommunicable, especially in women. While culture of gonococcus has its limitations and potential errors, it would appear that in each hundred cases cleared as gonococcus-free by direct smear, about 15 will be found still to have organisms if the material is subjected to culture. A complement fixation test is used, as auxiliary to cultures, in good clinic practice, but because of complexity its application is somewhat limited.

The routine use of sulfa drugs and later the antibiotics rather completely changed the public health aspect of the problem of gonorrhea. Complications are minimized, infectiousness is shortened, and recovery is comparatively prompt in the majority of cases. Though not ordinarily practicable in civilian life, there is reason to believe that penicillin, taken before intercourse, will serve as a reasonably effective prophylactic.

Chancre and Chancroid. "Chancre," sometimes called "hard chancre," is the initial sore of syphilis. It is therefore but a local lesion in a generalized condition. It produces but little destruction of tissue locally.

"Chancroid," sometimes called "soft chancre" is a local condition, due to a bacillus generally known as the Ducrey bacillus, but now officially named *Hemophilus ducreyi*. It does not lead to a generalized condition, but usually causes considerable local destruction of tissue. Its prevention is simple: thorough washing of the genitals with soap and water after intercourse. Chancroid is seen more often in the unclean than in the clean. It should always be remembered that a given genital sore may be of mixed nature: it may be both chancre and chancroid, and the careful clinician must exert every effort, in every case of chancroid, to determine whether or not syphilis is also present.

A skin test is available, and the antibiotics shorten the period of communicability of chancroid.

Granuloma Inguinale. This is a condition spread by sexual contact. It involves the skin and mucous membrane of the genital region, causing rather nasty ulcerations. In the lesions are found *Donovan bodies,* believed by most to be the causative agent. Granuloma inguinale is not widely distributed as are gonorrhea and syphilis, being somewhat limited to tropical climates. In the United States it is sometimes seen in the subtropical areas.

Lymphogranuloma Venereum. This disease is sometimes designated as *lymphogranuloma inguinale*. It is not the same disease as *granuloma inguinale*. Lymphogranuloma venereum is believed to be due to a virus. It is more a tropic than temperate zone disease, but has a wide distribution, occurring not infrequently in the United States.

The disease begins with a mild lesion, on the penis in the male, the vulva in the female. Extension of the condition in the male is essentially to the inguinal glands, which become large and matted and which may break down to sinus formation. In the female, extension is to the pelvic lymphatics, and from these, rectal sinuses and rectal strictures may develop. Clinical diagnosis is aided by the Frei test, an intradermal procedure depending upon an allergic response. The material used is the sterilized pus from unruptured buboes. Infected mouse brain has been used for the same purpose.

As is the case in some of the other venereal diseases, the antibiotics contribute to checking the disease and shortening the period of communicability.

Usual Measures Undertaken in a Program for the Control of Venereal Diseases. These programs approach the problem from a number of different angles. General measures may be classified as follows:

1. The promulgation of laws and regulations designed to benefit the situation.

2. The search for sources of infection and control of known foci of spread.

3. The repression of prostitution.

4. Education of the public.

5. The provision of free laboratory service for such use as clinics and private physicians care to make of it.

6. Popularization, in the medical profession, of the serological test as a routine procedure even where syphilis is not suspected, as in pregnant women, cases of heart disease, or persons given a general examination.

7. Provision of free drugs and antibiotics for use of clinics and private physicians when patients cannot afford to pay.

8. Establishment of clinics to provide free treatment of venereal diseases when the patient cannot pay for treatment.

9. Provision of free silver nitrate solution, or other material for eyes of the newborn; widespread use of this safeguard.

10. Study and research for obtaining greater knowledge as to methods of diagnosis and treatment of the individual and for better administrative handling of the situation as a whole.

The Public Health Laws and Regulations Regarding Venereal Diseases. These vary from state to state. The minimal requirements are these:

1. That venereal diseases shall be reported promptly to the health department. Most states permit reporting by serial number, rather than by name and address.

2. That the physician shall furnish the health department with the name and address of a patient if the latter, while in the communicable stage, discontinues treatment without notifying the physician that he is obtaining it elsewhere.

3. That a case of venereal disease in the communicable stage shall be isolated, as in any other communicable disease, if the person fails or refuses to observe the precautions necessary for the protection of others.

4. That the health department provide free clinics for treatment of those unable to pay.

5. In the past few years an increasing number of states have supplemented the above by passing laws requiring (a) premarital serological tests for syphilis, (b) that each physician have a serological test made on all pregnant women coming under his care.

Certain difficulties are encountered in enforcing venereal disease regulations, and the diseases are poorly reported to health departments. Even when reported, investigation of sources of infection is difficult because of secrecy on the part of the patient. Those infected are generally ambulatory, go where they wish, do as they please—and infect others.

However, since treatment for the venereal diseases has become simpler, less long-drawn-out, and more effective, the patient is in an infectious stage for a much shorter time than heretofore and goes on to cure. This, while a great accomplishment from both the individual and public health standpoint, has a serious implication: once the person is cured, he is as susceptible as ever before to contract syphilis or gonorrhea anew. There is no truly effective vaccine against either of these diseases. The only person truly immune to syphilis is one who has the disease.

Another aspect of simpler and more effective treatment is that it may be given in the physician's office. While the highly specialized clinics will perhaps have to be maintained for some time to come, there is a tendency in health departments to decrease such services as the case load of those unable to pay grows less.

The private physician, however, cannot undertake the difficult chore of tracing the source of a given venereal infection, and modern public health practice demands as complete and careful epidemiological investigation of syphilis and gonorrhea as in diphtheria or smallpox. By such painstaking search, a surprising number of foci are brought under treatment and made noninfectious: persons from whom a given case might have received the infection, others to whom he might have transmitted it.

Finally, health department appropriations for venereal disease work have, in the past, been quite inadequate. This still applies in relation to state and local appropriations, but the federal government notably increased its appropriations in this connection. Part of these appropriations must be listed as temporary, having arisen incident to problems of World War II. However, as most of these funds are distributed as grants-in-aid to states, congressmen and senators are likely to look with favor on continuing assistance of this sort.

Society's Attitude toward the Venereal Diseases. There is wide difference between the attitude of the uplifter on the one hand, and the public health worker on the other, as regards venereal diseases and their control. To the uplifter, the *moral delinquency* of the venereally infected person looms large. The fact that the individual has gonorrhea or syphilis is quite likely to be regarded as but evidence of sin. The public health worker is not particularly concerned with this phase of the question. To him the venereal diseases are *communicable diseases,* with large numbers of individuals daily exposed, and with serious morbidity and mortality. As in any other communicable disease, the health worker attempts to institute such measures as will prevent infection and, where necessary, bring about recovery.

It is difficult to measure the effectiveness of prophylaxis against venereal diseases. Heretofore, these consisted of mercury inunctions of the genitals and urethral injections of silver salt solutions, or mechanical protection through use of condoms. Some success, but not complete, has been reported by the armed services. The extent of civilian use of prophylaxis and its results are not known, though there is reason to believe that mechanical protection is practiced considerably by the more intelligent and unhurried. The prophylactic use of oral penicillin has been found to be effective in controlled groups. In this connection it should be emphasized that many persons and organizations would oppose such a procedure, as in their opinion it would tacitly offer protection to the delinquent in his or her dereliction.

The Problem of Prostitution. No one really knows the results of efforts designed to repress prostitution, though there is a plethora of dogmatic opinion. On the one hand, and aside from the question of morality, it is contended that the presence of a house of prostitution or of a red-light district is but an invitation to the male to expose himself to a woman who, in all probability, is infected with one or more of the venereal diseases. Against this, it is argued that the male needs no invitation of this sort; that prostitutes, clandestine or otherwise, are always available regardless of whether or not there is a segregated district. It is further contended (with very good evidence) that breaking up red-light districts pushes the prostitutes into hotels and rooming houses; and (with no evidence at all) that deprived of the red-light district the male will turn to rather pitiless seduction.

Those who are in favor of maintenance of prostitutes in segregated districts, advance arguments, in addition to the above, to the effect that the district and the prostitutes can be put under rigid medical inspection and police regulation. This contention does not stand up practically, since medical supervision and police regulations have been but empty gestures except in a few instances when prostitutes have been segregated under military control and confined within barbed wire, when the visiting males as well as the resident females were examined, and when prophylaxis was immediately practiced.

Periodic medical examination of the prostitute does good to this extent—a certain number, obviously diseased, will be discovered and may thus be removed temporarily as foci of infection. On the other hand, it gives a false security, since failure to discover evidence of a venereal disease, especially in a woman, does not mean that the disease is not present. Further, the physician examines, say on a Monday, and finds no trouble. Then on Wednesday, a gonorrheal infection received a week or so before comes to the end of its incubation period and enters the stage of communicability. In these circumstances, this prostitute becomes a uniquely dangerous focus of infection: only 48 hours before she has received a written statement of health, and she could and would utilize this certificate of medical inspection as an item of salesmanship.

Sex Education. Conscious efforts along these lines are made by two principal groups—parents and schools. There is considerable difference of opinion as to which is the proper one for such an undertaking, and as to the correct method of imparting information of this sort. Also, and incident to a venereal disease control program, many health workers welcome the opportunity to make speeches, show moving pictures, and distribute literature to high school students.

Regardless of who does it and when, sex education and information about the venereal diseases should be, or at least should appear to be, incidental. A father, for instance, should never draw shades, lock doors, create an atmosphere of sanctity and secrecy, and otherwise make an isolated event of a talk to his son on sex or venereal diseases. The poor youngster is tremendously embarrassed, perhaps secretly disgusted, possibly receives what will prove to have been a nasty psychic wound. What the father and mother should do with both son and daughter is to convey information naturally and casually, as part of a general conversation or discussion. The mother is going to have a baby, or the cat is going to have kittens: let it be discussed good-humoredly, perhaps decently humorously, but not obviously. As the children grow older, these parents can speak of syphilis as easily and casually as they would of tuberculosis or heart disease.

The same common sense should apply in schools. The children can learn reproduction as a part of botany or zoology or physiology; the high school boys and girls can get their information on venereal diseases as part of the regular course in hygiene or whatever it may be called and by the regular teacher. If this cannot be done because of mixed classes, ineptitude of the teacher, or religious disapproval, then it is not something to be taught in that particular school. In other words, an artificial situation is created when classes have to be separated, special lecturers imported, and information on venereal diseases made a portentous event.

The effectiveness of sex education in preventing the spread of venereal disease depends to a great extent upon what is taught. It is doubtful that either the boy or the girl informed thoroughly on sex matters is any more likely to avoid exposure to venereal disease because of the moral issue than is the youngster not so instructed. Pride in and the maintenance of chastity does, of course, act as a powerful protective factor; but virginity is not so much a matter of sex education as it is the observance of a code; and observance of a code does not necessitate an understanding of it. These two things—sex information on the one hand and chastity on the other—are quite separate. If they were not, the bars of chastity would be let down in a far greater proportion of the uninformed or those who majored in the arts, than, say, in college graduates who had majored in biology. There is no reason to believe that this is the case.

The person who is informed as to the danger of infection from casual sexual intercourse will certainly be more conscious of the chances of contracting venereal disease than will the uninformed and will have a greater fear of diseases of this kind. Will this fear act as a deterrent to exposure? Probably, to some extent, in a certain number of persons who would otherwise have exposed themselves. But there is no animal fear which will not be subjugated under the appropriate urge; and unleashed sexual desire is one of the strongest urges in living beings. While no one may speak authoritatively on certain phases of the matter, and it is a peculiarly difficult one on which to obtain facts, it seems not reasonable to believe that the mere fear of contracting a venereal disease will eliminate or even appreciably decrease the incidence of these diseases.

Is there then, *any* virtue in sex education and is there no possibility of preventing infection? The answer is that one who is properly informed can, as a result of this information, reasonably effectively protect oneself (assuming that a certain amount of exposure in the population is inevitable) by prophylaxis, antibiotic or mechanical, either or both. Though society is not yet ready to include this sort of instruction in sex education, it is to some extent and incidentally, practiced on the basis of sex education obtained from associates.

The Place of the Public Health Nurse in the Venereal Disease Control Program. The public health nurse occupies a peculiarly important position in the venereal disease control program. She serves in the clinic, she conducts interviews as to possible source and spread contacts, follows up in epidemiological investigations in the field, routes suspected cases to the clinic (or to private physician) for examination, checks on clinic cases to ensure regular attendance, is not infrequently the person who draws blood for serologic test or obtains other specimens for laboratory examination. Under medical direction she treats cases of ophthalmia neonatorum, and vulvovaginitis in young girls, gets the syphilis-infected prenatal case in for treatment and proceeds similarly with the infant, and engages in productive health education in relation to the venereal diseases.

If, and as, additional duties develop she will assume them. Next to the competent clinician, she is the most important element in the venereal disease control program. At that, she sees the mass problem while the clinician is, not infrequently, concerned only with the individual.

Effectiveness of Venereal Disease Programs. The results of programs directed against the venereal diseases cannot be measured in exact and concrete terms, but appreciable results have been attained in three directions.

1. Through the widespread use of silver salts in the eyes of newborns, the incidence of ophthalmia neonatorum has been decreased at least two thirds. It is possible that penicillin may replace silver salts.

2. Through active and effective free clinics for venereal diseases, hundreds of thousands of cases which otherwise would not have obtained treatment are made practically noninfectious or have been cured.

3. Partly as a result of the educational features of venereal disease control programs and partly because society at present regards it as smart to be unshockable (whereas a generation or two ago smart society was a prude), the subject of venereal diseases is more out in the open and therefore can be better dealt with.

REFERENCES

American Public Health Association: *The Control of Communicable Diseases in Man.* The Association, New York, 1955.

American Social Hygiene Association, Association of State and Territorial
    Health Officers, American Venereal Disease Association, and the
    U.S. Public Health Service: *Venereal Disease Today*. The American
    Social Hygiene Association, New York, 1955.
Maxcy, K. F.: *Rosenau's Preventive Medicine and Hygiene*, 7th ed. Apple-
    ton-Century-Crofts, Inc., New York, 1951.

chapter 8

Mental Health

PROBLEMS OF MENTAL health are widespread and ill-defined. To a greater or lesser degree, millions have mental health problems, varying from violent disturbances to mild eccentricities. Basic scientific knowledge is not abundant and practice is largely empirical. Because of the nature and extent of the mental health problem it seriously affects the public health.

Mental disease has long been a problem. How sufferers from such diseases are regarded by society has varied through the ages, with gradual betterment. Treatment in some conditions is more effective as well as more humane, but in others the outlook is discouraging. At least the filth and neglect and cruelty of the ancient asylums have been abolished in the more modern and better managed hospitals for those who are mentally ill.

There has been a further advance through recognition that problems of mental health are found in many persons outside of hospitals; that vast numbers of people, seemingly in good health, proper in behavior, and productively employed, actually lead miserable, apprehensive, and confused existences. And with this recognition, measures designed to help such people have been visualized. They are inadequate and halting, and sometimes unrealistic, but the mere recognition of this aspect of the problem gives assurance that, sooner or later, better, more adequate, and practicable measures will emerge.

Terminology and Classification of Mental Diseases. Modern terminology of mental diseases derives from and moves around the word *pysche,* of Greek derivation and meaning mind or spirit. Thus a *psychosis* is a disease of the mind; *psychiatry* is the science dealing with disease of the mind. A *neurosis* is generally considered to be a functional disturbance, without organic disease of the nerves concerned. For borderline or combination cases, there is the term *psychoneurosis.*

By common agreement and usage, these terms have general acceptance, yet such terminology means no more than would the use of the word *somatosis* to describe all diseases of the body. Doubtless a better terminology will develop with greater knowledge.

The old common term *crazy* is now never used in the medical profession, and even the public has pretty well given it up. *Insane* is essentially a legal term. In effect, one who is insane is without mind, incapable of handling his own affairs, unable to distinguish between right and wrong. Most people interpret insane to indicate a seriously disturbed, mentally ill, perhaps violent person. But a quiet idiot, in a legal sense, is also an insane person.

In an effort to offset the stigma usually attached to mental disease, there is a tendency to soften designations as much as possible. There is even an inclination to avoid use of the term mental disease. Instead, one is described as being mentally ill. Apparently one suffers no embarrassment in having a neurosis, and to be psychoanalyzed has become quite fashionable.

There is not complete agreement as to classification of mental diseases. The general trend appears to be to put those mental diseases not known to have a physical cause in one group and those with a known physical cause in another. Thus dementia precox or schizophrenia and the manic-depressive states occupy the first group, while such psychoses as are incident to cerebral arteriosclerosis go into another category. Somewhere in between are listed conditions such as epilepsy, Mongolism, feeblemindedness, psychopathic personality, the neuroses, etc.

Causative Factors. A first essential in understanding and treating or controlling any disease is a knowledge of its cause. Until that is known, the physician or the public health worker is sailing an uncharted sea. It is obvious, too, from the considerations presented above, that the term mental disease covers a number of diverse conditions, not all of which are due to one cause.

For purposes of brevity, it may be said that the central core of the mental disease problem is the mental disturbance without known physical cause. As time has passed, many conditions believed to have no physical cause have been shown, in part, to have such bases. An outstanding example here is what was known as general paresis of the insane, now referred to as paresis. This is a condition in which the sufferer is seriously disturbed, irresponsible, perhaps dangerous; and there was no known cause. It is now recognized as due to syphilis. Further, in mental disturbance associated with pellagra, the latter was overlooked, and the psychosis was regarded as without physical cause. Subsequently came recognition of the true cause. Developing knowledge suggests that such conditions as feeblemindedness, epilepsy, and Mongolism may arise from chemical or physiological deprivations in the uterus, or from prenatal or natal accidents. In effect, schizophrenia and the manic-depressive states are the only frank mental diseases where there is but little light as to physical cause, if such exists. How closely the neuroses and psychoneuroses are related to the more frank manifestations is not clear, but they too are not known to have physical causes.

Psychiatrists generally account for the psychoses on the assumption that the individual has been unable to integrate into his personality the shocks and the pressures of life. In an effort to control fears or instincts, and impulses that society frowns upon, with sex playing a strong part, he breaks under the struggle through which other persons pass successfully. Inherent in this concept is acceptance of the thesis that some personalities are more sensitive than others to the abuse and unhappiness of existence, and that some encounter more and worse buffeting than others. A little trouble, thus, might disorient and disturb seriously one who is of "weak" personality structure; and even the most serene individual might become unbalanced under continuing intolerable conditions.

Unfortunately, many of these terms are difficult to define, either inclusively or exclusively. Personality, for instance, has various connotations. Integrate, too, is somewhat vague. Further they offer no explanation easily understood by the man on the street or by one trained in the physical sciences, as to why some individuals are unable to integrate what others take in their stride. There are, of course, psychological explanations dealing with experiences in childhood where there was overprotection by the mother, or overaffection by the father, or rejection of the infant or child by one or both parents, or jealousy or insecurity, etc. There is some tacit admission that psychoses and allied conditions appear more frequently in some families than others, but these conditions are not believed to be inheritable as such; it is rather a tendency toward them that is inherited.

It can be seen that there are assumptions and rationalizations in the presently accepted concept of mental diseases. Psychiatrists generally and the public are more nearly satisfied with these explanations than are scientists concerned primarily with disturbed physiology and pathology. The latter, and some psychiatrists, are inclined to look for a physical cause: not necessarily gross pathological lesions, but rather a physiological unbalance, as in metabolism, the hormones, salt balances, etc. None would deny the effect of stress and early unpleasant or shocking experiences on the individual, but there is growing inclination to reach for those underlying physiological, biochemical factors that make one individual more susceptible to these pressures than are others. There is thus an increasing inclination for a fresh approach and for more inclusive research in mental diseases, and for inclusion of physiopathology as well as Oedipus and Narcissus in such research.

Feeblemindedness. To express the child's innate intelligence, the "intelligence quotient" (IQ) is used. This quotient indicates the relationship between a child's real or chronological age and his mental age. To determine the mental age, the examiner uses a series of tests, problems and questions, readily solved or answered by a child of normal intelligence at the age under consideration. Only experts should attempt to perform and interpret these tests. Having determined the mental age of a given child, it is compared with his age in years and parts of years, and expressed as a per cent. Thus a child whose actual age is 10 years might be found to have a mental age of 8 years. The quotient here would be expressed as $8 \div 10$ or .80.

In grading feeblemindedness, the scale usually observed is *idiots* (infantile in intelligence and actions), *imbeciles* (intelligence-reaction attitude of a child under school age), and *morons* (intelligence sufficient to permit them to get along, but in a very restricted capacity).

The U.S. Bureau of the Census gives a more exact separation of the grades of feeblemindedness, as follows:

Idiots: Mental age less than 3 years; an IQ of less than 20 in a child.

Imbeciles: Mental age of 3–7 years; an IQ of 20 to 49 in a child.

Morons: Mental age of 8–11 years; an IQ of 50 to 69 in a child.

The extent of the problem of feeblemindedness or mental deficiency is difficult to determine. Recognition of mental deficiency depends to a very considerable extent upon the community facilities for testing the intelligence on a routine basis. Various studies of the prevalence of mental deficiency have indicated a marked relationship to age and social class. In population studies that have been conducted the highest rates are usually found in the 10–14 age group, with rates as high as 50 per 1000 of the population in that age group showing evidence of mental deficiency of some degree. Reported prevalence rates among adults are usually considerably lower. This is probably due to the lesser tendency to test adults than school children for, after all, these adults are but the children of yesterday, and if they were feebleminded then, they are still feebleminded as adults. Certain studies have indicated a higher prevalence of mental deficiency in rural populations than in urban groups; however, more recent studies do not bear out this finding.

Extent of the Problems of Mental Health. There have been various estimates as to the number of persons in the United States in need of guidance, advice, or treatment because of mental problems of one degree or another. It is not easy to establish a reliable figure in this connection. The number of persons in hospitals for mental disease can be stated fairly exactly. However, there are always some who should be in mental hospitals, but have never been there. Others are on a sort of leave status. Guesses, with some basis of fact, proclaim that 1 person of every 10 (or 16 or 20) will spend some part of his or her life in a mental hospital.

Similar data can be obtained for epileptics in hospitals, and the feebleminded in institutions. These perhaps represent only a small part of those affected, for families are more likely to keep a feebleminded person, especially a child, at home than they are to keep one who exhibits more dramatic evidence of mental illness.

A study carried out by the National Institute of Mental Health in 1954 revealed the fact that 137,979 mental defectives were under supervision, of whom 121,995 were patients in hospitals for the mentally defective. This is believed by the National Association for Mental Health to represent less than 10 per cent of the mentally deficient in the total population.

When one moves from these farily well definable and recognizable conditions to the psychoneuroses, neuroses, psychopathic personalities, behavior problems, alcoholics, and deviates of other kinds, estimates as to the size of the problem take on the characteristics of speculation.

A recent study of a random sample of the population in an urban community was carried out and indicated a prevalence rate of 1% showing some form of mental illness.

The introduction of electroshock treatment has tended to decrease the amount of hospitalization necessary for persons suffering from some forms of mental illness.

Going beyond these individuals who without great difficulty can be recognized as mildly disturbed persons, there are found those encountered in everyday life who might be called mentally or nervously unfortunate: ill-natured and querulous, tense and fearful, sour in personality, overaggressive or timid, suspicious, boastful, or otherwise personally objectionable. The number of these people is legion. They are found everywhere, even among readers and writers of books, and psychiatrists. Their relations with others are bad; they make their wives or husbands and children unhappy and themselves get but meager satisfaction from life. There can be no vaccine or pill that will cure these people, but the world will be a better place when their number or proportion is lessened. This can come about only through a long and continuing process of better understanding and practice of principles of mental health.

The Epidemiology of Mental Illness. From the preceding discussion, it will be apparent that one cannot present an epidemiological picture of mental illness as can be done in connection with tuberculosis or cholera where cases are fairly easily recognized, and where generally the occurrence of each case is reported and recorded with details as to age, sex, race, occupation, economic circumstances, environment, date of onset, and similar relevant data.

Because mental disturbances are apparently due to a number of different causes of which none is clearly and objectively established, except in those having a physical basis, an epidemiological approach is handicapped at the outset. Further, diagnosis of the two major mental diseases, schizophrenia and manic-depressive types, is largely subjective. Diagnosis, therefore, is likely to be tentative, dogmatic, or confused in some instances. This does not mean that there is often danger of saying that one is mentally disturbed when he is not, unless there is skillful and coached malingering, but the exact classification may require long and careful consideration. Further, a considerable number of persons brew their mental disturbances very quietly and never get into the hands of one competent to make a diagnosis.

Inasmuch as an epidemiological study depends largely upon knowing the number of events, or cases, and because there must be certainty that all cases supposed to be included are included and that all noncases have been excluded, the deficiencies in diagnosis, reporting, and recording loom large as deterrents to outlining an epidemiological picture.

In spite of these difficulties, a few simple data have come to light and are worth considering:

Schizophrenia. There have been various estimates as to the magnitude of this problem; approximately 175,000 persons were hospitalized with the diagnosis of schizophrenia in 1951, a rate of 147 per hundred thousand population. There are, of course, many patients with this disease who are not hospitalized, perhaps as many as are in the hospital at any one time.

The incidence of this condition, that is the number of new cases in a given time period, say a year, is naturally much lower. In 1951 36,000 new cases were admitted to mental hospitals. If this can be accepted as an indication of the incidence of the disease, it would indicate an attack rate of 23 per 100,000 for cases severe enough to require hospitalization. The total incidence rate may be considerably higher but accurate estimates are not available.

About the only clearly cut subitem of epidemiological interest in schizophrenia is that this is largely a disease of early adult life. Most cases occur under 40 years of age. There seems to be no preponderance of cases in one sex. Some believe that cases more often arise in those disadvantageously placed economically. This may or may not prove to be true. Season apparently plays no part, and infection is not believed to be an operative factor, although persons with brain damage from communicable diseases may exhibit some of the symptoms of schizophrenia. Patients with schizophrenia constitute the most permanent part of the hospital population.

Manic-depressive Psychoses. This is the second most important of the so-called psychogenic disorders, that is mental illness without discovered physical foundation. Data collected indicate that of all first admissions to hospitals about 6 per cent are diagnosed as having manic-depressive psychosis. It manifests itself at a later time than does schizophrenia and occurs more frequently in women than in men. No specific causative factor or pathogenesis has been established. The inheritance of a tendency to this mental disturbance is thought possible, but what this inheritance is, its mechanism, how it may be recognized or measured is not known. The effect of environment and the pressures of life are not generally believed to play so great a role as in schizophrenia. Socioanthropological studies now under way in many places and under varying cultures may throw new light on this question.

Other Psychoses and Related States. There seems to be no necessity for discussing in detail the epidemiological aspects of psychoses definitely associated with known physical disturbances, since the incidence of the psychosis is limited to, though not necessarily always present in, those who have developed the underlying pathology. Thus, while not everyone with syphilis develops paresis, true paresis occurs only in those who have syphilis; arteriosclerotic psychoses depend upon the underlying sclerosis of the cerebral arteries, and thus these psychoses most often occur in older persons. Senile dementia, closely related to the latter condition, has the changes incident to old age as its basis. Admissions to psychiatric hospitals because of the psychoses of old age have increased rapidly in recent decades and now approach 40% of all admissions.

Chronic alcoholism is now regarded as the result rather than the cause of mental disturbance. It is not known whether there is one unique cause, or many, for the million chronic alcoholics in the United States.

From the above consideration of the epidemiological aspects of mental illness, it is seen that the picture is dim in outline, not sufficiently distinct to serve as a guide in a mass attack for control. But epidemiology is a tool that may contribute to elicitation of cause or causes and should therefore be used unremittingly in mental illnesses in spite of handicaps. Certainly a much clearer picture will be obtainable if and when the conditions dealt with can be diagnosed more sharply and objectively.

Treatment Facilities. From a practical standpoint the first essential in caring for those with mental illness is that there be hospitals for proper treatment. From a long-range standpoint, however, the first essential should be prevention. But how to prevent is not known, and in the meantime there are about a quarter of a million new patients annually who must be cared for and some 100,000 who must come back to mental hospitals as readmissions. In addition to providing hospitals there is the problem of clinic service for those only mildly disturbed, for mental hygiene advice to parents, for the juvenile delinquents, for schools, for those discharged to home care, etc.

To the need for these facilities must be added the demand of an increasing number of older persons needing psychiatric hospital care, and the fact that there is a dearth of pyschiatrists and allied specialists. Further, treatment is time consuming and expensive, both in hospitals and clinics, and in private practice. These demands far exceed the facilities available.

Bed Facilities in Mental Hospitals. It is estimated* that there are some 586 mental hospitals in the United States. This includes all sorts: public, veterans, private, wards in general hospitals.

On the average day these hospitals accommodate about 740,000 patients, some of them under badly crowded conditions. Because of discharges, deaths, and new admissions, the total number of different patients who pass through mental disease hospitals in a year is much greater than the above figure. Thus the state hospitals, which have an average daily occupancy of approximately 475,500 patients, handle nearly 700,000 persons per year.

The magnitude of the mental hospital population is reflected in the fact that, in the United States, it constitutes nearly one half (47 per cent) of all patients in all hospitals for all causes. This is exclusive of those in institutions for the feebleminded and epileptic.

One of the great and significant differences between the hospital population in general and that in hospitals for mental disease is that the latter stay a very long time. In a study of patients in New York State hospitals some years ago it was found that only 16 per cent stayed less than one year, whereas another 16 per cent had been there from 15 to 24 years. In the schizophrenia group, which makes up about half the total population in hospitals for the mentally ill, about 16 per cent had been in the hospitals from 25 to 44 years, and 37 per cent for more than 15 years.

The present general goal in hospital beds for the mentally ill in the United States is 5 beds per 1000 of population. This would necessitate adding about a quarter of a million beds to those existing in 1949.

In 1956 the trend toward increasing numbers of psychiatric patients hospitalized was interrupted for the first time. It remains to be

* Most of the figures used here and subsequently in this chapter are taken from data published by the National Association for Mental Health and the U.S. Public Health Service. See end of chapter for more precise identification.

seen if this will prove a significant change or merely an interruption in the rise.

Cost of Operating Mental Hospitals. The cost of operating public mental hospitals in 1956 was $662,146,372. The average cost for the care of a patient per day was $3.26. In general the cost of veterans' hospital care is much higher than that in state hospitals and in 1956 was approximately $9.00 per capita per day. In many private institutions the costs are even higher. It is estimated that the cost of the care of psychiatric patients including maintenance and capital cost amounts to an average of $3.74 for each person in the general population.

Most states require that some part of the cost of caring for patients be charged back to the county or jurisdiction from which each comes. In turn, an effort is made to collect from a patient's estate or responsible relative some part of the cost of his care. Fortunately, questions of finances seldom act as a barrier to admission of cases. Apparently only about one out of five pays partially for care in state hospitals.

Hazards in Populations of Mental Hospitals. Mentally ill patients must be watched carefully lest they injure themselves or others. Trained hospital administrators, staff, and attendants exercise every care to reduce these hazards to a minimum. But over and above the hazard of accidents, suicide, occasional abuse by an unfit attendant, etc., mentally ill patients in large groups tend to show a tuberculosis rate much higher than that of the general population, and outbreaks of gastrointestinal diseases are encountered from time to time. Seriously disturbed patients and those who have markedly deteriorated do not practice personal hygiene, and the pressure under which a shorthanded staff must work contribute to the health hazard of both inmates and attendants. From time to time unfortunate notoriety and blame come to hard-working and underpaid superintendents and staffs. When such episodes make the headlines, a chief executive or member of an appropriating body will, not infrequently, rise in seemingly righteous wrath because of the conditions brought to light, to which he has contributed through niggardliness or lack of previous interest. Constant alertness, the highest standard of hygiene practicable, and a competent medical service, as well as a psychiatric staff, help to find physical disabilities or infections at an early stage.

Commitments to Hospitals for the Mentally Ill. Reduced to its simplest terms, commitment of a mentally ill person to a hospital is a process designed to obtain proper care for the patient in the shortest practicable time, and, if necessary, to protect others. However, because of the stigma attached to mental illness, because the person is deprived of liberty for an indefinite period, and because he is usually incompetent to handle his own affairs, definite legal issues are involved. Rather precise and sometimes cumbersome and unfortunate proceedings are required.

Present laws in connection with commitments, which are state laws, represent somewhat of a compromise between medicine and the law. Psychiatrists generally feel that the processes are too legalistic; lawyers are insistent that there be proper protection of the person concerned and due process of law, even though cumbersome.

The worst type of commitment law was that in which, by tradition, mental illness was handled as a crime: arrest, jail, the charge of insanity, jury trial. This process has been considerably softened and accelerated through provisions for commitment in emergency on the basis of physicians' or health officers' certificate, with judical hearings rather than jury trials in ordinary cases.

The laws of the different states vary as to commitment procedures, but in general the admission of a mentally ill patient to a hospital is on one of four bases: (a) involuntary commitment, (b) emergency commitment, (c) observational commitment, and (d) voluntary entrance. The first of these, *involuntary commitment*, is the old and formal practice involving petition to the courts (by relative or others), medical certification, hearing in court, and final action. In some states formal notice must be served on the mentally ill person, and it may be required that he be formally arrested on a warrant. Practically all states provide that there may be a jury trial if requested by the person concerned or his friends.

The *emergency commitment procedures* are provided in order to meet those situations where an individual becomes suddenly and seriously disturbed, perhaps violent. In these cases the judicial process is waived temporarily, and patients may be admitted to hospitals for the mentally ill on the formal certification of the health officer. Patients so admitted can be held only for a week or ten days, pending action for more formal commitment procedures if justified.

Somewhat similar to emergency commitment is short-term *commitment for observation and diagnosis.* But, whereas emergency commitment is only for a period of days, and formal commitment may be for life, observational commitment is from one to three months. On the basis of study of the patient in this period, diagnosis and plans for future care and treatment can be made.

The term *voluntary admission* or *entrance* of a patient into a hospital for the mentally ill explains itself. One of the great advantages is that the patient does not, by the process of entering the hospital, go into the records as one mentally disturbed. Theoretically, it provides an opportunity for the individual, feeling himself under serious mental strain, to have himself treated. Practically, few persons on the edge of a mental breakdown will be able to make this decision. Therefore they sign the necessary application, which signing they must do themselves, under the persuasion of relatives or friends. A protection to the patient thus admitted is that he may not be kept confined against his will. He must be released within a specified time, not more than two weeks in most states, after he asks for release. Obviously, if release would entail danger to himself or others, procedures for formal involuntary commitment may be set in motion.

As mentioned above, the state laws in relation to mental illness vary. Some are good, some antiquated. There is growing public and professional sentiment for their improvement. The U.S. Public Health Service, through the National Institute of Mental Health, has provided a draft document that embodies the more modern concepts of such laws which, it has been hoped, would aid the several states, as was done in connection with the vital statistics laws. (See page 27.)

The Release of Patients from Hospitals for the Mentally Ill. As indicated above, those patients who enter hospitals in any circumstances other than formal involuntary commitment must be released in a relatively short time unless additional action involving court procedure is instituted. However, the seriously disturbed patients or those who were once seriously disturbed are under formal commitment, and it is with these, the bulk of the hospital population, that the question of discharge arises. Some die, some remain unimproved, or grow worse, some get better. With improvement, or apparent recovery, plans are made for discharge.

Under most state laws, the decision to discharge a patient is the responsibility of the medical director of the hospital, or of a board. Doubtless under pressure to find beds for new cases, some hospital authorities let patients go who should be kept; others, finding a patient to be a good worker, and faced with shortages in attendants, or gardeners, may let a few remain longer than necessary. Generally, however, those responsible exercise fine judgment. Patients are given trial leaves, from a few days to a month, to see how they stand up to outside conditions. Or they may be given much longer leave, reporting back for re-examination on a sort of outpatient basis. Some states even board out quiet homeless individuals. Some may be discharged without qualification other than a vague follow-up hope.

In spite of the care exercised, unpleasant and sometimes horrifying consequences follow the release of patients from hospitals for the mentally ill: rape, murder, etc. In retrospect, it becomes easy to see that they should never have been discharged, and there is quite justifiable public indignation. The hospital director is given no credit for the thousands of times that his judgment was correct in discharging patients, nor for his acumen in discovering danger in those whom he continues to hold. There is room for improvement in present practices and standards for discharge, but the problem is difficult. Newer knowledge, more adequate staff, and better administrative procedures will doubtless give some aid, but since the decision to discharge a patient rests to some extent upon his assumed future actions, judgment can never be perfect.

The Federal Government in Mental Health. As mentioned previously, the laws relating to commitment of mentally ill patients are essentially state laws. The federal government enters into this aspect of the problem and movement only to a limited extent: in the District of Columbia, and in connection with members of armed services, veterans, federal employees, wards of government, etc. Certain veterans' hospitals are assigned for psychiatric cases, and St. Elizabeth's Hospital in the District of Columbia is maintained to meet civilian federal needs. The federal government also maintains hospitals for narcotic addicts, particularly federal prisoners. In these hospitals there is provision for voluntary entrance of civilian applicants in limited numbers.

In recent years the federal government has given most valuable impetus to the mental health movement along a number of new lines. This new force became more effective when, in 1946, the National Mental Health Act became operative. This law did not relate to hospitalization but rather to a nationwide mental hygiene movement on a community basis. There is provision for research, for training of workers who will serve outside the hospitals, and for grants-in-aid to states in their development of statewide and local programs in mental health.

The National Institute for Mental Health of the U.S. Public Health Service provides quiet guidance for this national program. It conducts research, administers grants to universities, hospitals, and other competent investigators, administers a strong and sound fellowship program. With states and other authorities, the Institute carries forward studies and demonstrations, and collects, analyzes, and publishes information pertinent to mental health problems.

In the grants-in-aid provisions, the Public Health Service deals with the mental health authorities of the respective states. This is not always the same state authority that administers the mental disease hospitals of the state (see "State Organization and Administration," below). In 1957 the federal government, through the U.S. Public Health Service, assisted the states in their community mental health work to the extent of some $4,000,000. For each dollar that a state thus receives, it must provide two dollars from state and local sources, for use in the extrahospital mental health program.

State Organization and Administration in Mental Health. Some aspects of this subject have already been discussed in relation to hospitals for the mentally ill, but a modern mental health program encompasses far more than hospitalization, and there must be a mechanism for carrying forward those most important parts of the program that relate to the emotional, mental, and nervous problems of those outside hospitals. It is in these situations that such measures as exist for prevention may be applied. And it is preventive measures in mental health upon which rests some hope for the decency, peace, and happiness of the world.

There are many different patterns of administration of mental health services in the United States. Hospitalization of the cases of serious mental illness has been accepted generally as a state responsibility but there is no uniformity in the administrative mechanism provided by different state laws. In one state, for example, all state institutions, including prisons and hospitals, are administered by a department of institutions and agencies. In other states mental disease hospitals are under the control of a department of mental hygiene, although community mental health services are the responsibility of the department of health. In many states the department of welfare has the responsibility for the hospitalization of the mentally ill. In a few states mental hospitals are administered under a board of mental hygiene, having no departmental status within the state government.

There has been a tendency in recent years to clarify the responsibility at the state level. Because of the magnitude of the problem and as a result of incentives under the federal grants program an increasing number of states have well-defined major departments of government charged with the responsibility for hospital care of the mentally ill.

In the development of community services for the non-hospitalized mentally ill person, and for the detection and prevention of mental illness more than half of the states have designated the health department as the authority responsible for this stage of the program. A few states place this responsibility in the department responsible for the hospital care of the mentally ill and in a few states this responsibility is that of the department of welfare. State health departments in increasing numbers are developing major divisions of mental health to provide out-patient clinic service and preventive services in the field of mental health.

Viewed administratively, the above situation is not a sound one.

The purpose of providing hospitalization is to improve, or at least provide professional care for, the mentally ill. Merely because both hospitals for the mentally ill and penitentiaries have to make vast purchases of food and clothing or operate a farm is not sufficient reason to lump together the responsibility for controlling criminals on the one hand and caring for the mentally ill on the other. And because care of the mentally ill is a medical problem, it would seem a matter of administrative convenience, rather than of function, to place this authority in a department of welfare.

Finally, a board as an administrative agency has but little to commend it. Boards are extremely important in the establishment of policy, standards, regulations, and in advisory and liaison capacities. However, both experience and common sense indicate that a board which meets once each month, or every other month, cannot administer a large and complex undertaking. Its members are preoccupied with other affairs, cannot be informed in detail, are not present to meet day-by-day situations, and their performance in administrative matters are likely to be *pro forma*—in contrast to the great service they can render along broad advisory lines and in formulating policy.

The present trend gives reason to hope that in the not too distant future the responsibility for administration of state hospitals for the mentally ill will rest in a department of state government whose function and competence lies in this field; that such a department will be complemented by a board or council, which is not concerned with administrative matters but rather with broad duties as indicated above.

As to whether or not hospitals for the mentally ill as well as community mental health programs (see below) might properly and advantageously be placed in the department of health is a controversial question. Most psychiatrists rather vehemently oppose the idea. The public health people are reluctant, if not apprehensive, as to the implications of the proposal. Perhaps this reluctance and fear could be overcome with coaxing.

State programs for community health are not, in all cases, operated by the same group concerned in hospitals. The National Mental Health Act required that each state, when applying for federal grants-in-aid, designate an agency for administering the mental health program; and the act, by its language, indicated that this would be the state health authority unless there were already a state mental health authority concerned in community mental health. Some 29 states indicated the state health department (or board of health) as the state mental health authority for purposes of the community-wide extrahospital program.

This program has been conducted along the broad lines of training and education, recruitment of professional personnel, educational activities, clinics, demonstrations and research, with prevention strongly flavoring the whole undertaking.

There is a growing tendency for health departments, working in close cooperation with the mental hospital, to provide some supervision of discharged cases. In a few states the department of health is charged with the responsibility for ambulatory care for the mentally ill. The public health nurse is assuming an increasing role in the mental health program, assisting in case finding by referral of patients to health department clinics or to hospital outpatient departments and in providing a follow-up service for discharged patients. With the increased use of chemotherapeutic agents in the treatment of the mentally ill, patients may be discharged much earlier if there is some form of continuing observation and supervision in the home.

Community Programs in Mental Health. These are spotty and sparse, but tending to grow. In larger cities, most hospitals have some provision for temporary care of those violently disturbed; in many smaller communities such unfortunates must be kept in jail for a day or two. Large hospitals conduct services in the psychiatric field as part of their outpatient clinics. Usually there is a long waiting list.

Local health departments have not generally operated mental health services as they do child health conferences, etc. Whether they will, or should, or can do this is a moot question. Certainly however, no service of the health department which involves contact with people should be operated without due respect for and appreciation of the mental components of the persons whom they serve. Well-oriented physicians and nurses can, and in some places do, render excellent mental health service in clinics for tuberculosis, venereal diseases, the chronic illnesses, prenatal cases, and mothers and infants. Health departments too should recognize that regardless of by whom administered, mental health constitutes a vast public health problem, and no inconsiderable part of health education should be in this field.

REFERENCES

Lemkau, Paul V.: *Mental Hygiene in Public Health.* McGraw-Hill Book Company, Inc., New York, 1955.

The National Association for Mental Health, Inc.: *Facts and Figures about Mental Illness and Other Personality Disturbances.* The Association, New York, 1952.

The National Committee against Mental Illness: *What Are the Facts about Mental Illness.* The Committee, Washington, D.C., 1957.

The National Institute of Mental Health: *Patients in Mental Institutions, 1954,* Part I. Government Printing Office, Washington, D.C., 1957.

U.S. Public Health Service: *Mental Health Statistics, Current Reports.* Government Printing Office, Washington, D.C., 1951.

chapter 9

Environmental Health

Sanitation

THE HUMAN BEING was not always even decently clean, either in his person, his house, or his town. He recognized these things neither as necessities nor possibilities. In the same conversation in which John Wesley piously, perhaps sonorously, declared "Cleanliness is indeed next to godliness," gruff old Josiah Wedgwood, the potter, echoed, "and next to impossible." Gradually, under the urge of aesthetics, convenience, and hygiene, the self-respecting person or community has come to be reasonably clean. But hygiene as it relates to the individual and sanitation as it relates to the community demand a great deal more than a clean skin and good municipal housekeeping.

It is perhaps fortunate that many of the most effective measures in sanitation contributed to the convenience and comfort of the individual. If, in cities, it had not made life easier and more pleasant to have an indoor toilet, water in the kitchen and bathroom, and the prompt removal of garbage, it is doubtful that these things would have been done so promptly or so completely on merely hygienic grounds. Certainly progress has not been so marked along lines where sanitary necessity has been the only urge, as in replacing the rural insanitary privy by one sanitary but no more convenient, or as in drainage of swampy areas, or ratproofing, or housing. But on the whole, regardless of the impelling force, tremendous strides have been made along all lines of sanitation, and work of this sort is an important part of every health program.

Usage of the Words "Hygiene" and "Sanitation." There is no universally accepted, clearly cut difference in the meaning of these words, as at present used.

"Hygiene" is of Greek origin, "sanitation" from the Latin, and on the basis of these derivations, the two words would be interchangeable in usage. However, custom has tended to limit the use of "hygiene" to the individual—his person and intimate surroundings and practices; and to use the word "sanitation" more in connection with the out-of-doors affairs and the community as a whole. Not infrequently, in order to be sure that one is conveying the thought intended, the term "personal hygiene" or "environmental sanitation" is used. To complicate further an already confusing situation, the word "hygiene" is often used in a broad generic sense to cover the whole field of health—just as the word "medicine" is used to include surgery, x-ray, and various other procedures in diagnostics and therapy.

Problems Incident to Communal Living. To a modern-minded visitor, probably the most striking aspect in ancient primitive settlements would have been the accumulation of rubbish, carcasses of animals, perhaps offal, and a largely indiscriminate deposition of excreta. Usually in such villages or even in cities, the streets were ill-defined, narrow, with rivulets of filth and islands of maggot-ridden decaying organic matter. Flies swarmed as a matter of course and rats were abundant. It is reasonable to believe, and records indicate, that from this waste arose foul odors not in themselves dangerous but unpleasant.

Homes in these primitive settlements were mere hovels, windowless, chimneyless, floorless, and therefore dark and smoky and dirty. Pigs and chickens, flies and various other kinds of insects, competed with humans for tenantry of the huts; and the human family was lousy. Lack of refrigeration made it necessary that one develop a taste for tainted meat, and such milk as was drunk, coming from the grime-smeared cows, milked by foully polluted hands, was neither tempting nor salutary. Drinking water was necessary then as now. The source was the nearby stream or spring; and the person of an investigative turn of mind would have been able, perhaps, to follow the drainage from Foultown rather directly into the sources of drinking water. Such an environment would contribute to the indirect spread of disease through the avenues of excreta-polluted water, milk, food; through excreta-smeared fingers, through flies and fleas and lice and mosquitoes.

Even in modern times, communal living tends to facilitate both direct and indirect transmission of disease from person to person. One may gain an appreciation of the part played by density of population and the spread of communicable diseases, by comparing events in two equal population units, say of 100,000 each. One of them, the section of a city, occupies an area of 2 square miles. The other 100,000 population is scattered over a rural area 50 miles long and 40 miles wide—2000 square miles. Assume further that except for density of population, *all other things are equal.* In these circumstances, the potentialities for spread of communicable diseases would be much greater in the concentrated population for the following reasons:

1. The number of cases and carriers would be 1000 times more concentrated in the urban than the rural area.

2. The same degree of concentration would apply to susceptibles.

3. In the dense population there would be greater probability of direct contact between some case or carrier and some susceptible.

4. In the dense population there would be concentration and accumulation of excreta and garbage, greater probability that infected persons would pollute the food or drink of others; and that insects carrying infection (flies, fleas, lice, mosquitoes) would more quickly encounter susceptibles and infect them.

5. Individuals in a center of population, because of its commercial importance, would have more intercourse with the outside world than would the same number of individuals distributed sparsely over a rural area; thus the hazard of introduction of disease from without.

6. As years passed, the operation of these contributory factors would produce a greater number of foci (cases and carriers) in the dense population than in the scattered one. The number of susceptibles in the former would become less than in the latter, through hav-

ing had these diseases. However, this favorable factor would be offset by the concentration of susceptibles already mentioned.

It should be noted that in the above discussion the conditional "would" has been used consistently; and it should be noted also that between the dense and the scattered population *all other things than population concentration are assumed to be equal.* Actually, other things are never equal. Cities have instituted precautionary measures which quite effectively offset many of the hazards peculiar to concentration of population.

Sanitary Measures Usually Instituted in Cities. Naturally, these vary with the city, but those actually existing with more or less completeness are the following:

1. Sewer systems, designed to dispose of human waste, wash water, and drainage.

2. A system for the collection, disinfection, protection, and distribution of a safe water supply throughout the city.

3. A system for the collection and disposal of garbage.

4. Regulations for, and supervision of, the production, processing, and distribution of milk.

5. Regulations for, and supervision of, the sanitary condition of swimming pools, industrial plants, food establishments, school buildings, and of certain other areas or buildings where large numbers of people congregate.

6. Regulations as to housing, including rodent control.

7. Procedures for abatement of nuisances and in connection with miscellaneous sanitary matters.

The essential purpose of a sanitary measure is to interpose a barrier in some channel of infection; to block the path between a focus of infection (case or carrier) on the one hand and susceptibles on the other. Specifically, the sanitary measure may: effect the disposal of potentially infectious material, as in the sewer system; bring about the purification of already polluted drinking water; obtain the maximum elimination of the hazards in milk; destroy insects capable of transmitting pathogens; or provide proper ventilation. In any event, at one extreme is the actual or potential focus of infection; at the other, susceptibles. Interposed between the two is the sanitary measure. An auxiliary sanitary purpose is the provision of generally healthful surroundings, as in housing.

It is much easier to dispose of refuse and excreta and to furnish pure water in the city than in rural areas. In cities one central authority can institute one sewer system or one safe water supply for all homes and pay for it out of the city treasury; whereas in rural areas, persons live so far apart that a common sewer system and a central water supply are impracticable. Every farm home must have its own excreta disposal unit and its own well or spring; and the provision of these facilities at each individual home depends upon the intelligence, knowledge, and financial ability of the particular family owning, or living in, the home. Even aside from the fact that a large proportion of rural families will make no unusual effort to provide sanitary facilities at their homes, the possibilities of sanitary excellence of rural excreta disposal units or wells are limited unless there is a considerable outlay of funds.

Excreta Disposal by Sewers. In connection with sanitation, one should bear in mind the difference between "sewerage" and "sewage." The word "sewerage" refers to the system provided for the disposal of sewage; "sewage" is the matter carried in the sewer system. Sewage is made up of excreta, bath and dishwater, and discharge from industrial plants. In addition to the system for domestic sewage, there are sometimes supplementary sewers for storm water and surface drainage. Most sewer systems empty into the nearest large body of water. Though such an adjacent river or lake is the natural outlet for the system, it is, at the same time, the most easily available source of an ample water supply. The measures taken to minimize the dangers of pollution of streams by sewage are along the following lines:

1. There must be a margin of safety in the stream's ability to absorb, oxidize, and transport sewage as compared with the amount of sewage emptied into it.

2. Emptying sewage into the stream is not ordinarily permitted unless the sewage has been "treated."

3. Sewer outlets from treatment plants from a given city enter the stream at points *below* the place where the water supply is taken. In nonflowing water, as in lakes, the outlet of sewers and the intake of water are removed as far as possible from each other. Their relative positions depend upon topography of lake bed, currents generated by prevailing winds, and other local factors. In such situations, of course, the objective is to direct the water carriage of sewage away from the intake of water.

Steps Usually Carried Out in the Treatment of Sewage. These measures vary with different localities. All have as their objective the prevention of odors and as rapid as possible destruction of pathogenic organisms. In localities where the amount of sewage entering a stream is small in comparison with the size and flow of that stream, less treatment is required than when the opposite conditions exist. The breakdown of the organic matter in sewage is essentially a biochemical process, depending upon the presence of oxygen. When the demand for oxygen is greater than the amount present in the water, this breakdown of organic matter is slowed up. Scum forms, foul odors arise, fish are killed. This oxygen necessity, in any given situation is known as the *biochemical oxygen demand,* usually abbreviated as BOD.

In the ordinary operation of a sewerage system, the sewage is (1) *screened* to remove sticks, cloths, etc., and then passed through one or more large concrete tanks where (2) *by sedimentation* inorganic material such as sand, brought in by street washing, settles out; and (3) where organic matter, by aerobic and anaerobic *bacterial action,* is decomposed. The number of pathogenic organisms is decreased by these processes, and is frequently carried further by (4) *filtration.* Occasionally, the process is carried on through one more step, (5) *disinfection.* In the latter procedure, various disinfectants such as chloride of lime, or chlorine are used.

When there is no nearby body of water, most of the processes of sewage treatment, described above, are carried out rather completely, and the final product is allowed to flow into disposal fields for absorption by the soil. These disposal areas can be used only intermittently, and a tremendous acreage is necessary to meet the needs of large cities. A sandy, porous soil is a requisite.

Excreta Disposal in Unsewered Areas, as in the Rural Home or Schoolhouse. The method adopted usually depends upon whether or not water is piped into the building and upon the financial circumstances and what might be called the hygiene and aesthetic culture of the persons concerned. In excreta disposal without a sewer system, some type of privy must be adopted; where a water closet is installed in such circumstances, disposal is as described below under *septic tank* and *cesspool.*

The following are the different kinds of sanitary privies used:

1. *The Box and Can Type.* This is somewhat like the old-fashioned commode. The flyproof seat box contains a receptacle, usually large enough to last 4 or 5 days, when, unless there is a scavenger service, it must be emptied by the householder, the contents covered over in a previously prepared furrow, the can washed and disinfected. Properly operated, it is a safe method, but its decent maintenance requires more care than is usually given. Objectionable odors are quite common.

2. *The Pit Type.* This consists of a flyproof privy box, which is above a pit dug in the earth. The pit is 4 or 5 ft deep, about 4 ft from side to side, and some 3 ft from front to back. Its sides are lined with boards to prevent caving. If the pit is in sandy or sand-clay soil, does not connect with rock crevices, and is at least 100 ft and downhill from a well, it is a satisfactory type of privy. It is inexpensive, and requires but little care. When the pit is nearly full, a new one is dug, the privy house, which is usually quite light, is placed over it, and the old pit filled and covered with earth. This is the most common type of sanitary privy seen in rural areas.

3. *The Vault Type of Privy.* Instead of an earth pit under the seat box, this type of privy has a watertight vault made usually of concrete. The vault must be cleaned once or twice a year and is to that extent inconvenient.

4. *The Septic Tank Privy.* This is a small tank quite similar in principle to those used in municipal sewerage systems. Droppings fall

into the tank and undergo decomposition through bacterial action. An outlet from the tank is provided and its final product, the effluent, is discharged into the soil through porous field tile, placed in a slight slope, lying from 18 to 24 in. underground. This type of tank can be used either with a water closet or as part of an outdoor privy. With the latter, a bucket or two of water must be added each day. Only toilet paper may be used.

5. *The Chemical Type Privy.* This consists of a flyproof seat box, in outdoor privy or in bathroom, beneath which is a metal tank so treated as to resist chemical corrosion. This tank contains a strong caustic solution which disinfects and liquefies excreta. A valve is provided so that the contents of the tank may be discharged into the soil as it fills. It is a quite satisfactory system, but cannot be made at home and is expensive both in first cost and maintenance.

From the above it may be concluded that the essential requirements in sanitary privies are:

1. That the privy contents be protected from flies.
2. That dangerous pollution of soil, either surface or subsurface, be avoided.
3. That there be reasonable freedom from odors.
4. That first cost be not excessive.
5. That maintenance costs be low.
6. That unremitting care be given.

The usual rural privy is quite objectionable. Excreta falls upon the surface, under the privy. It is exposed to flies, rats, pigs, chickens. The flies are quite likely to establish a fairly orderly circuit—privy, kitchen, dining room. Chickens, with fecal-contaminated feet, tend to pollute the rope of the well bucket and the top of the well. In poorer rural homes, especially those in juxtaposition with clumps of bushes, there may be no privy of any sort.

In rural dwellings with an indoor water closet, the sewage is finally disposed of by a tile sewer which may empty into a nearby stream, or into a septic tank or a cesspool. When the stream is only a ditch, an insanitary situation is created. The septic tank has already been described. The cesspool is a pit 8 or 10 ft deep, 6 to 8 ft in diameter, without watertight sides or impervious bottom. Just below the ground surface it is covered over with heavy timbers or logs, these in turn being covered with earth. The contained matter undergoes decomposition and liquefaction, and is absorbed into the surrounding soil. Cesspools, where distance from the well is great and where soil is porous, are reasonably satisfactory. They should not be used in limestone areas nor in small towns where water supply is from individual shallow wells.

Diseases Which May Be Spread through Improper Disposal of Human Excreta. In a discussion of this subject it should be borne in mind that excreta is not dangerous because it is excreta. Its improper disposal creates a nuisance, aesthetically offensive, but only a small proportion of it carries organisms capable of producing specific infection. It is the presence of these specific organisms in *some* excreta which constitutes the menace, and in order to remove this menace, even though it is present in only a relatively small proportion of excreta, *all* excreta must be disposed of as carefully as if all actually contained pathogenic organisms.

The diseases which may arise incident to improper disposal of excreta are: cholera, not at present a menace in the United States; typhoid and paratyphoid fevers; dysentery, both amebic and bacillary; hookworm disease, ascaris infection, and, less frequently, other types of intestinal parasites. The virus of poliomyelitis has been found in sewage, as have tubercle bacilli, but this does not mean that human excreta is the principal medium through which these diseases are spread.

Water and Water Supplies. A factor of importance from the public health standpoint is the so-called self-purification of streams. It should be borne in mind that this is essentially a relative term. This purifying action depends upon many processes, varying in each situation; and there is no scientific basis for the popular belief that all streams purify themselves in a certain number of miles—three, five, or seven. Important considerations in this connection are: (1) the amount and character of pollution; (2) the volume of the stream—dilution of pollution; (3) the oxygen content of the stream—destruction of bacteria in water depends largely upon the presence of oxygen; (4) the temperature—cold water can absorb and maintain about twice as much oxygen as warm water, but typhoid bacilli survive longer in cold water; (5) the depth of the stream, character of the bottom, incline or fall of the stream—shallow streams, with rocky beds, flowing rapidly* produce wavelets and rapids toward the bottom of the stream which tend to keep a high oxygen content in the water; (6) sunshine—disinfecting action near surface and its favorable influence on the growth of algae, which assist in maintaining oxygen content; (7) the length of time the purifying factors have had to act upon the pollution.

City Water Supplies. The usual measures taken by a city to provide a safe water supply are, in general, as follows:

1. Effort is made to obtain initially as pure a supply as possible, and, within the limits of practicability, to protect the watershed from which the water comes. This can be done in relatively small lakes; it is impracticable in most streams and large lakes.

2. If a city receives its water supply from a river, this supply is taken only *above* the city's own sewer outlets.

3. The water is partially purified and clarified through natural processes in storage reservoirs (sedimentation, sunlight, action of harmless organisms on harmful).

4. Further sedimentation is accomplished by treatment with alum and other coagulants.

5. Filtration removes any remaining turbidity and bacteria.

6. Disinfection, usually by chlorine, destroys any bacteria which may have escaped the other processes.

7. Cross connection between the pipes of the purified supply and the pipes of an untreated water supply is prevented, the latter being provided in many cities for emergency fire protection purposes, or in connection with certain industries.

The amount of alum used in bringing about flocculation and sedimentation varies from 150 to 500 lb of aluminum sulfate to a million

---

* The opposite conditions, where bacteria are carried down and destroyed through sedimentation, are important factors in the purification of water.

gallons of water. Through alkalis in the water or added to it, the sulfate is changed to the hydroxide, which forms a "floc," settling gradually and carrying to the bottom a considerable proportion of the bacteria and inorganic material contained in the water. The proper amount of alum to be used varies with the water treated, and even in the same water supply the amount used must be changed from time to time to meet varying factors.

Speaking generally, filters are of two sorts: slow and rapid. Both consist of sand and gravel, the former being layered upon the latter. At the bottom of the filter are outflow pipes for the clear water. Each process removes more than 95 per cent of bacteria from water. Slow filtration is more effective in this function than is rapid. In each instance, the effectiveness of the process is increased by the formation of a gelatinous film on the particles of sand and gravel, this making a tighter and more effective filter. The slow process, which does not ordinarily include previous coagulation with alum, yields daily from $2\frac{1}{2}$ to 4 million gal of water per acre of filter surface. Rapid sand filters yield from 100,000,000 to 150,000,000 gal per acre per day. Slow sand filtration is the older of the two methods. Rapid sand filtration is the more common procedure in America. Care of filters, washing, repair, etc., are highly technical processes and exceedingly important.

Other things being equal, the most important factor in purification of a city's water supply is disinfection by chlorination. Chlorine, compressed in tanks equipped with an automatic release apparatus, is discharged into the water supply as the last part of the purification process. The amount in the water is infinitesimally small, from two tenths to five tenths of one part of chlorine to a million parts of water. It is not injurious, and in these amounts gives no objectionable taste to water. To determine whether or not water contains the necessary amount of chlorine, the orthotolidine test is used. This reagent is added, in proper amount, to the water to be tested. A light canary yellow results when the water contains from 0.3 to 0.5 parts of chlorine per million parts of water. Lighter or darker yellows indicate under- or overchlorination.

Various special and collateral methods are used in water treatment under special conditions. Odors, tastes, color, hardness, must be removed if present to an objectionable degree. See page 273 for reference to fluoridation of public water supplies.

Rural Water Supplies. Users of individual water supplies, as in rural areas, cannot be assured of the mass protection available in cities. The essential danger is from pollution by human waste containing pathogenic organisms. The character of this pollution is that of fecal contamination, rarely by urine. The source from which it comes is the insanitary privy or some other point where excreta is deposited. The manner in which the pollution occurs is either subsurface, through fissures in soil or rock, leading from privy to well; surface, where privy contents are washed into well; or otherwise indirect, as by contamination of well rope by polluted human hands or feet of animals. When chickens smear the well top, this material is subsequently washed into the well through cracks in the top, when water is spilled. There is no such thing as a "typhoid well." If a well has been the source of typhoid fever season after season, it means that human excreta containing typhoid bacilli has continued to pollute and repollute the water in the well. The danger in the well is, therefore, not an inherent one, but is due to infectious material brought to it.

These hazards in individual wells may be offset by the institution of a sanitary method of excreta disposal. Recognizing, however, that sanitary disposal of excreta is relative and not absolute, protective measures should be instituted in connection with:

1. Depth of well: deeper wells draw from water which usually has undergone more filtration than is the case in shallow wells.

2. Casing of well: an impervious lining in the well prevents shallow levels of ground water from seeping into it.

3. Curbing of well: a shelving concrete collar around the upper part of the well prevents ingress of surface washings.

4. Top of well: a tight top prevents material brought by feet, animals, etc., from dropping into the well.

5. Drawing water from well: pumps are more nearly safe than

buckets since the latter necessitate some opening in the top of the well and involve the use of a chain or rope which is open to contamination.

Contrary to what the public believes, water analysis is not designed to discover typhoid or dysentery organisms, but colon bacilli. The latter come mainly from intestinal discharges and the presence of this organism in water strongly suggests pollution; and the pollution may contain typhoid and dysentery bacilli.

Milk as a Problem in Sanitation. The principal diseases which may be transmitted by milk are diphtheria, dysentery, "milk sickness," scarlet fever or streptococcal sore throat, tuberculosis (especially bovine), typhoid and paratyphoid fevers, and undulant fever. Milk has been indicted as one of the routes through which poliomyelitis might spread, though probably it is an unusual one. Foot-and-mouth disease of cattle, seen only rarely in man, may be spread through milk.

The parts played by the cow, by milk, by human agencies, vary in the different diseases:

Diphtheria. The milk is polluted by some human being after it leaves the cow. It is possible, though extremely unlikely, that abrasions on the teats and udder may develop diphtheria lesions from human contamination.

Dysentery. The milk is polluted by the hands of the milker and occasionally through water used in washing containers in which milk is placed.

Milk Sickness. Toxin is in the milk as it leaves the cow. It is derived from certain kinds of snakeweed eaten by the cow, causing in the latter a condition known as "trembles." This is not an infectious process.

Scarlet Fever and Septic Sore Throat. The teats and udder of the cow may be infected with the organisms which cause these conditions and they may be in the milk at the time of milking. Human agencies may also introduce this infectious material in otherwise safe milk.

Tuberculosis. Cows are subject to the bovine type of tuberculosis, and if teats and udder are infected, the organisms will pass into the milk. Bovine tuberculosis may also get into the milk through flakes and dust of infected manure. The organisms of human tuberculosis may be introduced accidentally into milk by human agencies. The latter type of organism is not nearly so frequently encountered in milk as is the bovine.

Typhoid and Paratyphoid Fevers. Cows do not have these diseases, and even though they drink polluted water, the organisms do not come through in the milk. When milk contains these bacilli, it is because it has been polluted after leaving the cow, by organisms on the hands of the milker, or on the teats of the cow, or in water used in washing receptacles.

Brucellosis. This disease of cattle and goats, also of swine, produces an infectious abortion in these animals. The organisms are in the milk as it comes from the cow or goat. Infected hands may contaminate milk during milking or subsequently.

Essentials in Milk Sanitation. To provide safe milk it is essential:

1. That the milk come from cows which are healthy, known to be tuberculin negative and free of brucellosis infection.

2. That milkers and others handling milk be free from communicable diseases, and not carriers.

3. That all utensils used as milk containers be sterilized after each usage.

4. That milking be done with clean hands or clean machines from clean teats and udders into small-top pails and in an atmosphere as free from dust as possible.

5. That immediately after milking the milk be chilled and kept at a temperature not over 50° F, preferably lower; and milk on the delivery wagon not exceed this temperature.

6. That bottling and capping of milk be done in a sanitary manner.

7. That milk be sold to the consumer only in the original bottle.

8. That milk be pasteurized.

To carry out these requirements, there is needed at the dairy farm reasonably dry pastures and barn lot. Barns should be well lighted, airy, cleanly painted or whitewashed on the interior, and as free from dust as possible. It is generally required that barn floors be of impervious material, usually of concrete, with sloping channels for carrying off drainage; there is also needed adequate, easily available water for flushing floors. Recent studies suggest that clean milk may be produced in the pen-type stable without impervious floor but with fresh dry bedding added daily. Barns also should provide facilities for washing and disinfection of hands, and for similar cleansing of teats, udders, and flanks of cows. An ample supply of clean milking clothes is a necessity. Small-top milking pails, and a clean, easily cleanable, screened milk house, separate from barn and farmhouse and in as dust-free atmosphere as possible, are essentials. In the milk house there must be an apparatus for rapid cooling of milk, and an icebox or refrigerator for temporary storage. No dairy farm should be permitted to operate without a sterilizing outfit for utensils—steam or chemical. In addition there must be provisions for sanitary disposal of excerta, stable manure, and other waste on the farm, and a safe water supply.

Supplementing these more or less physical things, it is vital that there be an understanding and a conscience on the part of dairy workers and management. If those responsible for facilities and methods are not themselves intelligent and conscientious, no amount of regulations and requirements will be completely effective.

Bottling, pasteurization, and subsequent maintenance of low temperatures in milk up to the time of delivery to consumer are not usually responsibilities of the dairy farm.

Pasteurized Milk, Certified Milk. Pasteurization consists in treating milk so that all parts in a given container or vat reach 142° F, this degree of heat being maintained for ½ hour. It is to the city's milk supply what chlorination is to the water supply.

Pasteurization should not be used as a means of disinfecting dirty milk; only decently clean milk should be accepted for pasteurization. The process destroys the pathogenic organisms with which milk is sometimes contaminated: brucella organisms, bovine tubercle bacilli, streptococci, diphtheria organisms, typhoid and dysentery bacilli. Properly pasteurized, milk does not have a disagreeable taste, nor is the quality of the milk changed to any extent. Vitamin C is destroyed, but there is not usually sufficient vitamin C even in raw milk to meet the infant's demands, and supplementary vitamins, rather than milk, should be relied upon in this connection.

Certified milk is milk produced and sold under the supervision of a medical milk commission appointed by the local medical society. The rules and regulations under which milk may be certified are quite stringent, but in the system there is the ever-present weakness that between medical examinations of personnel, a worker may develop, and fail to report, some acute communicable disease; or some carrier of typhoid fever or diphtheria may remain undiscovered in spite of examinations. After all, certified milk is nothing more than a high-grade raw milk, and raw milk necessarily carries a potential danger.

The quality of milk, as delivered to the consumer, is checked by laboratory tests. Its food ingredients are tested by chemical and physical means for solid contents (to detect "watering"), for proportion of cream, etc. Bacterial counts are made to determine its general cleanliness. Certified milk requirements permit no more than 10,000 bacteria per milliliter; the maximum number of organisms permitted in other milks vary with the ordinance in operation in the different cities. Usually, bacterial counts must not exceed 100,000 to 200,000 bacteria per milliliter of milk before pasteurization and not more than 30,000 after pasteurization. In this connection it should be borne in mind that even more important than the number is the kind of bacteria in milk. A small number of typhoid bacilli is more important than a large number of nondisease-producing organisms.

An important adjunct in milk control is the *phosphatase test,* designed to determine whether or not milk has been effectively pasteurized. The process of pasteurization destroys the enzymes phosphatase and amylase in milk. If these enzymes are present in milk supposed to have been pasteurized, it is evidence that the process has not been effective.

Food Poisoning as a Sanitary Problem. Foods other than milk may convey infectious material, and the prevention of such food-borne outbreaks is to no small extent dependent upon the care, refrigeration, and proper handling of the food itself. Not infrequently one hears of illness in an individual or group of people where some common foodstuff, such as meat, fish, fruit or vegetable, or some product or combination of these articles seems to have been the agency responsible.

Outbreaks of this sort may be due to ingestion of pathogenic bacteria or other infectious agents, or to the ingestion of some bacterial toxin preformed in the food; or to some chemical poison introduced in the manufacture or preparation of the food; or to some organic poison incident to the physiology of the meat or vegetable eaten.

The organisms believed to be most often responsible, where actual bacterial infection is the cause of the illness, belong to the *Salmonella* group, S. *typhimurium* and S. *enteritidis* being most frequently identified. Meats and meat products are the kinds of food often associated with salmonella infections. It would appear that the presence of the organisms may be due either to a disease of the animal from which the meat was obtained, or, more frequently, the result of human contamination. Rats and mice may be infected by *Salmonella,* and their possible role in food contamination must be admitted.

A condition in which the causative agent of the disease is present in the animal from which the food is derived is *trichinosis* due to the *Trichinella spiralis* which is conveyed through infected pork not adequately cooked.

Clostridium botulinum and the *staphylococci* appear to play the principal roles in producing preformed toxins which occasion violent illness. Cases of botulism are largely associated with canned foods, which have been improperly sterilized. Not much is known of the role played by food in introducing staphylococcus toxin, though milk has been implicated. Custard-filled foods, hollandaise sauces, and other materials which act as a good culture medium for *staphylococci* have also been implicated in outbreaks of staphylococcus toxin poisonings. Most often, the food is contaminated by a human being.

Chemical poisoning due to the poison's presence in food is not ordinarily seen, though there have been many instances in the past where arsenic, lead, and other inorganic agents have caused widespread illness. A silver polish containing cyanide caused outbreaks at first assumed to be due to bacterial infection.

In plant poisoning, mushrooms have been most often indicted, though there are a number of others occasionally operative—potatoes, rhubarb leaves, and plants eaten accidentally or by children. Poisoning from animal food, especially fish of certain kinds, is reported from time to time. While poisoning from vegetables and fish undoubtedly occurs, it should be borne in mind that true bacterial infection may be the real operative factor in many cases, and that personal idiosyncrasy, allergy, may be responsible for others.

The health department gets reports on but a small proportion of food poisoning. As a rule, it is only where food was consumed at a public place with subsequent illness of the guests, that disturbances associated with vomiting, purging, and prostration come to public attention. If the same thing occurs in the home, little is said about it. In botulism, where fatalities are not infrequent and when the clinical picture is far more dramatic than in the gastrointestinal type of disturbance, reports are more likely to reach the health department.

Investigations of illness apparently due to food need to be made exceedingly carefully, both from an epidemiological and bacteriological standpoint. Very careful and exact case histories are essential, and specimens of the various possibly concerned foods, and of vomitus and stools of the patients, should be obtained for immediate laboratory examination. Even though the period between ingestion of food and onset of symptoms is generally quite short—from 12 to 48 hours—food specimens are difficult to obtain.

In those cases where the symptoms consist of vomiting, diarrhea, and abdominal pain, persons attacked usually believe that they have "ptomaine poisoning." Not infrequently the attending physician concurs in this diagnosis, and occasionally, also the uninformed investigator from the health department. The ptomaines might conceivably cause illness, but they are essentially products of decomposition, not usually present unless strong, repellent odors are emanated. Food of this sort is not likely to be eaten. "Ptomaine poisoning," as a diagnosis, is in the category with "acute indigestion"—popular but not well founded.

In order to offset so far as it is possible the danger of infection and illness from food, health departments have instituted various regulations for, and inspections of, establishments concerned in food distribution, such as abattoirs, food processing plants, bakeries, butcher shops, vegetable and fruit markets, and similar places. Carrying out inspections of this sort involves a considerable amount of time and expense, perhaps more than the apparent results justify. On the other hand, there can be no doubt that food infections, intoxications, and other types of poisoning and adulterations would occur much more frequently than is now the case were the matter left entirely to the conscience, care, and intelligence of the millions of persons concerned only in the commercial handling of a nation's food.

Garbage Disposal. Garbage, per se, will not cause any particular disease, although it furnishes good feeding ground for flies and rats; and accumulated, decomposing garbage gives rise to objectionable odors. In most cities, its collection and disposal is not directly under the health department, but is a responsibility of some street cleaning service. The average citizen sees this service only in its negative aspects—when something goes wrong. He seldom thinks of the vast mass of garbage produced by a city of a quarter million population and he seldom wonders what the garbage trucks do with the stuff which they collect. Actually, the modern handling of a city's refuse is a far cry from medieval days, when the pedestrian in the city streets not only had to watch his step, but had to keep an eye aloft because of the slop and garbage hazard.

There are a number of ways in which garbage is finally disposed of by cities. These may be sumarized as follows:

1. The oldest method for the disposal of garbage and trash is to dump it into low places. These dumps may create most unsightly suburban areas, attract flies, rats, and garbage pickers, emit evil odors, and have a tendency to catch fire by spontaneous combustion. When the latter occurs and the wind is just right, the city pays for its penuriousness by being enveloped in foul-smelling gases. However, with modern practice of covering and packing each day's garbage as dumped, this method has proven quite satisfactory, converting many swampy areas into land usable for industry, playgrounds, etc.

2. When garbage is disposed of by dumping at sea it is carried in specially constructed barges from 10 to 25 miles out to sea. There is always the chance that tides and winds may return floating garbage

to its home port, and if bathing beaches are near, they are likely to be the final repositories of some portion of the city's refuse.

3. Feeding to hogs requires organization somewhat along the lines of a large industry. At the household there must be separation of garbage from paper, cans, etc., and a collection system capable of making long hauls to a hog farm where there is a sufficient number of hogs to consume the garbage brought. In exceptional circumstances the system is satisfactory, but it is not generally practiced. It has the distinct economic advantage of converting waste material into pork; however, remember that garbage-fed hogs have a higher incidence of trichinosis than do grain-fed hogs. The garbage should be boiled.

4. Incineration is a modern, though somewhat wasteful, method of refuse disposal. Trash and rubbish is used to burn the more moist garbage in specially constructed furnaces.

5. Reduction plants, by appropriate methods, are able to salvage from garbage 2 or 3 per cent of grease. This is later utilized in the manufacture of soaps and glycerin.

Sanitary Measures for Prevention of Insect-borne Diseases. Reference has already been made to the different relationships which hosts in general bear to their parasites. In this connection, it should be noted that insects may act as agents in the transmission of disease in one of two capacities: (1) when the organism or virus finds life in the insect a biologic necessity, and (2) when the organism or virus is but a passenger in or on the insect. Further, the insect may serve in the dual role of host and parasite, i.e., the host of an organism or virus and at the same time a parasite of the animal from which it draws blood (ectoparasite).

Sanitary measures for control of insect-borne diseases may be applied along one or more of the following lines:

1. Directly against the insect.
   a. Destruction of the adult insects, as in trapping and swatting flies, fumigation of ships to kill fleas and mosquitoes, louse powders, spraying of interiors of airplanes and dwellings.
   b. Protection against adult insects, as by screens.

    c. Prevention of breeding, as in drainage of swamps, or oiling or poisoning of ponds to kill mosquito embryos.

2. Destruction of the host, other than human, to which the insect is a parasite.

    a. Destruction of the adult host, as in trapping and poisoning rats.

    b. Attack on the environment, as in ratproofing, thus making feeding and breeding difficult.

The more important insects concerned in the transmission of disease in this country are flies, fleas, ticks, and mosquitoes. Lice, important in the transmission of typhus fever abroad, are a potential rather than an actual danger in the United States.

Flies. The common housefly, *Musca domestica,* may carry infectious material on the legs, around the mouth, in the excreta, or in vomitus. Probably a great many diseases may, occasionally, be thus transmitted by the fly, but the ones of particular concern to the public health are typhoid fever, trachoma, and dysentery.

Swatting, trapping, and screening against the fly are at best only supplementary measures. The spraying of walls with DDT has not proven to be continuingly effective. Real control can come only through prevention of breeding. Flies breed by choice in stable manure and privy vaults. Flyproofing of the latter and proper disposal of the former are essentials. From deposition of eggs to emergence of fly requires from 10 to 14 days, depending to some extent on environment. If, therefore, manure is cleaned out, spread thin or treated with a disinfectant (borax solution) once a week, the larval and pupal forms are killed. In cities, the exclusion of cows and the replacement of the horse by the automobile have done much to decrease the fly population. In rural areas, while proper disposition of manure is theoretically possible, practically it is neglected.

In certain sections other flies are of importance in the transmission of disease, such as *Chrysops discalis* in tularemia, and the tsetse fly in the spread of African sleeping sickness.

Fleas. This insect acts mechanically in transmitting both plague and the type of typhus fever seen in this country. The flea appears to carry the infective material in the digestive tract. This, regurgitated or defecated, is rubbed into the itching wound of the flea bite. The Indian rat flea, *Xenopsylla cheopis* and the rat flea of this country and Europe, *Ceratophyllus fasciata,* are the ones of most concern.

Sanitary measures against the flea are directed mainly against the rat. Control measures consist in: destruction of wild rodents in areas where they are known to be plague infected; local rat destruction campaigns through trapping and poisoning; ratproofing of buildings, particularly warehouses and around water fronts; proper supervision and methods at garbage dumps and slaughterhouses to prevent rat harborage; fumigation of ships from plague ports, to kill rats and fleas; and rat guards on mooring lines.

Ticks. The tick appears to play the role of a true biologic host to the parasites of Rocky Mountain spotted fever and tularemia. *Dermacentor andersoni* and *Dermacentor variabilis* are the two species known to be important in transmission of these diseases. Control measures, other than avoiding tick-infested areas and personal care, are difficult. The infected tick does not transmit his infection until after he is rather thoroughly engorged; hence after exposure to tick-bearing bushes, etc., careful examination of clothing and skin is effective. Strictly speaking, ticks are not insects.

Mosquitoes. Mosquitoes may transmit disease only if they have themselves taken in the parasites or virus of the disease. Bloodsucking is limited to the female.

The diseases in which these insects are primarily concerned are dengue, malaria, yellow fever, filariasis, and some forms of encephalitis.

The malaria-carrying mosquitoes are members of the genus *Anopheles.* The most important species in this country is the *Anopheles quadrimaculatus.* The following are important characteristics of these mosquitoes:

1. They are relatively large and dark, with heavily shaded or spotted wings, with the palpi, or feelers as long as the proboscis.

2. They bite mainly at night—hence the old idea that malaria came

from the night air, and they give the appearance of standing on their heads when biting or at rest.

3. Anopheles do not ordinarily breed in tin cans, cisterns, etc., but choose natural accumulations of water—ponds, slow-moving streams, etc.

4. The larvae or wigglers lie parallel to the surface of the water, and tend to remain close to the surface even though disturbed. This is in contrast to the larvae of other mosquitoes.

5. They are rather hardy, and infected mosquitoes live through the winter in sheltered places.

The common house mosquito is known as the *Culex*, of which there are several species. Aside from being a nuisance, the *Culex* population is capable of transmitting the virus of dengue and the filaria embryo, the causative factor in elephantiasis (filariasis). The mosquito important in the spread of yellow fever is the *Aedes aegypti*. This mosquito may also transmit dengue. Both of these mosquitoes are domestic. They breed by choice in domestic water receptacles, near their source of food. A species of *Culex, Culex tarsalis,* has been shown to be a vector of the encephalitides.

Sanitary measures for permanent control of mosquitoes are designed to prevent the breeding of mosquitoes, rather than to destroy the adult insects. Against the latter, bed nets and screening have been the principal protections in settled communities.

The more modern attack on adult mosquitoes, especially the *Anopheles,* has been through the use of DDT. These initials represent the complex chemical name of a white powder: dichloro-diphenyl-trichloroethane. When dissolved and sprayed on walls, a residuum toxic to mosquitoes for some months is left. Such spraying is highly effective in villages, etc., and is widely used. Unfortunately flies develop a resistance to it and perhaps some mosquitoes, but rarely the *Anopheles.* DDT has also been used in poisoning mosquito larvae. This material is highly poisonous to many other forms of insect life and only slightly toxic to man. It must, however, be used with some caution.

The ordinary mosquito sprays and aerosol bombs, used as a temporary protection against present mosquitoes, contain pyrethrum which is obtained from flowers of the chrysanthemum family and are highly effective in selected conditions: rooms, airplanes, camp quarters, etc.

Reasonably effective mosquito repellents provide temporary protection to the individual who must venture into mosquito-infested areas from time to time.

The main points of attack on the breeding places of mosquitoes are as follows:

1. Drainage of ponds and swampy places. Mosquitoes must have water for development of larval forms—no water, no breeding.

2. Elimination or proper safeguarding of wells and cisterns, destruction of tin cans, the prevention of standing pools in house gutters, etc.

3. Oiling. Where it is impossible to drain, a film of oil is spread over the surface of the pond. This oil prevents the larvae (wiggletails) from breathing and they perish.

4. Dusting of pond and swamps with insecticides. This brings about poisoning of larval forms. In large areas difficult of access this dusting is done from airplanes.

5. Stocking of ponds and streams with minnows (*Gambusia affinis*). These minnows feed upon the mosquito larvae, and are quite effective in destroying them. For best effects, brush and weeds must be kept cleared from banks at the water line, otherwise the minnows cannot get at the larvae.

Housing and the Public Health. It is difficult to determine exactly the effect of good or poor housing on the public health. As a factor in sickness and death, poor housing, per se, is confusingly associated with economic status, overcrowding, undernutrition, exhausting or dangerous occupations, poverty in general, perhaps ignorance. Because these variable factors enter into the housing situation and because many of them are essentially economic, health departments in this country have tended to neglect housing as a public health problem. Such standards and regulations as exist heretofore have been responsibilities of various other city bureaus, such as plumbing, or building, and activities are carried on in a more or less unimaginative routine.

The necessity for decent housing is sufficiently great, from a pubilc health standpoint, to demand intelligent, constructive, carefully planned, and far-reaching programs. It is not enough to require that new homes, tenements, etc., comply with proper regulations, it is necessary that slum clearance be undertaken seriously as a major activity in the health department. Such a program should include the provision of low rental quarters, preferably city-owned; and legislation and public attitude should be such that the inevitable opposition of owners of high-income, low-grade property can be brushed aside.

Better housing will not develop immediately everywhere, and an undertaking of this sort bristles with difficulties and deficiencies. In spite of this, no thoughtful student of public health can absolve himself of responsibility by a negative attitude.

Industrial Health

Medical and sociological interest in the health and disease of persons engaged in industry is not new, though in recent years these interests have been intensified and expanded. The older medical literature contains frequent references to diseases peculiar to workers of various types, and in the last century many of the factory and housing laws, particularly in England, related to the health of those whose occupations placed them in industrial work.

It should be noted that two terms are employed here, "occupation" and "industry." The first relates to the particular kind of work an individual does. He might be a welder, a riveter, a carpenter. The second term refers to the kind of industry in which he pursues this occupation. He might be in the automobile industry, in meat packing, in coal mining, in drug manufacturing. By virtue of his occupation he might be subject to peculiar hazards, as from injury, infection, irritating dust, or poisonous fumes; or as a result of the industry in which he is engaged, he might be jeopardized by excessive fatigue, poor illumination or ventilation, insanitary plant environment, or even the general disadvantages of low income, inadequate diet, poor housing.

Medicine has been inclined to approach the subject in terms of occupational diseases; public health has had a broader approach, regarding workers as individuals who, because of the combined hazards of occupation and industry including economic disadvantages, constitute a group for which special precautions must be exercised. The precautions applied relate to those hazards peculiar to a given occupation or industry, or both, plus ordinary public health practices in such fields as nutrition, tuberculosis, syphilis, etc., being concerned not only with working conditions but with the worker's home and its environment, with his family, their recreation and health education, and their ability to obtain medical, nursing, dental, and hospital care.

The Population Concerned in Industry. The size of the population which one designates as industrial, depends to some extent upon how inclusively the word "industry" is defined. This is not uniform or on a national basis, nor consistent in practice. An individual who makes wearing apparel is usually regarded as being an industrial worker, but the clerk in the store who sells it is not so regarded unless it is a large store with unionized workers.

Aside from this theoretical question of definition, the proportion of the nation's population actually engaged in industrial work at any given time will be influenced by many factors: the place of industry in the nation's economy, depressions and booms, war necessities, foreign trade, etc.

Government's Role in Industrial Hygiene. A number of interests and responsibilities have brought the federal government into the field of industrial hygiene. In reality, the U.S. Public Health Service owes its origin to a responsibility of this sort, for when its nucleus was established in 1798 its essential duty was to furnish medical care to a particular industrial group, the sailors of the Merchant Marine. In more recent years, the Bureau of Mines in cooperation with the U.S. Public Health Service, has conducted important research and practical education in this subject. The Department of Labor, particularly through the Children's Bureau, has brought about federal legislation in relation to working conditions of women in those industries engaged in interstate commerce, and in regard to child labor. Of most importance is the work of the U.S. Public Health Service. This program expanded tremendously to meet the industrial hygiene problems arising out of World War II, and both in research and in practical aid to states and industries renders commendable service.

The interest of state health departments and of departments of labor in the subject of industrial hygiene has increased in recent years. Where this interest arose primarily in the health department, the industrial hygiene program is carried on by that agency of state government. Where the problem has been approached primarily as incident to labor relations and conditions, industrial hygiene stems from the labor department of the state. The trend is to have such programs carried on by the state health department with necessary integration with activities of the state department of labor or some similar state governmental agency.

In general, the industrial hygiene program is designed to protect the workman on his job: by law or regulation or contract, long hours of exhausting work are guarded against, the ordinary sanitary facilities and protections are ensured, special physical or chemical hazards are obviated as far as possible, proper light and ventilation are provided, as are first aid and emergency care of the injured.

Some states require that physicians report particulars as to persons suffering from occupational diseases and industrial accidents. Inasmuch as definitions of these two terms depend largely on the compensation laws in force, and because these laws vary from state to state, reporting of occupational diseases in the nation as a whole is neither uniform nor complete.

The development of industrial hygiene programs in the United States has been largely in factories, manufacturing plants, mills, and in general where large groups are congregated under one management. Small industries, as a rule, receive only inspectorial services designed to ensure observance of state or city regulations as to minimum standards. Many large groups, such as farm workers where each unit is an independent one, are not reached by industrial hygiene programs as such; nor are great numbers of persons who, though in occupations of industrial importance, are scattered widely.

Workmen's Compensation Laws. These vary from state to state, as federal laws of this sort relate only to civil employees of the United States government. The earlier laws providing compensation to workmen were concerned only with industrial accidents. Practically every state in the Union has a law providing compensation for injuries in industry. A later trend has been to provide compensation for occupational diseases as well as for accidents. About half the states have laws of this sort, and each law has its own definition of what constitutes an occupational disease. In one state, compensation is paid only for such diseases as are peculiar to the occupation or industries, such as silicosis, lead poisoning. In others the provision is much broader and includes conditions possibly incident to occupation, but not peculiar to that occupation: tuberculosis, hernia, or similar conditions that arose or were recognized during employment, that might or might not be related to that employment.

In general, compensation is in an amount equal to about two thirds of the worker's wages and medical care is provided. Often there is a period of one or two weeks' waiting before compensation funds become available, this being designed to discourage malingering. In some states the employer designates the physician, in others the workman may choose whatever physician he wishes. The trend is to permit the patient to choose his doctor from a panel of physicians developed by the compensation commission. Some states have a limitation on the length of time one may obtain medical care; others cover this point only vaguely. Adjustments and decisions are reached by commissions rather than through courts.

When an accident or disability occurs, the workman in most states is free from the burden of proving negligence on the part of his employer and of defending himself against contributory negligence or carelessness. This, from a legal standpoint, makes the Workmen's Compensation Law somewhat of a phenomenon. The cost of compensation and medical care is borne by the employer, but only temporarily; he passes it along to the public in the price of his products.

The Staff in an Industrial Plant. The number and character of workers engaged in the industrial hygiene program in any given establishment will vary with the number of persons employed, the kind of industry, the demands of the workers, and the attitude and interest of the management.

In the small plant, there may be provisions only for first aid, or for a physician to be called in emergency; or there may be a full-time nurse who does dressings, and perhaps gives advice as to personal hygiene. Larger industries provide rather complete dispensaries, and infirmary, eye and dental clinics, x-ray and laboratory service, a visiting nurse service in workers' homes, and even a cooperative insurance scheme for ordinary medical service. Such large medical staffs are usually supplemented by the work of sanitary engineers particularly skilled in air conditioning, ventilation, illumination, noise elimination, and in safety devices designed to protect the employee from machinery, heat, dust, fumes, explosives, etc.

Pre-employment and Preplacement Examinations. Most plants require that prospective employees pass a physical examination before employment. This procedure was formerly designated as a *pre-employment examination*. To many interested in labor, this term connoted a protection of the employer at the expense of the worker and was objected to on that ground. The term now popular is *preplacement examination*, the implication being that its purpose is to find a place suitable for the individual, adapted to his handicaps if there are any such disabilities.

The scope of the examination varies, as would be expected. Hearing, vision, perhaps color vision, freedom from active tuberculosis, communicable diseases, hernia, disabling heart disease, crippling arthritis, or an incapacitating deformity are the essentials. Active venereal disease would justify exclusion, but the mere presence of a positive Wassermann test should not.

Disabilities Arising in Industry. The industrial worker is, naturally, subject to the same accidents and illnesses that affect persons in general, plus those disabilities which arise from his industry and his occupation.

It is difficult to measure quantitatively and qualitatively the force of these hazards. The criterion generally observed is time lost from work because of illness or injury, no consideration being given to illness or minor injury insufficient to prevent work. When this criterion is used and proper records are kept one may undertake a study of how many illnesses the worker has per year, the nature of the disability, the frequency with which disabilities occur, the length that each lasts, with subdivisions as to men and women, old and young, etc., and, to a limited extent, whether or not the disability arose because of the nature of employment. Gafafer* has analyzed data on absences of one day or longer due to sickness and injury in employees in a public utility and presents interesting data.

He found that the annual number of absences per 1000 persons was 919 for men and 1851 for women. The number of days lost per year was 8.2 for males and 11.9 for females; the average number of days per absence was 8.9 for men, 6.4 for women.

Gafafer's detailed data indicate that in the group studied, industrial injuries caused 22.4 absences per 1000 men, with an average of 30 days for each absence; 4.5 absences of about 9 days each per 1000 women. In nonindustrial accidents, each 1000 men had 43 per year, averaging 9 days each; women had 81 nonindustrial accidents per 1000 women per year, each accident averaging 15 days absence from work.

Sickness caused 854 absences per 1000 men per year, the corresponding figure for women being 1766. The average number of days absence per illness was 8 for men and 6 for women. Still referring to Gafafer's figures on the particular group studied, the kind of sickness was as follows: nearly two thirds was due to respiratory diseases, of which colds were the most frequent; a little less than a fifth of the sickness was due to digestive diseases, with the remainder being caused by miscellaneous conditions.

From the above summary which fairly well reflects the general situation, it can be seen that nonindustrial injuries are five times as frequent as injuries arising in industry, that sickness causes seventeen times as many absences from work as do accidents, that in men nonindustrial injuries were about twice as frequent as industrial injuries, nearly twenty times in women. Here one must remember that men

* Gafafer, W. M.: *Manual of Industrial Hygiene.* W. B. Saunders Co., Philadelphia, 1943.

are, by nature of their work, more exposed to injury in industry, and that even though working, women are more subject to household accidents. One must also bear in mind that the force of the various factors that cause disability may not be measured entirely by the number of absences: the length of each absence and other factors must also be taken into consideration. For further details in this connection, the reader is referred to texts and monographs on this subject.

Special Industrial Hazards. Some industries and occupations have no peculiar hazards. Others have one or more. Among these are dusts, fumes, vapors, poisonous liquids or solids, infectious material, skin irritating substances, radiant or radioactive material, high temperature, low temperature, rarefied or compressed air, monotony, fatigue, noise, and various physical hazards, as in timbering, fishing, mining, etc. Most of the terms just used are self-explanatory, except in the case of fumes, gases, etc. These have been carefully defined for purposes of regulations and standards by various authorities concerned. In effect, it may be said that *dust* is made up of solid particles, suspended in the air or resting upon surfaces. They may be organic or inorganic in character, depending upon the source from which they arise. Such sources may be rock, wood, hides, etc. *Fumes* also consist of solid particles which condense after being in a gaseous state, the gaseous state in turn having arisen from a metal in molten form, or undergoing chemical action. *Vapors* represent the gaseous state of materials ordinarily solid or liquid; *gases* are substances normally in a gaseous state.

Not all dusts, fumes, gases, and vapors are harmful. Many factors, such as chemical nature, concentration, size of particles, etc., determine this point. As industry and manufacturing processes expand, new and sometimes dangerous substances must be handled by workers. Adjustments, safety devices, establishment of standards, and elimination of the highly dangerous, demand the constant vigilance of those responsible for industrial hygiene.

The Prevention of Disabilities Peculiar to Industry or Occupation. Most of the conditions that arise because of the hazards or exposures of a given occupation are preventable. To prevent, however, there must be rather complete coordination of effort between management, workers, and the industrial hygiene staff. The latter must be possessed of a wide and detailed knowledge as to the processes and materials used in the industry. They must know, for each step in a manufacturing procedure, the potential hazard from this solvent or that high temperature, the physical and chemical changes induced that may generate toxic or irritating by-products from a substance harmless in its original form. They must know, too, the concentrations at which a given vapor or gas becomes dangerous, the maximum atmospheric dust load in which it is safe for one to work, and have an appreciation of the practical differences in hazards where the dust particle is of one sort or another or of different sizes. The engineer must possess skill to offset dangerous concentrations and exposures by mechanical devices such as ventilation, respirators, ducts, and vents. The physician must be prepared to make the various laboratory tests which indicate beginning disability in a worker, and must be particularly qualified to trace back to its source such manifestations as industrial dermatose, lead poisoning, silicosis, anemias, and even the nervous disturbances which arise from monotony, noise, and the pressure of the production line.

In a similar manner, management and labor must cooperate. The former must regard the provision of protection and services as both an obligation and an investment; the latter must participate with understanding and good spirit.

Women in Industry. The coming of the machine age has in many instances changed the character of work done in industry. While mining, smelting, etc., still require strong backs and big biceps, many industries are so completely mechanized that the hard work is done by electric power. The worker need do no more than push a button or pull a lever. Thus the highly specialized skill and strength of the mechanic is not always necessary, and women are increasingly employed as workers in industry. Their presence in factories inevitably creates new problems, some of which are minor, while others necessitate readjustments. Women with families are likely to have more absences for reasons other than personal illnesses: emergency shopping for children, sickness in the family, excessive fatigue from a job at home as well as in the factory. Menstrual disturbances may cause periodic incapacity. The industry finds it necessary to provide separate toilets, lavatories, shower and dressing rooms, and special rest rooms for women. Laws must be observed as to leaves of absences for pregnancy. These things are mentioned not in criticism of women in industry but as factors which enter into the industrial situation.

Costs of Industrial Hygiene Programs. These vary from place to place with the type of industry, with the number of persons employed in the plant, with the adequacy of the health program, with salaries paid to physicians, nurses, engineers, etc. In two different-sized plants, with industrial hygiene staffs proportional to payroll, the industrial hygiene program in the smaller plant would be relatively more expensive because of an irreducible overhead. Many small plants get around this by providing only the skimpiest industrial hygiene service or none at all.

From various studies that have been made as to costs, divergent data have arisen. Part of this is because expenditures themselves have varied and part because of different systems of allocating costs. There is a general tendency to break program costs into three main headings: medical service, safety programs, and industrial hygiene. Medical service is by far the most expensive, averaging annually around $5.00 per year per person employed in the industry. Safety programs cost something over $3.00, with a similar amount for that part of the program designated as industrial hygiene. Such expenditures of from $10.00 to $15.00 per year for each person employed must prove itself to be a good investment if the businessmen concerned are to engage in or continue it. Fortunately, careful cost studies indicate that it costs much less to have such a program than to do without it.

Radiological Health

Radiological Health Hazards. Since first he came on this earth, man has been exposed to certain natural sources of radiation. Thus cosmic radiation would have a serious effect upon him were it not for the protection provided by the atmosphere surrounding the earth; and natural radiation from the radioactive elements present in the earth's crust would harm *Homo sapiens* and other species but for the nature and circumstances of these deposits. However, for good or ill, man has learned how to concentrate radioactive elements, as in the production of radium, and this creates potential hazards to life and health. The production of x-rays or gamma rays by Roentgen in 1895, immediately and subsequently used as a most valuable diagnostic tool, has since been recognized as having grave harmful effects if not properly controlled. The more recent development of atomic or nuclear fission for the production of weapons and for peacetime power production has captured the immagination of mankind; but it has also created new and serious problems of health protection.

The Health Aspects of Ionizing Radiation. Soon after the development of radium by the Curies and the x-ray by Roentgen, the harmful effects of these types of radiation were recognized. Innumerable physicians, the early users of radium and x-ray, suffered from over exposure to these types of radiation. The radiologist with fingers missing as a result of x-ray burns and with carcinoma and leukemia resulting from over exposure to radium, became well known. The disastrous effects of the atomic bomb explosions in World War II thoroughly demonstrated the lethal effects of large doses of ionizing radiation. Fortunately infrequent, but serious, accidents in laboratories where experimental studies in ionizing radiation and nuclear fission products are being carried out also focused attention upon the grave health hazard that was at least potentially present.

One cannot escape the almost certain conclusion that with the future development of atomic energy, both for weapons and for the generation of power, the hazards of radiation will multiply. At the same time there is evidence that, since radiation effects are cumulative, harmful results may be expected from this increased exposure unless great precaution is taken. Perhaps of greater importance than the observable pathological effect of radiation on the individual is the potential genetic effect. There is, unfortunately, inadequate direct information concerning the genetic influence of ionizing radiation on man, but there is general agreement that radiation does induce mutations, some of which are certain to be deleterious, and there is increasing reason to believe that all mutations produced by ionizing radiation are undesirable.

The public health approach to the hazards of radiation will have to take a number of different directions. First there must be maximum control of ionizing radiation from such sources as radium used in medicine, and in the use of the x-ray for diagnosis and treatment. There must be adequate provision for protection of the population from hazards related to nuclear reactors used for the production of power; and there must be arrangements for the proper disposal of radioactive wastes associated with the production of nuclear energy. The disposal of such wastes already constitutes a problem of some magnitude.

In dealing with the problem of x-ray radiation, there are several approaches that can be made by physicians, hospitals, clinics, and health departments. First, all unnecessary x-ray radiation should be eliminated. Certainly the use of x-ray for the fitting of shoes should be prohibited. Second, there should be regulations concerning shielding of all x-ray equipment, both for the protection of the patient and that of the operator or physician. It has been estimated that the largest source of ionizing radiation for the population, even when those engaged in work at atomic energy projects are included, comes from diagnostic x-rays many of which were undoubtedly unnecessary or duplication. As in many other fields of public health activity, public and professional education will be important. The public education program should be designed to give the citizen an understanding, not only of the hazards of radiation, but of the values to him of x-ray in diagnosis and treatment. Another approach will be through professional education, particularly of medical students and the physician who uses the fluoroscope and x-ray occasionally in the routine of his practice.

As mentioned above one of the most serious problems in the development of health safeguards in the atomic age is the disposal of radioactive wastes. Nuclear energy produced by the disintegration of heavy elements such as uranium creates a particularly difficult problem. Industries using this form of power produce waste which gives off radiation. Although fission liberates large amounts of energy, the fission products are equal in quantity to the original element. Up to the present time no general use has been found for these by-products, and they must be disposed of in a safe manner. The by-products of a nuclear reactor consist of radioactive substances in solid, liquid, and gaseous forms. The extent of the health hazard of these by-products is not fully understood, but it is unquestionable that they present serious potential hazards to health of the population. No entirely satisfactory method of disposal has as yet been devised. The problem of waste disposal from nuclear energy reactors includes all of the standard waste disposal problems. Gaseous wastes are produced that must be disposed of in a safe manner, and methods of purification will undoubtedly have to be devised. There is evidence that gases discharged from plants in which uranium ore is crushed, or from nuclear reactors cooled by air which becomes radioactive, have contaminated vegetation which eventually resulted in the ingestion of radioactive food by the people of the community. Constant vigilance will be necessary in such installations to prevent serious hazards to the surrounding population.

Highly contaminated liquid wastes and solid wastes are also difficult to dispose. Liquid wastes from reactors in which cooling is accomplished with water presents a serious problem, in that not infrequently large volumes of water become contaminated and are difficult to dispose of in a safe manner. In situations where there may be disposal into the ocean, in the hope of attaining infinite dilution, there is the problem of contamination of fish and seafood that ultimately will be consumed by the people of the community. At the present time, highly contaminated solid wastes are being stored with presumably adequate shielding protection. But such a process as this cannot go on indefinitely because of the cost of storing with these safeguards.

From this very brief summary, it will be recognized that the disposal of radioactive substances bids fair to become an acute problem of great magnitude; and the public health worker of the future will find the matter of ionizing radiation among the most vexing and menacing monsters that man has yet created.

Atmospheric Pollution and Health

Atmospheric pollution was not considered primarily of health significance until relatively recently. Many cities, particularly industrial cities, have been concerned with atmospheric pollution primarily from an esthetic or economic standpoint. Efforts have been made through regulations to limit air pollution in the area surrounding industrial plants because of the general unpleasantness created by heavy pollution with smoke, noxious odors, soot, and fly ash. With the increasing industrialization of the country the problems of air pollution have increased markedly. In the early 1940's the atmospheric pollution in and around Los Angeles, the so-called "smog," became a serious problem and health authorities began to question the effect of this heavy air pollution on health and began to take steps to control air pollution in that area. The dramatic episode in Donora, Pennsylvania in October of 1948 focused attention on the health aspects of air pollution more acutely than ever before in the United States. The Donora episode clearly demonstrated that under certain atmospheric conditions a normally tolerable air pollution may become so accentuated as to produce illness and even death. This and similar experiences throughout the world have focused attention on the influence of air pollution on health and have stimulated extensive studies and serious efforts to control air pollution. Many health departments have established regulations concerning the discharge of various noxious substances into the air and have developed requirements for the treatment of gaseous discharges from industrial operations.

REFERENCES

Breslow, Lester: "The Epidemiologist Looks at Smog." *Pub. Health Rep.*, 70:1140–43, 1955.

Hollaender, Alexander, ed.: *Radiation Biology.* McGraw-Hill Book Company, Inc., New York, 1955.

Manufacturing Chemists Association: *Air Pollution Abatement Manual.* The Association, Washington, D.C., 1954.

National Air Pollution Symposia: *Proceedings*. Stanford Research Institute, Los Angeles, published annually.

Stern, B. J.: *Medicine and Industry*. The Commonwealth Fund, New York, 1946.

U.S. Atomic Energy Commission: *Control of Radiation Hazards in Atomic Energy Programs*. Government Printing Office, Washington, D.C., 1950.

chapter 10

The Individual
and His Hygiene

PERSONAL HYGIENE, IN its broader sense, includes those practices, habits, and precautions on the part of the individual, which, assumedly, will tend to protect him from disease and maintain him in the highest degree of health. It demands personal cleanliness, good dietary habits, adequate sleep, a nice balance between rest and exercise, between work and recreation, an unharassed mind, dental care, precautions to avoid spreading infection to or receiving infection from others, and perhaps a few more. The principles and practices of personal hygiene, theoretically, are based upon established scientific facts. Actually, many assumedly hygienic procedures have no such foundation and overlap the field of aesthetics.

Bathing. Bathing is a practice to be commended, but little is known about its effect upon the health of the individual. Its benefits vary, but may be separated somewhat as follows: (1) physiological, (2) psychological, and (3) aesthetic.

The physiological effect of the cold bath is to produce a preliminary constriction of the surface capillaries, followed by their dilatation. This brings a feeling of warmth to the skin, is associated with some increased activity in the circulation, including the cerebral, making the individual more alert. The warm bath, through the effect of immersion and heat on the skin, joints, muscles, and perhaps indirectly the nerves, brings about a phase of relaxation and tranquillity. Perhaps the least physiological benefit derived from bathing is the removal of grime and secretions from the body as a whole. Formerly it was believed that this detritus must be removed, lest it "choke the pores." This probably is not true, as there is no scientific basis for a belief that an oft-bathed person lives any longer than a seldom bathed one. However, an excess of ectoparasites (lice, ticks, etc.) would be removed mechanically by soap and water, perhaps with a corresponding dilution and removal of bacteria, molds, fungi, etc., which are normally present on the skin. These, plus friction and abrasions, might contribute to local infections unless periodically decreased or removed by bathing.

Psychologically, one is "set up" by a bath. A decent ritual has been performed, and one is entitled to sit with one's peers. One feels better, cleaner, and from a psychological standpoint as regards this particular situation, is better and cleaner. The dirty individual is likely, mentally, to feel his uncleanliness and to reflect it in his attitude. In either instance, however, bathing or failure to bathe is more likely to be the effect, rather than the cause, of one's mental attitude. Precept and example in those with whom one associates have much to do with the bathing habits one forms.

Aesthetically, close, comfortable, and continuing association of man with his fellow man, depends largely upon how frequently the fellow man bathes. This is vaguely though definitely recognized by society and even influences the bids of commercial organizations for clientele. Thus the cost of admission to movie theatres are in inverse proportion to the human odors one encounters. Unfortunately, unwashed humans become objectionable rather than ill.

The high standards of living in most of the United States, including as they do easy access to bath tubs, contribute toward a relatively well-bathed population. Public health education in schools and the fact that the well-to-do are well bathed tend to spread the habit of body washing among all those who aspire to better things. Generally speaking, the rising generation of each family observes in adulthood this aesthetic amenity more carefully than did the parents, though a good deal depends upon parental precept and example.

Hand Washing and the Public Health. Hand washing comes into a category entirely different from "bathing." The hands are often contaminated with pathogenic organisms, and are constantly carried to the nose, eyes, and mouth. Frequent washing of the hands is therefore definitely of help in preventing the entrance of communicable disease organisms into the body. Children should be guided to acquiring the hand-washing habit after visiting the toilet, before meals, on arising and retiring, and when obviously soiled or after contamination with offensive material. Hand washing may not be substituted for proper disinfection of hands, since the effect is a mechanical removal of almost all contamination rather than a destruction of all pathogenic organisms. But this should be remembered: Thorough, prolonged scrubbing of the hands, with the use of a nail brush, is more effective than a mere dip of unwashed hands in a disinfectant solution.

Dental Hygiene. The more important measures to be observed in dental hygiene are a balanced diet for the mother during the prenatal period; ample amounts of lime- and phosphorus-bearing foods containing vitamins at all times, but especially during infancy and childhood; regular brushing of teeth, at least once, preferably twice, a day; regular examinations by a dentist, at least once, preferably twice, a year; and corrective measures as advocated by the dentist.

The soundness of the teeth and their resistance to decay depends largely upon diet, both past and present. The permanent teeth are rather completely formed many months, some of them years, before they erupt through the gums. If during this formative stage materials for tooth building are not brought by the blood stream or are not properly utilized, sound teeth cannot be developed. Recent experiments lend support to the view that a tendency to decay in teeth may be accelerated or retarded even by the current diet of the individual. Loss or impairment of function of teeth through the condition ordinarily described as pyorrhea is not completely understood in terms of cause or cure. There is some reason to believe that the underlying cause is general rather than local.

Brushing or otherwise cleansing the teeth, aside from the decency of the custom and the resultant appearance of the individual, is of distinct benefit. It may be compared to the painting or surface protection of a house. Good construction deserves this sort of protection and if the construction is not sound, surface protection will aid, even though it cannot completely offset the decay incident to poor or flimsy materials.

Dental caries is probably the disease most widespread among the American people. Although it has been recognized that restriction in the consumption of sugars and other carbohydrates will reduce the incidence of tooth decay and although this knowledge has been widespread, it has not resulted in any appreciable effect upon the diet of people of the country. Further efforts through education to change dietary habits may well be justified.

Interesting and important new light was thrown on the subject of dental caries when it was found that in certain parts of the country there was a high incidence of mottled enamel, a discoloration of the teeth; and epidemiological studies carried out in areas where mottled enamel was a frequent finding revealed the fact that in those same communities dental caries occurred with significantly less frequency than in communities where mottled enamel was not found. Further studies showed that in those communities where mottled enamel was frequently observed there was a relatively high fluoride content in the water. Chemical analysis of water throughout the country showed traces of fluorine in varying amounts in almost all waters examined in the different areas. It was demonstrated that there was significantly less dental caries in communities whose water supply contained 1 part per 1,000,000 of fluoride than in communities having less than this amount, and that mottled enamel did not occur in those communities in which the fluoride content was between 1 and 2 parts per 1,000,000. These findings of the importance of fluorides in the prevention of dental caries led to two new developments. First, topical applications, in which the teeth are painted with a 2 per cent solution of sodium fluoride. While this gave encouraging results, it was found to be time consuming and not entirely satisfactory, although it is still in use.

The second development rests on the fact that the addition of small amounts of sodium fluoride to public water supplies will materially reduce the incidence of dental caries in the populations consuming such waters. Thus water fluoridation, carefully carried out to supplement the natural fluoride to approximately 1 part per 1,000,000, has been shown to produce a marked decrease in dental caries in the cities whose water supply had been so treated. Studies of the general effect of this amount of sodium fluoride in the water supply has revealed no evidence of any harmful effect on general health either in those communities in which the fluoride content is high naturally or in areas where fluoride has been added.

The Mass Effects of Poor Dietary Habits in a Population. The mass effect of dietary faults may show itself very much as would an outbreak of a communicable disease. There is, however, this difference: the latter arises because of the transfer of an actual substance directly or indirectly from one person to another; the former is not due to any transfer of material from the sick to the well, but rather to common participation in error. Considering diet in its broadest sense, to include water, and to relate to contained deleterious, nonmicrobial substances as well as to deficiencies, mass effects are seen in mottled enamel of the teeth, simple goiter, in beriberi, in pellagra, in scurvy, in night blindness, in rickets. Aside from these dramatic, epidemic-like manifestations of dietary faults in the mass, there occur others so common that they attract but little attention: decay in the teeth, undernourishment, obesity. In addition are many persons with what might be called borderline dietary deficiencies, some of which are recognizable as such only through complex laboratory and clinical studies. Few of these are recognized for what they are.

The small stature of the inhabitants of certain countries, ordinarily considered as a racial characteristic, probably is to some extent related to diet. The fact that in this country many children of small immigrants are distinctly taller than their parents is suggestive of better balanced and more abundant food.

The subject of nutrition is an exceedingly complex one, and no attempt may be made to discuss it here. It would be advantageous, however, if the student and the public would recognize this complexity and would put faith in the writings of conservative scientists rather than in the statements of those who are more enthusiastic than sound, or who have something to sell. The role of diet in health is exceedingly important, and the newer knowldege of the role of mineral salts and vitamins opens up vistas for a better public health. However, many absurd and false claims have been made, and one needs be a little cautious in accepting slogans and clichés.

The Popular Term "Malnutrition" as It Relates to Diet. Properly speaking, the nutritional status of an individual is the end result of body metabolism, which in turn depends upon a number of factors, somewhat as follows:

1. *The intake of food and water:* with amount, quality, and balance in proper ratio, and other factors normal, the nutrition is at the optimum.

2. *Muscular activity, rest, sleep, growth periods:* intake of food, ordinarily satisfactory, may be offset by excessive activity, lack of rest, or growth demands.

3. *The endocrines:* imbalance of the endocrines may result in either too slow or too fast a rate of metabolism, with overweight or underweight. Metabolic disturbance may relate to only one type of food or to more than one.

4. *Functional and organic disturbances in the digestive tract:* chronic or acute gastritis, duodenitis, pancreatitis, ileocolitis are conditions which interfere with proper digestion or assimilaton of food.

5. *Toxemias:* these produce directly or indirectly either an interference with food intake and assimilation or an overactive metabolism, or both; e.g., the undernourishment following acute febrile diseases, the wasting in tuberculosis, the continuing malnutrition in chronic malaria, hookworm disease, and diseased tonsils.

Undoubtedly, these five factors combine and interact in many instances, and it is therefore not enough to determine that malnutrition exists. Its cause must also be determined. Determination of the nutritional status of an individual must depend upon many considerations to be interpreted by the clinical judgment of a physician. Too often public health workers lead mothers to believe that underweight in a child means malnutrition and that all malnutrition can be corrected by food. This is not necessarily true.

Although not dramatic, one of the most serious disturbances of nutrition is overweight. It is so commonplace that not nearly enough attention is given to it. Yet it stands out sharply and clearly that certain types of heart disease, hypertension, diabetes, etc., are more often associated with overweight than with normal or underweight. Life expectancy, too, is definitely less in the overweight.

Women, in recent years, have tended to give far more attention to weight than have men. It is quite likely that this concern is to meet the demands of fashion rather than of hygiene, but the results are nevertheless beneficial. The fat man, however, through some mysterious rationalization, tends to regard his big belly as being of solid muscle and a matter of pride—and lives a shorter life than he could.

Fatigue and the Public Health. Physiological studies of fatigue have been concerned essentially with chemical changes in the tissues, lessened functional capacity of the muscles, etc. But fatigue must be viewed more broadly than this. It must be considered as including repeated nervous, mental, or emotional, as well as physical exhaustion of the individual. When this happens only occasionally, the individual gets back to normal before a repetition of this exhaustion. When it happens every day, that individual's physical efficiency, his judgment, peace of mind, and happiness are jeopardized. This problem is of public health importance because fatigue appears to be increasing step by step with the complexities of modern life. The monotony of narrowly specialized industrial work, the strain of ever-increasing competition, the confusion of crowds, speed of one sort or another, the noise of elevated trains and honking automobiles—all contribute to a daily recurring fatigue, involving a very large proportion of the population. The problem is one for which there is no immediate remedy, but demands serious consideration.

Posture. The first and greatest violation in posture is permitting the abdominal muscles to sag and lengthen. With this is associated drooping of the shoulders and flattening of the chest. Slack, protuberant abdomens develop because these girdle muscles are seldom used and consequently possess poor tone; or from an overadipose omentum; from indifference and habit; from a chronic lack of body poise incident to low morale; and in mothers, as the result of oft-repeated overstretching in pregnancy. Age also appears to lessen the ability of the abdominal muscles to withstand the pressure from within.

Mental state and posture seem to interact one on the other. The individual who feels fine, who still regards the world as conquerable, who looks alertly toward whatever problems may come up, is quite likely to reflect this mental alertness and poise in his posture. But if life has pretty well licked him and if he has accepted this as a fact, correspondingly will he reflect it in his posture. On the other hand, the person with a naturally erect posture, or a carelessly, chronically assumed poor posture, seems to be, as the psychologists say, "conditioned" to the development respectively of good or poor morale. The tramp who is down at the heels feels himself to be a pretty shoddy individual and slouches along accordingly. It is not probable that a poor carriage has any effect upon longevity or resistance to disease. It does, however, have some bearing upon mental and physical alertness, upon efficiency in general, and upon morale.

Muscular Development. There is no reason, other than assumption, to believe big muscles will make one live longer or protect him from disease. If man, as an animal, still had to depend upon his physical prowess for survival or even for leadership, then powerful muscular development would be distinctly an asset. But this is not the case, and the natural physical exercise incident to games, indulged in by children, youths, and decreasingly by older persons, is probably more nearly optimum than is an artificial regime designed to produce big muscles and increase the chest expansion. So far as is known, the physical condition of one who has lived a life of muscular strain is no better at the age of 50 than of one whose exercise has been quite mild and incidental. Actually, incomplete data suggests that a life involving unusual muscular effort lessens the life expectancy of the individual. And resistance to or recovery from infection, freedom from heart disease and cancer, soundness of the teeth, mental fitness, or resistance to venereal infection, seem not to be in any way dependent upon the size or strength of the skeletal muscles.

Probably the main value to be found in exercise is mental relaxation in doing something which gives pleasure to the individual, and which, at the same time, takes him out of the daily routine. A secondary effect of exercise is the utilization of muscles ordinarily not used, the increase in metabolism, the sunshine, outdoor air, increased appetite, etc.

Effects of Hygiene: Summary. Out of the above various considerations of cleanliness, food, and exercise, one may say quite definitely that the observance of dietary rules, the maintenance of an even temperament, the avoidance of frequently repeated fatigue or emotional exhaustion, and similar measures will tend to keep the individual in excellent condition and will offset diseases incident to faulty diet, and be of some protection against those conditions which seem to be associated with exhaustion and exposure. On the other hand, such measures are not generally effective in preventing degenerative diseases and the acute infections. The cleanest skin, the greatest muscular development, the most beautifully balanced physiological processes, are of no avail if one gets tetanus spores in the deep recesses of a suppurating wound; tonsils may become diseased regardless of personal hygiene; arthritis or heart disease appear just as likely to arise in the clean as in the dirty. Thus, though personal hygiene has its values in preserving health, it should not be offered to the public as a panacea; it should be borne in mind, too, that certain types of personalities will evolve into cranks on the subject of what they consider "hygiene." They may become vegetarians, or fresh air fiends, develop an abnormal fear of germs, or become introspective, or constantly apprehensive of sickness for themselves or family.

Periodic Physical Examinations of the Adult. In considering this question one must make certain sharp differentiations: differentiations between the ideal and the practicable; between what is desirable and what is possible; between what human beings ought to do and what they will and will not do, and how they react.

The rationale and objectives of the annual physical examination movement are well founded and clearly cut: a regular inventory of the human body for discovering disease processes in their early stages, and providing the maximum correction or curbing of such conditions. That is the ideal. Unfortunately, from a practical standpoint, there are these obstacles: (1) the human being is not so constituted that he will, in any great numbers, present himself periodically for such an examination, even though it might cost him nothing; (2) even fewer will present themselves and pay a fee in keeping with a worthwhile type of examination; (3) the average physician is not particularly interested in this type of work and has not the equipment to make a searching examination of the various organs and systems; (4) because of the latter two factors, the type of examination made is comparatively a superficial one; (5) limitations imposed by the type of examination done, and even the limitations of the most complete type of examination, plus limitations of knowledge, necessarily leave a residue of unrecognized pathology.

The value of periodic examination of adults has not been sufficiently accepted to influence the public health. But in spite of the fact that the number of persons receiving and benefiting from this practice is infinitesimal as compared to the needs of the total population, there have been many instances where benefit to the individual was striking: the discovery of early diabetes, syphilis, tuberculosis, focal infections, etc.

It is possible that, as medicine advances, more practical procedures than now exist will be developed. Certainly the periodical physical and mental check-up offers a great opportunity in preventive medicine, at least theoretically. The so-called multiphasic tests are perhaps a step in this direction; yet even here, there is a danger that short cuts may be introduced to the detriment of more complete procedures. Finally, in promoting periodic examinations, great care must be exercised lest people become health conscious to the extent that everybody worries about his health. There is much to be said for living happily rather than apprehensively.

Ventilation. It was formerly thought that the essential factor in ventilation was "freshness" of air. This conception of ventilation requirements lost sight of a number of other elements which are now known to be of great importance. These are: temperature of air, the amount of moisture contained, and air movement. Formerly too, the danger of accumulation of carbon dioxide in air breathed and rebreathed was strongly emphasized. "Crowd poison" was believed to occur in any indoor group not protected by good ventilation. The more modern conception of ventilation is as follows:

1. The carbon dioxide concentration of breathed and rebreathed indoor air does not nearly reach a dangerous degree of concentration; nor is there danger of exhaustion of oxygen content of air through breathing and rebreathing in ordinary circumstances. Oxygen depletion may occur through its excessive consumption by some heating or other flame-bearing apparatus.

2. While expired air appears to contain small amounts of organic matter, this has not been shown to be toxic.

3. The deleterious effects of poor ventilation appear not to operate through the process of respiration, but because it prevents effective heat radiation from the surface of the body.

4. The factors in air which produce discomfort and distress in the individual are excessive humidity, elevated temperature, and lack of air movement. Experiments have shown that if an individual's body is surrounded by air possessing these characteristics, he obtains no relief from his distress even though, through a tube, he breathes an ample amount of fresh air. And if his body is surrounded by reasonably cool air, or air with low moisture content, or air with some motion, he can for some hours breathe so-called vitiated air, through a tube, without ill effects.

5. High surrounding temperature produces slowing of radiation of heat from the body and greater perspiration in the individual. If in these circumstances the air surrounding the body contains a relatively large amount of moisture, it has but little ability to absorb perspiration; if there is lack of air movement, it is impossible for an interchange of high moisture air with air of lower humidity in other parts of the room to occur.

These are all factors in preventing the individual from getting rid of heat by radiation and the evaporation of perspiration. Very low surrounding temperature with strong air movement, as in a winter blizzard, results in too marked lowering of the individual's body temperature.

The moisture content of air is usually expressed in terms of *relative humidity*. By relative humidity is meant the relationship between the amount of moisture actually contained in the air and the total amount of moisture the air could contain at the existing temperature. Temperature markedly influences the amount of moisture which air can hold: the higher the temperature, the greater load of water vapor it can carry. Considering complete saturation of air with water vapor as 100 per cent humidity, then if it is half saturated the relative humidity is 50. If three fourths saturated, the relative humidity is 75.

Computation of the relative humidity in the air is most easily and practically made by use of the sling psychrometer. This instrument consists of two thermometers. The bulb of one of the thermometers is covered with a moistened cloth. Preliminary temperature readings having been made, the two thermometers are whirled rapidly. As the moisture in the cloth over the wet bulb evaporates, the bulb is cooled and the temperature recorded by that instrument is lower than on the preliminary reading. This decrease in recorded temperature, when compared to the thermometer used as a control, is an index of the amount of moisture absorbed by the air from the cloth over the bulb. In accordance with an established scale, the relative humidity is determined.

General Requirements in Good Ventilation. These are:

1. An ingress of fresh air at the rate of about 1800 cubic feet per hour per person.

2. Temperature maintenance in a zone between 65° and 68° F.

3. A middle ground in humidity, usually a relative humidity between 50 and 75.

4. A gentle air motion, not strong enough to cause a draft but sufficient to keep the air moving.

5. Freedom from irritating or toxic gases, fumes, etc., and from an amount or character of dust particles which might prove irritating or injurious.

Each of the above elements in good ventilation is so closely related to the other that absolute standards may not be laid down for any particular one of them except perhaps the last. Elevation of surrounding temperature, for instance, may be offset to a great extent by air motion or vice versa.

Supplying ventilation for large buildings and for spaces without outside windows must be done through devices providing apparatus for circulating, cooling, and in certain instances for washing or filtering the air. In less complicated situations, as in private residences, thermostatic control of heating devices and windows with deflectors serve quite satisfactorily. Home air conditioners, although relatively costly, are reasonably effective for summer use.

Lighting. The amount of light on any given surface is expressed in terms of *foot candles*. A foot candle is the amount of illumination which exists one foot distant from a light equal to one candle. Thus the intensity of light on a desk would be expressed as so many foot candles. The instrument for measuring light is designated as a "foot-candle meter" or "illuminometer." The instrument is quite small and its use is simple. It is placed on the surface to be measured and the reading is taken from a scale. In the older type of instrument it was necessary to make a comparison between gradations of illumination generated by a storage battery within the instrument, and the illumination being measured. In the newer type of foot-candle meter, the process is photoelectric and the reading is quite easy.

Natural Lighting. The requirements in schools are discussed in Chapter XIII. In industries, particular problems are created because the width of many workrooms is so great as to interfere with diffusion of light. In many industries, too, light diffusion is decreased by dust on walls and ceiling. Sometimes shadows and cross shadows result. The problem of how to provide adequate daylight in any given workroom is one which must be solved individually, if solvable. The amount of light necessary at any particular point depends upon the kind of work to be done: one foot candle would be sufficient in most passageways, twenty foot candles would be necessary in work requiring fine measurements and adjustments. Glares, either incident to facing a too bright sky, or reflected from bright objects, are particularly to be avoided. They lead to eyestrain, and may contribute to accidents in industry.

Artificial Lighting. The following general features are agreed upon as desirable:

1. For reading or other reasonably close work, there are needed at least 15–20 foot candles of light.

2. The source of light should be steady, without flickers, and guarded from the direct field of vision.

3. Light should fall from above and from slightly behind the individual.

4. Indirect lighting, in which light does not strike a surface directly but is diffused upon it from ceiling and walls, reduces shadows to a minimum; direct lighting tends to throw sharp shadows.

5. Indirect light, being diffused, may fall upon both the worker or reader and the object handled, but direct light should be so controlled as to fall only upon the object—never into the eyes.

chapter 11

Childbearing
and Its Relation
to the Public Health

EVEN THOUGH CONTINUATION of its kind is the essential purpose of
each species, there is a definite hazard in childbearing; and the death
of the mother not only removes a reproductive element from the
race but decreases the chances of survival of the newly born infant.
If these hazards can be eliminated or reduced, it seems logical to do
so; and aside from logic or other cold-blooded perspectives, society,
with such kindliness as it possesses, demands that lives be saved
wherever possible provided it does not cause society too much trouble
or cost society too much money. Thus there has developed an interest
in the health of the expectant mother; and the more the situation is
studied, the more it becomes apparent that if available knowledge
could be applied and reasonably adequate care provided in every
pregnancy and confinement, many deaths incident to childbearing
could be prevented. Measures directed toward this end constitute the
hygiene of maternity.

Deaths Incident to Childbearing. Deaths classed under this heading are those that occur from the hazards of pregnancy, childbirth,
and the puerperium. Obviously if a pregnant woman died because

of an automobile accident or murder, such a death would not be considered as part of maternal mortality. On the other hand, if such a woman died from heart disease, or a long-standing nephritis, etc., it would be necessary to consider the degree to which her pregnancy contributed to the fatal outcome.

The major causes of death in childbearing and their relative frequencies have changed considerably in the last few decades. Maternal mortality as a whole has decreased more than 80 per cent in the last 25 years. Among white mothers it has decreased much more rapidly than among nonwhite mothers. The three major causes of maternal death are hemorrhage, infection, and toxemias of pregnancy. These three causes account for approximately two thirds of the total maternal deaths. Until recent years sepsis was the principal cause of maternal mortality, but with use of the antibiotics, sepsis has declined more rapidly than hemorrhage as a cause of death. At the present time toxemia is the most important single cause followed by puerperal hemorrhage and sepsis. A comparison of the number of women dying from causes associated with childbearing with the number of deaths from the more common communicable diseases shows the seriousness of pregnancy, delivery, and the puerperium as a hazard. In the United States in 1956 there were 1702 deaths reported as associated with childbearing. From diphtheria 103 deaths were reported, 266 from whooping cough, 762 from meningococcal infections, 566 from poliomyelitis, and 530 from measles. In making these comparisons it should be borne in mind that deaths from childbearing occur in only one sex and in the female reproductive period, essentially in the age group 15 to 45 years of age.

In the age period 20 to 29, a smaller proportion of women die from these causes than in the period 30 to 39; and there is a smaller proportion of deaths in the latter group than in women over 40. Of women under 20, a higher proportion die from childbearing than in the 20 to 29 age group. There is some reason to believe that one factor concerned in the under 20 group is that in this age period extramarital pregnancies, with attempted abortion, are proportionately more frequent than in older women.

The hazards of childbearing vary also with the health or disease of the individual. Especially unfavorable is the presence of any of the following: tuberculosis, nephritis, diseases of the heart and arteries, diseases of the liver, pelvic deformities, and mental instability.

Tuberculosis, latent before and apparently latent during pregnancy, may manifest itself by rapid extension after delivery.

Nephritis tends to become worse in pregnancy.

The strain of labor is serious in damaged hearts and thinned or brittle arteries.

Unusual burden is placed upon the liver during pregnancy, and a diseased organ withstands this increased metabolic strain poorly.

Pelvic deformities act as definite mechanical obstacles to normal delivery.

Mental instability tends to become accentuated and may evolve into permanent psychopathic conditions.

Where Deliveries Occur. The circumstances under which pregnant mothers are delivered and the professional skill available or exercised at this time have an important bearing upon her and her infant's chances of survival. Of some importance, too, is whether or not the pregnancy goes on normally to full term or is interrupted; and if interrupted, whether accidentally or with intent; and if with intent, whether under competent professional action, with nonprofessional action, or self-induced. As to the latter no exact figures are available, since events of this sort do not become a matter of public record. However, from clinic studies in various places it is estimated that approximately 15 per cent of pregnancies end in abortion, regardless of cause. That the risks of pregnancy increase when the outcome is abortion can be appreciated from the fact that about one out of each eight maternal deaths is associated with abortion.

Conditions and circumstances under which mothers are delivered of babies differ from place to place, and vary with economic influences, race, and whether urban or rural. All over the United States there is a general tendency toward an increased utilization of hospitals. Considering this country as a whole, it may be said that well over 85 per cent of all births occur in hospitals. In cities, about 94 per cent of births are in hospitals; in the rural areas, about 76 per cent.

These over-all figures vary greatly from state to state and among cities.

Midwives. Women, acting as midwives, attended the majority of deliveries until comparatively recently, and in many European countries they still perform routinely in normal cases. Midwives are therefore quite closely tied to the history of the human race. In this country, the bulk of midwife practice has been with the foreign-born and children of foreign-born, Negroes, and women who could not afford a physician. A considerable number of rural women, when no physicians are available, employ midwives. In the United States as a whole in 1956, only about 2.8 per cent of deliveries were by midwives.

Except in somewhat isolated areas, the activities of midwives have decreased markedly in the past few decades. The causes for this are numerous and include improvement of economic circumstances in those who must employ someone at delivery. Perhaps, however, the most important single force in nearly eliminating the midwife is the greater availability of hospital facilities. Inasmuch as the midwife is not admitted to hospital practice, she may serve only that decreasing proportion of women who remain at home for delivery. Thus, in recent years in New York City, where nearly all women are delivered in hospitals, only about a dozen midwives remain in practice. The number of women they attend in confinement is less than the number delivered in ambulances and taxicabs on the way to the hospital.

Most states recognize midwives, either directly or by implication. In some they must be "licensed," in others "registered," but the requirements for this licensing or registration are usually quite casual. They may not sign death certificates, must report births, and must instill prophylactic in eyes of newborn. Nearly all health departments exercise some supervision over midwives and attempt to teach them the principles of asepsis, when to call a doctor, and warn them of things they may not do.

The Role of Syphilis in Childbearing. Syphilis of the mother, of all diseases which do not destroy the mother's life, is one of the greatest hazards to the infant in utero. Early syphilis in the mother usually results in abortion or miscarriage. Fairly recent but latent syphilis usually produces a stillbirth. A history of repeated uncompleted pregnancies should arouse suspicion of syphilis; and no pregnant woman should be considered so free from the possibility of syphilis as to justify omission of a serologic test as a routine.

Some 42 states now require that the attending physician have such tests made on every pregnant woman under his care. As a further precaution in this connection, premarital serologic tests are required in an increasing number of states: 38 as of 1950.

Syphilis discovered and treated early in pregnancy can be so controlled that the woman goes to term with every probability of being delivered of a nonsyphilitic baby. Such babies, however, should not be considered to have escaped congenital infection except after rigid serological tests and observation.

The Maternal Mortality Rate. By "maternal mortality rate" is meant the number of deaths from pregnancy, delivery, and their complications, per 10,000 live births during a given period of time in a given place. There are bases other than "the number of live births" used in calculating maternal mortality, such as the number of deaths from these causes per 100,000 population. Certain agencies express the maternal mortality rate as the number of deaths per 10,000 total births, which includes stillbirths as well as live births. However, comparison of the number of maternal deaths with the number of live births is the ratio usually utilized.

As an illustration of the calculation of this rate the following data may be used: in 1956 there were 15,680 live births in the city of Smithton. In the same year, there were 12 deaths from the hazards of childbearing. The problem is to determine how many deaths occurred per 10,000 live births. Then if x represents this number,

$$x : 10,000 = 12 : 15,680$$

Since the product of the means equals, in such examples, the product of the extremes,

$$15,680x = 120,000$$
$$x = 7.6$$

The maternal mortality rate for Smithton, in 1956, is thus calculated to be about 8 deaths per 10,000 live births.

One of the great health improvements in the past quarter century is the marked reduction in this rate: the saving of women's lives. In the registration states of this country in 1925, the rate was 65 deaths per 10,000 live births. It was above 50 as recently as 1936. The rate for 1956 was 4.1.* The maternal mortality rate for nonwhite mothers is about three times the rate for white mothers.

The improvement is from no single cause, but rather from a beneficial combination of circumstances. One of these is better prenatal care for a greater proportion of expectant mothers. Another is to be found in better medical care. A third factor was the introduction of the sulfa drugs and later the antibiotics in preventing or controlling infection. Finally, an increasingly well-informed young womanhood plays no small part.

The Principal Elements in a Maternal Hygiene Program. The make-up of any public health program is largely determined by the objectives of that program. In maternal hygiene the objective is to conserve the life and health of expectant mothers and their developing infants. Consequently, the program is made up of the following elements:

1. Medical care for every pregnant woman who can be persuaded to obtain or accept it during pregnancy, delivery, and in the postpartum period. This care may most normally be rendered by the private physician of the woman's choice. When she cannot afford or arrange for private care, it may be obtained from an organized clinic, such as the outpatient part of a hospital, or from special physicians for the care of the indigent, insured, or low-income group.

2. Periodic nursing visits. This is often limited to prenatal and postpartum visits by the nurse but should include nursing care at the time of delivery if the woman is to remain at home. When the nurse is not to be present at delivery, she at least attempts, beforehand, to aid the woman in preparing for delivery by having supplies on hand and a neighbor or relative to assist the doctor.

---

* In comparing maternal mortality rates for and since 1949 with those of previous years, consideration should be given to the fact that, in the new classification practices required under the sixth revision (1948) of the *Manual of International Lists of Diseases and Causes of Death,* about 9 per cent less deaths of childbearing women are assigned to childbearing as a cause than heretofore.

3. A reasonably decent place for confinement: hospitalization for those women whose surroundings are so unfavorable, or whose condition is such that home delivery would be hazardous.

4. Ensurance that hospitals which receive women for delivery have proper equipment, facilities, and resources. This may be brought about only partly by legal requirements; high standards and perfection of detail in practice must rest upon self-discipline in individual hospitals and staffs and in the observance of exacting professional performance generally.

5. Legislation requiring a serological examination in pregnancy.

6. Inauguration and support of those measures designed to give the woman in industry such special consideration as is necessary during the latter part of pregnancy and the postpartum period.

7. Measures designed to create community understanding, especially among women, of the need for proper instruction and care of expectant mothers. This is done by means of pamphlets, news articles, speeches to women's clubs, and radio broadcasts.

8. Continued and wise health education of young women in general and expectant mothers in particular.

The Antenatal Clinic. No maternal hygiene program can be said to be satisfactory unless medical supervision and nursing care are pro-

TABLE 5

NUMBER OF DEATHS FROM DELIVERIES AND COMPLICATIONS OF
PREGNANCY, CHILDBIRTH, AND THE PUERPERIUM PER 10,000 LIVE
BIRTHS IN THE UNITED STATES*

Year	All Causes As Set Forth Above	Puerperal Septicemia	Other Causes As Set Forth Above
1956	4.1	0.7	3.4
1950	8.3	1.7	6.6
1940	38.0	15.0	23.0
1930	67.0	24.0	43.0
1920	80.0	27.0	53.0

* National Office of Vital Statistics: *Vital Statistics of the United States,* 1956. Government Printing Office, Washington, D.C., 1958, and corresponding volumes for preceding years.

vided for women who would not otherwise receive it. The antenatal clinic is an important element here, and the service rendered by such clinics may be summarized as follows:

1. A complete history is taken, usually by a nurse, supplemented later by physician's notes. This history goes into previous health, with the details of previous pregnancies, and includes data as to economic status and home conditions.

2. A general physical examination is made, the case being referred to special clinics if abnormalities outside of those incident to pregnancy are discovered.

3. A detailed pelvic examination is made to determine if pregnancy exists; the degree to which pregnancy has advanced; the condition of the cervix, uterine adnexa, and perineum; the position of the infant; and the pelvic diameters. The place and character of the fetal heart sounds are determined.

4. Urinalysis, serologic tests, chest x-ray, blood pressure are taken as routines, and special tests, such as blood chemistry, sputum, if indicated.

5. Instructions are given about general hygiene, food, exercise, and precautions; an appointment is made for a return visit to the clinic; and arrangement is made for a place of delivery.

6. A complete record is kept of all findings, of instructions given, of special orders, and of the place for delivery.

7. A schedule for home follow-up visits is arranged by the public health nurse, or sometimes by medical social service workers.

The Public Health Nurse and Maternal Hygiene. The general program of the public health nurse is under the direction of the organization which she represents. Her service to any given patient is in accordance with the standing orders of her organization, these to be modified in light of specific instructions given by the attending physician of that case. There is no question of competing with the physician in charge. She supplements, assists, and acts as his representative.

The purposes of the public health nurse's antepartum visits to the patient's home are:

1. To ensure continuing contact between the patient and the physician or clinic.

2. To ensure that the patient understands and carries out the physician's directions.

3. To report to the physician the patient's general condition and, in particular, any dangerous findings noted.

4. To provide the patient with general information as to diet, personal hygiene, rest, etc.

5. To assist the patient in making arrangements and providing supplies for the infant and for delivery if this is to be at home.

6. To instruct the mother in fundamentals of care of the newborn.

7. To persuade the mother of the need for good mouth hygiene and visits to the dentist.

8. To assist in every possible way in maintaining the patient's morale and equanimity.

Her purposes in a postpartum visit are:

1. To check upon the condition of the patient and report to the physician.

2. To teach the home attendant, by demonstration, how to care for the mother during this period.

3. To teach the mother the elements of infant care.

4. To get the mother, in future, to keep the infant under regular medical supervision.

5. To get the mother to report back to her physician for a final postpartum examination.

It is not always easy to ensure periodic contact between the antenatal case and her physician. Most women, except the more informed and intelligent, have been inclined to look upon the physician as someone to be called only for aid in delivery, or if some rather alarming symptoms arise. Further, where the woman is paying for her service, she considers each visit to the doctor's office as one more item of expense. The physician may instruct the patient to return every so often, but if she does not come back he cannot afford to pursue. For these reasons the public health nurse occupies the part of a most important connecting link between physician and patient.

The public health nurse in many ways assists the patient in carrying out the physician's directions:

1. By interpretation and explanation. In the excitement of the doctor's office or the clinic, the patient is quite likely to obtain only a hazy idea of just what instructions have been given.

2. By adaptation of general instructions to the particular conditions in the patient's home.

3. By demonstration to some member of the family of any particular measures which an attendant must carry out in the care of the patient.

In her report to the physician on any individual case, the public health nurse usually states, in summary, whether the general condition appears to be good or not. She reports in detail upon bleeding (even the smallest amount), persistent headache, dizziness, disturbance of vision, mental confusion, persistent vomiting, sudden abdominal pain, marked shortness of breath or edema, fever, syncope, convulsions. Where such danger signals are present, she puts the woman to bed, calls the physician at once. Records of blood pressure reading and urinalysis, sometimes of fetal heart sounds, are reported routinely.*

The report is made at the end of each visit, in writing, and is sent by mail. If any dangerous findings are noted the doctor is immediately communicated with by telephone, the written report following.

In the absence of specific orders from a physician, the public health nurse usually advises an ordinary three-meal-a-day balanced diet. This will provide the usual portions of proteins, carbohydrates, fats, mineral salts, and vitamins, found in the average food intake of a normal person. If there is need for special restrictions or for increase

* The practice of having public health nurses take blood pressure readings and make urinalyses varies in different places. The present tendency is to have the nurse include these tests in her work. There are no great mysteries or difficulties in carrying out either of these procedures, and they can be performed satisfactorily by any properly trained nurse, with instruction and practice. While the nurse will know in general the significance of albumin in the urine or a high blood pressure, the actual interpretation of these findings, and measures for their correction, must be left for the attending physician. The urinalysis done by the nurse is quite a simple one, seldom including a microscopic examination, frequently being limited to a test for albumin.

in some particular food element, such advice should be on the basis of the physician's decision.

The nurse should not advise the expectant mother that she must "eat for two." Ordinary appetite and food intake, under normal conditions, will provide for nutrition of both mother and developing infant.

The frequency of public health nursing visits depends upon the case and whether or not the woman is going regularly for medical advice. A pregnant woman should be seen by her physician, or in his absence by the public health nurse, about once a month through the sixth month, once in two weeks in the seventh and eighth months, once every week or ten days in the last month. A nursing visit of this sort takes from 25 to 35 minutes.

The public health nurse does not, as a rule, care for the expectant mother at delivery. As the nurse of a health department or visiting nurse association, she has many duties besides those in connection with maternity cases, and her schedule does not permit assistance to the doctor at delivery. Such service is highly important, is supplied to some extent through voluntary agencies, but those unable to pay for nursing service at delivery get but little of it. The public health nurse does, however, attempt to have the mother provide herself with supplies which will be needed at delivery, and further guides the mother in obtaining a layette. Local and state governments and the federal government provide pamphlets listing materials needed for home deliveries.

The value of the work of the public health nurse in preventing puerperal morbidity and mortality depends to a great extent upon the character of the hazard. As she is not usually present at deliveries, her ordinary service has but little effect in preventing puerperal sepsis or other situations incident to delivery. Through routine examination of urine, taking of blood pressure and alertness for symptoms of toxemia, however, the public health nurse can save many lives by getting early toxic cases immediately under the care of their physicians. Accidents of pregnancy may be prevented to some extent through instruction of mothers in simple hygiene, and precautions.

Hemorrhage in pregnancy may be early discovered, while it is but slight, by the public health nurse.

There are also a number of miscellaneous, though not fatal, complications which the nurse's advice may help: cracked or retracted nipples, varicose veins, dental decay, under- or overnutrition.

Incident to her service to maternity cases, the public health nurse makes a reasonably complete record of her findings, advice, and service. In such a record the following data are usually included:

1. Identifying data: name, address, color, age, of patient.

2. A record of such occurrences in past pregnancies as might be important in the care of the present pregnancy.

3. Significant data in present pregnancy: name of physician in charge, physician's orders, expected date of delivery, where delivery is to take place, result of serological test for syphilis, and record of current findings on each visit, with particular reference to blood pressure, urinalysis, dangerous symptoms, general hygiene.

4. A record of the dates of home visits, instructions given on each visit, date of the nurse's report to the physician, and other significant data of current nature.

5. Family and social data: economic level of the family, general environment of the home, and whether or not there is reason to suspect syphilis or tuberculosis in the patient's husband.

6. A brief summary of the outcome of pregnancy: where, when, name of attendant, whether stillborn or liveborn child, normal or instrumental delivery.

Many antenatal nursing records for maternity cases call for more detail than can be obtained with accuracy or are utilized even if obtained.

REFERENCES

Eastman, Nicholson J.: *Williams Obstetrics,* 11th ed., Appleton-Century-Crofts, Inc., New York, 1956.

Maxcy, Kenneth F.: *Rosenau Preventive Medicine and Public Health,* 8th ed. Appleton-Century-Crofts, Inc., New York, 1956.

chapter 12

The Hygiene of Infancy
and Young Childhood

THE NEWBORN INFANT has a greater probability of dying within a year than at any subsequent age up to the period 65–70 years. After reaching age 1 he has a much better chance of survival, for in the period 1–4 the death rate is only 1.2 deaths per 1000 population of that age, whereas in the period under 1 the death rate (1956) was 33.6 per 1000 persons under 1 year of age. From these data the intensity of hazards in early life may be appreciated. Obviously, the younger the child, the less firm is his hold on life. Thus, in the United States in 1956, of all infants who died under 1 year of age, 38 per cent died before completing 1 day of life; 64 per cent in the first week of life; 72 per cent in the first 4 weeks of life. Expressed in another way, it may be said that more then 3½ times as many infants die in the first month of life as in the next 11 months.

Common and conventional practice is to consider the age of *infancy* as including only children under 1 year of age. The *neonatal* period is a subdivision of infancy: children under 1 month (specifically, 28 days) of age. The *preschool* period extends from 1 year of age up to 6. The upper age limit of this period is so placed because most children enter school at about 6 years of age. However, it is a somewhat unfortunate dividing line, as standard population figures and data on morbidity and mortality are not provided on this basis, but for children under 5 years of age.

Factors That Enter into the Antenatal Period. The factors that determine the quality of infants born are many and complex. To a very great extent, the mental and physical make-up of an individual depends upon corresponding qualities in his ancestors. This, however, is not completely and invariably true, for it is possible that the least desirable genes from a generally sound mother may, in a particular fertilization, be combined with the least desirable genes from a generally sound father and result in an offspring possessing only the mental and physical liabilities of the parents, these liabilities in these parents having remained latent and uninfluential in their own lives. The exact reverse of this might happen, wherein poor stock might produce a child of unusual quality. Medical science has learned from the geneticist a great deal of the factors here involved, and there has developed an interest in eugenics.

Eugenics would consist essentially in selected matings, so that on the one hand there would be encouragement in improvement of racial stock and, on the other, there would be exercised deterrence to reproduction of the unfit. Unfortunately, it is not always possible, in fact, it is quite impossible, to say that the mating of certain individuals will assuredly result in desirable offspring; but it is possible in certain limited situations to say that a mating between two individuals would in all probability result in undesirable offspring. It must be borne in mind, too, that in human beings marriage and reproduction, or reproduction without marriage, are not amenable to control as is the case in the laboratory of botany or zoology or on the stock farm. The freedom of the individual enters strongly into the equation, and man and woman are notably reluctant to permit any organized system, marriage counselor, relative, friend, or acquaintance choose his or her mate.

The whole subjects of genetics, of eugenics and of inheritability of disease or tendency to disease, constitute vast fields within themselves and can only be touched upon here. In considering these subjects, however, one should make a distinction between *inherited* and *congenital* disease. An inherited disease is one wherein the infectious agent or the disability is to be found in the ovum or the sperm which fertilizes it. So far as is known, there are no infectious diseases in human beings that are truly inherited. There is reason to believe, however, that what may be called tissue weaknesses or tendencies may be inherited. Thus one finds a higher diabetic rate among children of diabetics than among children of nondiabetics, and hemophilia or bleeder's disease is one where males inherit the condition from the mother, manifest it, but do not transmit it in turn to their offspring; and where the daughter of the same mother does not herself manifest the disease, but transmits it so that it is manifested in her male children.

Anything deleterious that occurs in the developing embryo after the sperm has fertilized the ovum is designated as congenital disease. Thus the causative agent of syphilis (*Treponema pallidum*) may not be transmitted in either the sperm or the ovum, but if the mother has syphilis she may infect the embryo, resulting in the production of a syphilitic child. This is congenital infection. Other factors may cause congenital disease: inadequate or unbalanced nutrition in utero, lack of oxygenation of blood, unusual pressures, or certain toxins, such as the virus of German measles.

As in the case of the quality of children born, many influences act and interact to determine the quantity of children born. As previously mentioned, the rate of reproduction is designated as the birth rate and is expressed in terms of numbers of children born each year per 1000 population. One attempts to account for fluctuations in birth rates in terms of biological laws or the mass effects of civilization or both. One must here make another distinction, that is, between *fecundity* and *fertility*. Fecundity has been defined by the College of Fellows of the Population Association of America as the "physiological capacity to participate in reproduction." The same association defines fertility as "fecundity expressed in performance and therefore measurable." The one is a potential quality and is essentially biological. The other represents the net result of an interplay between ability to have children, efforts to have children, and efforts not to have children. Thus the fecundity of each of a married pair might be at a maximum but through abstinence, contraceptive methods, or interrupted pregnancies, this couple might remain childless. On the other hand, the fecundity of one or both of a pair might be comparatively low but the net results of their efforts to have children might be a fair-sized family. Complete absence of fecundity in either partner would, of course, result in no children.

The birth rate quite obviously reflects fertility. The general tendency of the birth rate is downward. One seldom encounters the large families of from 6 to 12 children which existed two or three generations ago. Also, as mentioned already, larger families are found more often among the poor than among the well-to-do.

About a generation ago, there arose a strong movement which operated under a general philosophy of birth control. The idea was to supply to married couples contraceptive information which would make it possible for them to limit the number of children. Some success was attained in individual instances, but probably not enough to have any influence upon the situation as a whole. Further, it was noted that, as contraceptive knowledge increased and contraceptive techniques and devices became more freely available, they were utilized more by those quite able to raise and educate children than by the group not so well placed economically. As a result of this, those interested in the birth control movement have evolved a broader philosophy, have designated their program as concerned with planned parenthood rather than with birth control, and are just as much concerned with the spacing and planning for an adequate number of children as they are with limiting the size of the family. This movement for birth control and planned parenthood has not gone unopposed. It has met religious opposition and legal barriers. Federal laws prohibit sending through the mail printed matter carrying contraceptive information or contraceptive devices. Opposition in some states remains so strong that it is illegal for a physician to advise a patient how to prevent pregnancy even though the physician knows that a pregnancy would in all probability result in death of the mother.

Assuming now that an embryo is in process of development, certain hazards must be recognized. Speaking broadly, these may be considered as hazards of development and hazards of injury. More specifically, there may occur: (1) defects in development, such as monstrosities, congenital deformities; (2) interference with circulation to and from the placenta; (3) toxemia in the mother, as an eclampsia; (4) infections in the mother, such as German measles, syphilis; (5) mechanical injury, such as injury to the mother; abortion, either therapeutic or criminal; or injury to the infant incident to difficult labor, i.e., exhaustion of the infant in the contracted pelvis, intracranial hemorrhage, injuries produced by forceps or otherwise by the obstetrician; (6) the death of the mother from any cause during the period of gestation. The outcome of these conditions may be abortion, miscarriage, stillbirth, or a liveborn defective child.

Some Data on the Normal Infant.

Average birth weight for males is from 7 to 7½ lb.

Average birth weight for females is from 6½ to 7 lb.

After the loss immediately following birth, usually about 10 per cent of weight, there is a fairly steady gain, averaging about 4 oz per week. At the age of 6 months, the normal infant will have doubled his birth weight, and will have trebled it at the end of a year.

The infant at birth is about 20½ in. long. Males are a fraction longer than females. Growth in length during the first year of life is from 8 to 10 in. Thus, at the age of 1, the infant is about 30 in. long.

The circumference of the head at birth averages 13½ to 14 in. This is increased in the first 6 months by 3 in., and from then on at a much slower rate. Up to the age of 1, the head is usually larger than the chest.

The posterior fontanelle is closed by about the third month. The anterior fontanelle is not closed until about the eighteenth month. Failure of the fontanelles to close may be indicative of rickets. Bulging fontanelles are seen in hydrocephalus and other conditions causing increased pressure in the cranium. The public health nurse should insist that the infant be at once carried to his physician when abnormalities in fontanelles, or in the skull, are noted.

At about 8 to 10 months the normal infant attempts to creep and, after a few weeks' experimentation, pulls himself up to various articles of furniture. About the end of the first year he commences to take a step or two. In a couple of months more he walks fairly well. He begins to associate names of persons and words shortly after 1 year of age. Gradually he strings words together.

From age 1, through the preschool period, gain in height and weight varies to some extent with the individual. Increases in height are about as follows: second year, 4 in.; third year, 3½ in.; fourth year 2½ to 3½ in.; fifth year, 2 in.

The Teeth in Young Children. There are 20 deciduous teeth. The first to appear are the 2 lower central incisors, which erupt when the infant is from 6 to 8 months of age. The other 18 teeth appear as follows:

In ninth to tenth months: 2 upper central incisors.
In tenth to twelfth months: 4 lateral incisors; 2 upper, 2 lower.
Early in second year: 4 anterior molars.
In latter part of second year: 4 canine (cuspid) teeth. By middle of third year: 4 posterior molars.

Thus a child 1 year of age will usually have 8 teeth; at 2 years he will have 16 teeth, and at 2½ years he usually has 20 teeth.

The first permanent teeth are molars. They are jaw teeth, 4 in number, an upper and a lower on each side. They erupt at about 6 years of age. *They do not take the place of any temporary teeth,* but come in behind the last temporary molars. They can be identified as the sixth tooth or teeth back. The grinding surface of this molar is broad and is thrown into ridges and depressions. Because of this complicated structure, pits and fissures not infrequently occur in the enamel, and there is danger of caries. Many parents, even when noting cavities in a child's first permanent molars, are not particularly concerned as they think of this tooth as a temporary one, to be replaced by another. Of course, it will not be replaced, and what is particularly unfortunate, if it is lost, irregularity of other teeth and possible underdevelopment of the jaw may result. Mothers need to be taught the importance of conservation of these teeth in their children, and in public health work there is an unusually good opportunity to advise parents in this connection.

The temporary teeth are completely formed before the infant is born. For this reason the nutrition of the mother, during the antenatal period of any given child, will largely determine the quality of that child's deciduous teeth. The nutrition of the infant and young child will, other things being equal, determine the soundness of the permanent teeth.

Mental Hygiene in Young Children. In the past, public health workers have accomplished very little in this field, except in isolated instances or in connection with special programs. The reasons for failure to accomplish more appear to be somewhat as follows: (1) though they should be prepared to deal with the problems of mental hygiene, general child hygiene programs, as operated, are not equipped to render this service; (2) there are difficulties in case finding; mental defectives and children with frequent and definite evidence of instability are easily found, but the milder cases of mental retardation, and children who present only occasional evidence of an underlying nervous or mental instability are discovered rarely; (3) relative scarcity of mental hygiene clinics necessarily limits the service; (4) the treatment of any particular case must be mainly through the parents concerned, and frequently these parents have not the intelligence, understanding, poise, and personality necessary in the circumstances; (5) causes of these disturbances are complex and difficult to discover; treatment is highly individualized, both as regards the case and the psychiatrist, and treatment must be long and continuing.

In spite of these limitations, the public health nurse, visiting the home, has excellent opportunity to teach mothers (1) that a child must be given a sense of security, of being loved, of respect for himself, the rights of others, and of decent human courtesy and courage; (2) that very young children are likely to imitate parental examples of temper, nervousness, rudeness, fears, queer food habits; (3) that they likewise tend to imitate even tempers, courteousness, brushing of teeth, taking of baths, and eating of balanced meals; (4) that these habits and attitudes, once established, for good or ill, are quite likely to remain fixed.

To offset negative or harmful attitudes, an attempt should be made to teach the mother that if nobody else in the family drinks milk, the child is not likely to enjoy it; that if others express dislike of green vegetables or of fruits, the child is likely to develop the same attitude; that if parents express apprehension of burglars, or evidence fear of lightning or what not, the child naturally expects a burglar every night or to be struck by each bolt of lightning; that an irritable, shouting parent will raise an irritable, shouting child; that threatening the child with dark closets and policemen has a viciously, and permanently, bad effect; that the equanimity and personality to be exhibited in adult life are largely fixed before school age; that it is better for the child to break an occasional leg, falling out of a tree, than to remain a shadowy personality, tied to the apron strings.

Common Physical Defects in Young Children. The kinds of defects found depend upon (1) the age group, (2) the types of examination given, and (3) the person examining. The most commonly seen defects in infancy are umbilical hernia and phimosis. Occasionally there are more serious defects, congenital in nature: congenital heart disease, deformities. Sometimes one encounters birth injuries. At the other end of this age group, in children in the fifth year of life, the picture changes. Most of the umbilical hernias have shrunken or disappeared; if circumcision has not been done, the phimosis usually remains. Poor nutrition of the mother during the antenatal period, and poor nutrition in the infant, may have contributed to decayed teeth. A small percentage of children have by now developed definitely diseased tonsils, though one must be careful not to consider these children's tonsils to be diseased merely because they are enlarged. In children of this age all lymphoid tissue, and the tonsils are mainly lymphoid tissue, tends to engorgement and temporary enlargement in response to mild, transient infection. As a result of upper respiratory infection, a small percentage of these young children have ear discharges. Orthopedic defects, remaining as residues of bone and joint tuberculosis, rickets, or poliomyelitis, are found rarely in comparison with the total number of children examined at a health conference.

The children most likely to receive attention for correction of their defects are those of intelligent, well-to-do parents, who have their children under the care of a private pediatrician; and children whose parents take them fairly regularly to a child health conference. The latter discovers the defects, and, though doing no curative work itself, arranges for clinic services for those unable to pay a private physician.

Children of parents in the upper economic levels and children of parents in rather poor circumstances, however, constitute only the smaller part of the group as a whole. Provisions for serving those who are able to pay only limited fees are quite inadequate.

Infant Mortality. The number of deaths under 1 year of age per 1000 live births, during a given period of time in a given place, is known as the infant mortality rate.

It should be noted that the basis of comparison is with the "number of live births." Stillbirths are excluded because there is no generally accepted definition as to how far uterogestation must be advanced before a prematurely expelled product of conception is regarded and reported as a stillbirth. To include stillbirths, as either births or deaths, in calculating infant mortality rates, would make it impossible to compare rates in areas operating under different laws and definitions in regard to that term.

As an example of how the infant mortality rate is calculated, it will be assumed that in a certain city in 1958, there were 3540 live births and 80 deaths under 1 year of age. What one needs to do is to translate the ratio $\frac{80}{3540}$ into terms of $\frac{x}{1000}$, finding the value of x. This value will bear to 1000 the same ratio that 80 bears to 3540, thus:

$$x : 1000 = 80 : 3540$$
$$3540x = 80,000$$
$$x = 22.6$$

The infant mortality rate in this hypothetical situation is, therefore, 22.6. In the United States in 1956 the mortality rate was 26.

The problem of the health of infants and children has changed both quantitatively and qualitatively. In 1915, the first year for which are available reasonably representative figures in infant mortality in the United States, the infant mortality rate was 100 deaths per 1000 live births; as of midcentury, this rate was about one third of that. In the earlier days of this century, over half the deaths in infants occurred after the first month of life; at present less than a third of the deaths are in infants from 1 to 12 months of age.

Expressed in another way, it may be said that the greatest problem in infant health and survival is in the first month of life: over 70 per cent of the infants who die are in this age period. And in the first month of life, the greatest hazard is in the first few days. One third of those who die in the first year of life die in the first day. Death rates in all ages of infants have been reduced, but there has not been as much reduction in the group under one month as in those between 1 and 11 months. Hence, though actually lower than they were, death rates in infants under 1 month of age loom larger in proportion to the total infant mortality than they did in the past.

In the first month of life the causes of death are mainly those which operated in the prenatal period or at the time of birth. Such factors, classed as *prenatal* and *natal causes,* account for more than four fifths of all neonatal deaths (deaths in the first 28 days of life), and for more than half of all deaths in the first year of life. The most important of these prenatal and natal causes is premature birth. Injury at birth, congenital malformations, syphilis, and certain other diseases or conditions, make up the balance of the prenatal and natal causes. Further details are provided in Table 6.

The range of the infant mortality rate in the United States is considerable: from 20.6 in Iowa to 37.9 in Mississippi in 1956. It is generally comparatively low in those states with only a small proportion of the population living under adverse conditions. In the South and Southwest, the high infant mortality rates prevailing among Mexicans and Negroes tend to produce a high rate for the states concerned. The nonwhite infant mortality rate in the United States in 1956 was about 42 per 1000 live births, as against 23 for white infants. Semitropical conditions contribute to gastrointestinal diseases. Infant mortality rates tend to be higher in rural than in urban areas.

It is an interesting fact that there are born more male than female infants, and that a greater proportion of male infants die under 1 year of age than do females. For every 1000 female births there are from 1050 to 1060 male births; for every 1000 stillbirths of females there are about 1175 stillbirths of males; for every 1000 deaths of females under 1 year of age there are about 1362 deaths of male infants in the same age group.

Objectives in Program. The objectives in infant and preschool hygiene service are, obviously, to protect and maintain the health of

TABLE 6

INFANT MORTALITY RATE FOR SELECTED CAUSES, BY AGE,
UNITED STATES, 1956*

Cause of Death	Total Deaths under One Year	Deaths under 28 Days	Deaths 28 Days, 11 Months
All Causes	26.0	19.9	7.1
Influenza and pneumonia, except pneumonia of newborn (480–493)†	2.1	0.0	2.1
Gastritis, duodenitis, enteritis and colitis, except diarrhea of newborn (545, 571, 572)	0.7	0.0	0.7
Congenital malformations (750–759)	3.8	2.1	1.7
Birth injuries (760, 761)	2.8	2.7	0.0
Postnatal asphyxia and atelectasis (762)	4.3	4.1	0.2
Pneumonia of newborn (763)	0.8	0.8	0.0
Diarrhea of newborn (764)	0.1	0.1	0.0
Hemolytic disease of newborn (erythroblastosis) (770)	0.6	0.6	0.0
Immaturity unqualified (776)	4.9	4.8	0.1
Accidents (E800–E962)	0.8	0.1	0.7

* National Office of Vital Statistics: *Vital Statistics of the United States,*
1956. Government Printing Office, Washington, D.C., 1958.

† The numbers in parentheses refer to the classification in the 1955 revision
of the *Manual of the International Statistical Classification of Diseases, Injuries,
and Causes of Death.* World Health Organization, Geneva, Switzerland, 1957.

infants and young children. In laying down a program to attain these
objectives, it is necessary first to determine, as nearly exactly as possible, just what the problem is and of what component parts it is made
up; and when, how, and in what circumstances they manifest themselves. It is on this basis that public health programs are, or should be,
organized.

The kinds of illnesses that infant and preschool hygiene is designed
to prevent, or mitigate, may be summarized as follows:

1. Conditions incident to antenatal life: syphilis; premature birth.
Preventive measures here are rendered as a part of maternal hygiene.
The prematurely born infant needs highly specialized and unremit-
ting care.

2. Disturbances of nutrition.

3. Gastrointestinal disease; those arising from unsatisfactory feeding; dysentery.

4. Respiratory diseases; the pneumonias.

5. Acute communicable diseases; diphtheria, scarlet fever, whooping cough, measles.

6. Physical defects; diseased tonsils, decayed teeth, defective vision.

7. Mental and nervous disturbances; tantrums, fears, shyness, sullenness, excitability.

8. Accidents.

The Private Physician in Child Hygiene. Although often overlooked, it should be recognized that the most important element in child hygiene is the private physician, particularly the pediatrician. Prevention is here practiced more than in any other area of medicine, and, increasingly, the pediatrician's time is given to well children.

Comparatively a few years ago this was not the case. Even intelligent and well-informed parents were not inclined to pay for services to keep their children well, but today that attitude represents the exception rather than the rule. Public health programs, therefore, should take cognizance of this trend and operate under policies that will keep children in the hands of the physicians of the parents' choice, catering only to those parents who would otherwise be unable to provide their children with preventive service.

The Pediatric Clinic and the Child Health Conference. As a rule, the pediatric clinic takes only sick children, the child health conference only well children. There is an ill-defined zone as in the child with mild rickets or slight diarrhea, where both serve. More frequently the clinic operates as part of a hospital, the child health conference as a part of a health agency. There is a growing tendency for pediatric clinics to render care of well children; and the health conference frequently will strap an umbilical hernia, puncture a bulging drum membrane in emergency, or paint something with iodine. It seldom goes further than this in treatment. Sometimes, in certain localities, the generic term "clinic" is used to include "health confer-ence."

An important part of the infant and preschool hygiene program is in connection with nutrition. Through medical direction and through home visits by the nurse, the public health agency attempts to teach the mother the fundamentals in feeding young children. Through providing regular child health conferences, the nutritional status of the infant or child is checked periodically. Such checks on nutrition must be on the basis of a medical examination. Weight alone is not sufficient. Through one arrangement or another, attempts are made to see that infants and young children, visiting the health conferences, are provided with a reasonably adequate amount of safe milk, and with auxiliary vitamin-rich foods, such as fruit juices, or cod liver oil. Special instruction is given to mothers' classes, to "boarding-home mothers," and others responsible for or interested in the care of children.

Operation of Child Hygiene Programs. Services for protecting the health of infants and young children are carried on by:

1. *Private physicians;* as mentioned previously, private physicians, especially pediatricians, make continuing and important contributions in this field.

2. *Voluntary health agencies;* this is a field in which many local voluntary agencies maintain excellent programs, operating child health conferences, nursing services, mothers' classes, health education programs, special hospitals.

3. *Health departments;* official agencies operate through health conferences, nursing services, special clinics, supervision of boarding homes, sanitation, housing supervision, etc.

4. *Hospitals and clinics;* institutions of this sort serve through special hospitals or departments for maternity, children's wards, pediatric clinics, etc.

5. *Welfare agencies;* social service agencies provide important aid, both direct and indirect. Day nurseries, kindergartens, parks, etc., are definite contributions. Aid in providing food, family guidance, em-

ployment, and medical care are of great importance to the health of young children.

The Public Health Nurse and Child Hygiene. Very important in the field of child hygiene and supplementing the service of the physician, is the work of the public health nurse. Her objectives may be summarized as follows:

1. To stimulate early and regular care of well children by their own physicians or by public child health conferences.
2. To ensure that mothers carry out medical advice.
3. To give the mother sound instruction in the principles of nutrition.
4. To obtain maximum practicable sanitary conditions in homes of infants and young children.
5. To demonstrate preparation of food, and infant and child care in the home.
6. To guide mothers in gaining entree to clinics or to help in obtaining medical care for the child when the parents cannot pay for these services.
7. To develop community interest, understanding, and action in connection with general phases of the child hygiene program.

In obtaining public support, the nurse popularizes more or less specific undertakings, such as: birth registration; vaccination against smallpox, diphtheria, whooping cough, and perhaps other diseases; education about the danger of exposure of infants to measles, whooping cough, tuberculosis; dental care; pure milk supply; the need for community assistance to safeguard the health of children of poor parents.

In connection with the artificial feeding of infants, the public health nurse emphasizes the necessity for absolute cleanliness in the preparation of the formula: the sterilization of milk, water, and of all utensils. She stresses the necessity for accuracy in measurements of ingredients and of amounts for feeding, and teaches the aftercare of prepared food, and of sterilized bottles, nipples, etc. She demonstrates the convenience of assembling as a unit those articles to be used in preparation of the infant's food.

Accomplishments in Infant and Preschool Hygiene. Many forces have operated and continue to operate in a beneficial manner, as follows: (first) community sanitation, safe water supplies, pasteurized milk, freedom from flies, and improvements in general cleanliness and housing; these measures have been particularly effective in the prevention of dysentery; (second) the advances in medical knowledge and its better application by physicians, especially pediatricians; infants and young children today are protected against or recover from diseases that caused high fatality a generation ago; (third) better economic conditions, less want and privation; (fourth) an increasing educational level of parents, particularly in health education in relation to infant care.

Vaccination against smallpox has nearly eradicated what was once a disease of childhood in the United States. Diphtheria toxoid has been most effective in preventing diphtheria. Pertussis vaccine provides a considerable degree of protection against whooping cough, and tetanus toxoid has quite largely replaced the use of tetanus antitoxin, particularly since the development of the so-called DPT immunization procedure in which a combined diphtheria toxoid, pertussis vaccine, and tetanus toxoid immunization program has been developed. Typhoid vaccine offers some protection for children not living in a sanitary environment and more recently the development of the poliomyelitis vaccine program has offered real hope of a conquest of this disease. Thus, though much remains to be done in the protection of the health of the infant and child, much has been accomplished.

REFERENCES

American Academy of Pediatrics: *Child Health Services and Pediatric Education.* The Commonwealth Fund, New York, 1949.

Freeman, Ruth B.: *Public Health Nursing Practice*, 2nd ed. W. B. Saunders Co., Philadelphia, 1957.

Schlesinger, E. R.: *Health Services for the Child.* McGraw-Hill Book Co., Inc., New York, 1953.

World Health Organization: *Administration of Maternal and Child Health Services.* WHO Technical Report Series, No. 115, Geneva, 1957.

chapter 13

School Health Service

COMPULSORY EDUCATION LAWS impose definite responsibility on local government as well as upon parents. If the child must go to school, then government on its part must supply the school; and if there are any health hazards peculiar to school attendance, it becomes the responsibility of government to exert every reasonable effort to offset these hazards. In the discharge of this obligation school health service has been developed. Such a service may be said to present three aspects: (1) the strictly medical, which involves the prevention of disease, the discovery of physical or mental conditions which might handicap the school child, and the institution of a program for correction of such defects; (2) the educational aspect, which relates to basic instruction in health matters for the child and, to some extent, his parents (health education); and (3) sociological aspects, which imply a community responsibility for provision of a sanitary environment in the school, and for provision of treatment facilities for those school children whose parents are unable to pay for private medical care.

It must be confessed that to a great extent the medical and nursing aspects of school health service and the procedures involved have been caught in the grip of routinism. Probably more time is given to it than its importance justifies, especially when this importance is compared with that of other health problems. But school children can be easily reached, congregated as they are in classes; and prin-

263

cipals and teachers constituting one professional group, and physicians and nurses making up another, act and react upon each other in a way that occasionally brings about routine gestures not always purposeful. For these reasons one needs to keep an even balance and a clear perspective. School health work is well worth doing, but its conventional methods and assumed results need the purge of objective consideration.

In general, the greatest concentration of school health work is with children in the first eight grades. Children in these grades are from 6 to 14 years of age and constitute not more than 15 or 16 per cent of the total population. There is great need for health supervision of pupils of high school age, but work with these older children is usually limited to first aid, and examination of members of athletic teams.

Professional Personnel Participating in School Health Work. There are four major groups:

1. *Physicians.*
    a. Those who perform routine physical examinations.
    b. Those who do corrective work, either in private or clinic capacity.
    These two groups are entirely separate.
2. *Dentists.*
    a. Those who perform routine dental examinations.
    b. Those who do corrective work.
    Though such dental corrections as are made are done largely by private dentists, and dental clinics, the school dentist who routinely makes examinations may do a certain and necessarily limited amount of corrective work.
3. *Nurses.*
    Usually the same nurse who assists in school examinations and other work in the school visits the homes of the children where necessary.
4. *Teachers.*
    a. Regular classroom teachers who give formal health instruction from a text and stimulate an interest on the part of children and their parents.

b. Special health teachers, who concentrate largely on physical education and in teaching personal hygiene and nutrition.

In the large school systems there must be added professional workers in the field of mental health: psychiatrists, psychologists, psychiatric social workers.

The doctors, nurses, and dentists may be employed either by the department of education or the department of health, more frequently and desirably, by the latter. Special teachers in health education and physical directors are usually employed by the schools. Under such an arrangement the health department is responsible for the medical, dental, and nursing elements in the program; the schools being responsible for providing proper understanding of hygiene. The "health educator" or the classroom teacher gives general health instruction to pupils in groups; the doctor, dentist, or nurse gives it as applied to an individual under observation.

The places where this professional personnel does its work may be listed in this way:

In the schools. In city schools a suite or room is set aside for the doctor and nurse. In rural schools, the principal's office or a part of the classroom, partitioned off by sheets, is used. Routine examinations, special inspections, conferences with parents, and first aid are carried on in the school.

In the home. The nurse visits the home for the purpose of advising parents as to defects in children, as to diet and practice of health habits by children, in connection with sick absentees, and as a part of communicable disease work.

In doctors' and dentists' offices, clinics, and hospitals. The correction of defects is carried on in places equipped to perform the service needed, and usually these places are not connected directly with either the department of health or the department of education.

To the above places where school health work is done might well be added "in the community in general," for, in certain instances, every community resource must be brought to bear: social service, churches, parent-teacher associations, and other civic groups. General community interest and support is highly important for successful school health work.

The Physical Examination of School Children. In some places each child is given an examination each year. In general, an attempt is made to provide two to four examinations during the eight years of elementary school. The trend is to decrease the frequency with which children are examined, and to provide more time for consideration of children whose physical, nervous, or mental condition is regarded as unsatisfactory by nurse or teacher. Such children are referred to the school physician, who may, in turn, refer them to special clinics.

The first grade is always examined. Others might be the second and sixth, or the third and seventh or eighth. The essential objections to examining every child every year are that (1) it uses up a great amount of time which might be employed more profitably otherwise, and (2) tends to cause pupils, parents, and teachers, and sometimes even the doctors and nurses, to believe that the examination is an end within itself. Actually, it is but a means of determining which child needs attention. Instead of going on year after year, "discovering" the same defects in the same children, the greater amount of money and time should be spent in getting corrections made.

Certain equipment is needed for examination of school children. Assuming that quarters, washing facilities, and lighting are satisfactory, there will be needed:

1. Beam scales and measuring rod.

2. Vision testing cards, standard and letter E.

3. Wood tongue depressors, and a place to throw used ones; glass slides, which are only occasionally needed; sterile swabs.

4. Stethoscope, otoscope, flashlight.

5. Alcohol or some other disinfectant for use after examining children with scabies, conjunctivitis, etc., and for wiping off otoscope and similar uses.

6. Other equipment in accordance with examiner's desires: some use head mirror, pleximeter, sphygmomanometer.

7. Forms for record of findings.

8. Spotlessly clean apron for nurse and equally spotless coat for physician.

The general procedure in the examination is as follows:

1. Groups of eight or ten boys or eight or ten girls, at a time, are sent from the classroom to the physician's school office.

2. A record form, showing name, date of birth, sex, parents' names and address, classroom number and grade, is prepared if there is not already such a record. This is done by a teacher, older pupil, a neighborhood worker, or the nurse.

3. In the dressing room, the pupils remove clothing to the waist, drapes being used for older girls, and remove shoes.

4. They go to the nurse, who measures and weighs each, tests vision, perhaps hearing, recording findings.

5. The physician examines the eyes, ears, nose, mouth, throat, chest, abdomen, joints, glands, and skin, more or less carefully. He records the findings.

6. If defects are found, there is prepared a "notice to parents," advising them of the condition and recommending that the child be taken to a physician of choice or clinic for correction. In some systems parents are notified of the result of the examination even though no defects are found.

7. The teacher is advised of the findings on her pupils, with special recommendations as to seating, rest, lunch, etc.

The physical examination given at the school is not a complete one. It is usually done rapidly, is limited, and is designed for the quick discovery of the more common defects, rather than for a diagnosis of unusual conditions. It should be supplemented by regular and more detailed examination by the family physician or at a clinic.

The actual incidence of the various defects differs to some extent from place to place and as to the age of the children examined. The difference in types of examinations, and interpretation by a large number of physicians, further tends to make comparison of findings difficult. The summary below is only approximate:

Defective vision is found in from 5 to 15 per cent of the school children examined.

Defective hearing is found in 1 to 4 per cent.

Diseased tonsils are found in 15 to 30 per cent.

Decayed teeth are found in 50 to 70 per cent.

There is the occasional occurrence of serious orthopedic conditions, heart disease, arthritis, nephritis, tuberculosis, nervous and mental disturbances; and quite frequently the examiner finds mild degrees of flat feet, poor posture, underweight, poor nutrition, otorrhea, or simple goiter.*

Vision and the Eyes. In routine work, vision is tested by the Snellen test card, or some modification of it. The card has rows of letters, but only the letter E in various positions for those who do not know the alphabet. There are a number of different letters in each row and all letters in any one row are of the same size: smaller than the row above, larger than the one below. These rows are designated as the 20-ft row, the 30-ft row, and so on. A child with normal vision should be able rapidly to read the 20-ft row from a distance of 20 ft. He is placed this distance from the card, which has a good light but no glare upon it. The eyes are tested separately. The eye not being tested is covered with a card; not with the fingers, as this gives too much pressure. There should be a pause before testing the second eye. Children who have difficulty are tried with the large letters on the 30-ft row, then the 40-ft row. Findings are recorded as a fraction, the numerator representing the distance the child stood, the denominator the line read, such as 20/20 or 20/40.

The more common visual defects found are:

Myopia is the most frequent and tends to become more accentuated in older children, Handicapping myopia is readily discoverable with the routine vision tests used in schools.

Hypermetropia is not so frequently encountered as is myopia. Only the more severe grades are discoverable with vision tests in schools.

---

* Where there is a soil or water deficiency in iodine, as in certain areas in the region of the Great Lakes and in some mountainous sections, simple goiter is found frequently. In young children, it responds quite satisfactorily to minute doses of iodine.

Astigmatism will be discovered depending upon the degree with which it impairs vision or causes symptoms. Some degree of astigmatism is quite common and not infrequently occurs with myopia or hyperopia.

Strabismus is discovered usually by inspection rather than by testing the vision.

In addition to those defects which cause disturbance in vision, there are encountered others, not primarily concerned with the function of sight.

Conjunctivitis is quite frequently seen in connection with colds, measles, and local infections. The condition known as "pink eye" occurs in school epidemics. Gonorrheal conjunctivitis is occasionally encountered, and the phlyctenular conjunctivitis of tuberculosis is sometimes seen.

Diseases of the lids: only rarely is trachoma seen, except in localities where it is prevalent. Folliculosis, affecting the conjunctiva of the lids, is not infrequently encountered. Styes are fairly common, especially in children in the lower grades in school. Chronic infection, involving the hair follicles, may cause redness, irritation, and loss of lashes, especially lower.

Evidence of trauma: irregular pupils from old injury or disease, corneal opacities, and the end results of gonorrheal ophthalmia are occasionally seen. These usually affect vision.

Hearing and the Ears. Many school physicians and nurses routinely make a rough test of hearing by means of the watch tick or some clicking instrument, by spoken voice, or whispered voice. These methods are of but little value. They seldom elicit information not already possessed by the teacher. A much more reliable method is by means of electric devices, which conduct standardized sounds and tones to pupils through headphones. This method is rather highly satisfactory if properly done and interpreted. Unfortunately, the device is quite expensive and is not in as frequent use as the less satisfactory watch and voice tests.

Measures taken to correct conditions found depend upon the degree of impairment of hearing and upon the cause. In congenital deafness, little can be done except to modify methods of teaching, institute lip reading, attempt to have the child gain an appreciation of vibration and its rhythm, and provide occupational education. Where the cause is otitis media, which, as a sequel to some acute infection, is the most common cause of mild and moderate impairment, local treatment by a specialist and favorable seating in class are the measures adopted. Accumulations of wax in the external canal sometimes cause mild and temporary impairment of hearing. It is easily discernible by use of an otoscope as part of a routine examination. Occasionally a child's poor work in class is found to be due to impairment of hearing rather than to mental slowness.

The Teeth in School Children. The number of teeth that one would expect normally to find in the mouths of school children of various ages are set forth below by school grades. It should be borne in mind that these numbers refer only to what is usually found. In a number of instances an individual child might shed deciduous teeth and erupt permanent teeth quite early or somewhat late. Again, in the statements given below it is assumed that when a deciduous tooth is shed the gap will be replaced immediately by a permanent tooth. This is not always the case. Finally, girls tend to erupt permanent teeth before boys do, and this must be taken into consideration. Ordinarily a permanent tooth appears in the lower jaw before its opposite appears in the upper jaw.

First Grade. The child in the first grade, from 6 to 7 years of age, usually has 24 teeth. Of these, 4 are permanent: the first permanent molars which come in behind the temporary teeth. These are sometimes referred to as the "six year molars."

Third Grade. The 8- or 9-year-old child in the third grade will be found usually to have 24 teeth, but differing from the first grade child in terms of ratio between permanent and temporary teeth. Of the 24 teeth it is likely that 12 will be deciduous teeth and 12 will be permanent, for in addition to the 4 permanent molars, the child probably has 4 lower and 4 upper permanent teeth: incisors, central and lateral. These erupted shortly after the permanent molars. The deciduous or temporary teeth that remain are the 4 cuspids (the upper of which are sometimes called "eye teeth" and the lower "stomach teeth") and 8 deciduous molars: two upper on each side, 2 lower on each side between the cuspids and the first permanent molars.

Fifth Grade. The child is by now 10 or 11 years old. About one-fourth of the children this age will have erupted second permanent molars, which do not replace deciduous teeth. Such a child will, therefore, have about 28 teeth. The number of teeth in the majority of instances, however, will remain 24 or be even less if some deciduous teeth have been shed and have not yet been replaced by permanent ones. In general the situation will be about as follows: four of the 8 temporary molars (immediately behind the cuspids) will have been replaced by permanent bicuspids; sometimes all 8 of the temporary molars have been thus replaced. If this replacement of temporary molars has been complete, the only remaining deciduous teeth are the 4 cuspids or the so-called "eye" and "stomach" teeth, and sometimes at this age, particularly in the lower jaw, permanent cuspids will have replaced temporary ones.

Seventh Grade. Unless they are precocious or retarded, these children will average 12 or 13 years of age. The number of teeth is now 28. The second permanent molars (4, one on each side, upper and lower), have come in behind the first permanent molars. In the great majority of instances the temporary cuspids will have been replaced by permanent ones, though in some instances children are late in the eruption of the permanent cuspids, and one might see a gap between the lateral incisors and the bicuspids.

The "wisdom" teeth, 4 in number, erupt at about 17 to 20 years of age. Sometimes they do not come through the gum tissue. For convenience, Table 8 showing eruption of teeth by child's age, is set forth below. In using this table, one should bear in mind that the permanent teeth of girls erupt, on the average, 4 to 6 months earlier than do those of boys. It should further be remembered that ages and sequence, as given, represent what is usually found. One may not expect each individual child always to follow the average.

Dental caries is the defect most frequently encountered in children of school age. Unless the child comes from a family of unusual intelligence, and of means, one finds unfilled cavities in most of the deciduous or temporary teeth which have not been shed. In older children,

TABLE 8

ERUPTION OF PERMANENT TEETH ACCORDING TO AGE*

Tooth	Lower Jaw	Upper Jaw
First molar	6– 7 years	6– 7 years
Central incisor	6– 7 years	7– 8 years
Lateral incisor	7– 8 years	8– 9 years
Cuspid	9–10 years	11–12 years
First bicuspid	10–12 years	10–11 years
Second bicuspid	11–12 years	10–12 years
Second molar	11–13 years	12–13 years
Third molar	17–21 years	17–21 years

* Adapted from Kronfeld, Rudolf: *Dental Histology and Comparative Dental Anatomy.* Lea & Febiger, Philadelphia, 1937.

by the time most temporary teeth are gone, some of the permanent teeth have cavities: the first permanent molars and the first bicuspids, in particular. In girls the permanent teeth erupt earlier than in boys, and, at a given age, caries will be more frequent in girls than in boys. This higher incidence of decay appears to be due to the fact that the teeth have been longer exposed, and not to a proneness of girls to suffer from caries. The cleanliness of the child's teeth depends largely upon home teaching and example, but school programs will help.

Mottled enamel is a condition occasionally seen in the permanent teeth. It is due to interference with the formation of enamel of the teeth. The teeth may be dead white, brownish, mottled, or blackened and corroded, more marked in upper front. It is seen in the United States only in certain sections, and in some foreign countries. It is due to an excess of fluorine in water drunk during the period of formation of the dental enamel. As the enamel of the temporary teeth is rather completely formed at birth, these teeth do not show the condition. In the permanent teeth, however, enamel is in the process of forming in any given tooth some 5 or 6 years before that tooth erupts, and this foundation of enamel continues until a year or so before the tooth makes its appearance. It is in this developmental period that a dele-terious substance in the drinking water has its effect. Once the tooth is erupted, no damage appears to be done. Prevention lies in the change of the drinking water supply to one not injurious. It is not the mere presence of fluorine in drinking water that causes the damage, but rather the amount present. Research and demonstration indicate that small amounts of fluorine in drinking water are beneficial in preventing caries, and it has been added to water which lacks it, in the infinitesimal amount (not to exceed 1 part per 1,000,000 in drinking water) necessary in nutrition. Most responsible medical, dental, and public health authorities have endorsed the proposal as beneficial and without danger. A number of cities have put it into effect.

Almost routinely, teachers make a valuable contribution to public health by attempting to stimulate their pupils to an interest in mouth hygiene:

1. Through direct instruction as to structure, formation, and care of the teeth.

2. Through instruction as to the relationship of diet to teeth.

3. Through attempting to see that, in one way or another, each child is supplied with a toothbrush.

4. Through obtaining interest and cooperation of the respective parents concerned.

Some school systems have dentists or oral hygienists for examination of the teeth of pupils. Others must rely upon the not expert inspection made by the school physician. Facilities provided for correction of dental defects are quite inadequate in comparison with needs.

Tonsils and Adenoids. Diseased tonsils and formidable adenoids occupy a large proportion of the thought and interest of doctors, nurses, and teachers working with school children. Perhaps too much attention is paid to the throat. It seems difficult to strike that balance which would eliminate consideration of conditions not needing attention and yet give proper care to those cases with tonsils actually diseased or adenoids really causing trouble. The decision as to whether or not a given pair of tonsils is causing trouble must rest upon more than the mere appearance of the tonsils, and such a decision is a matter of clinical judgment. It should not be undertaken by nurses or teachers, but only by physicians, and even they do not invariably come to the correct decision. The figures as to the reported incidence of diseased tonsils, given on page 268, are quite conservative. Rarely would one, tabulating a thousand records of examinations of school children, find less than 20 per cent of tonsils recorded as diseased; more likely the tabulation would show that in the examiner's opinion, almost every fourth child ought to have his tonsils removed. In the recent past there has been a tendency toward a more conservative attitude as to removal of the tonsils.

Actually diseased tonsils may cause toxemia, lassitude, anemia, or malnutrition. There is a suggestive association between frequently recurring tonsillitis and rheumatic heart disease. Naturally these things are to be prevented wherever possible, and it is undoubtedly better to remove a dozen innocent pairs of tonsils than to miss the troublemakers. On the other hand, it may, with justice, be said that the school health program has been too strongly focused on the pharynx.

Skeletal and Orthopedic Defects. Occasionally one finds skeletal defects dependent upon old rachitic disturbances: squarish heads, funnel or pigeon chests, bowed legs. These are not usually in the nature of handicaps, and, with better nutrition in infancy, have become less frequent. There are also encountered orthopedic defects incident to local infections in bones or joints: tuberculous hips, osteomyelitis. These, too, are becoming more rare. Results of poliomyelitis are usually seen as semiparalytic impairment in the lower extremities. Congenital orthopedic defects or those due to accidents are occasionally found by the school physician.

In the ordinary school population, only about three or four children per thousand will evidence orthopedic defects handicapping in character or extent. Such cases should be put into the hands of specialists. Through special federal grants to states, most localities are able to arrange for expert care of children thus handicapped.

Heart Disease in School Children. Probably not over 1 or 2 per cent of school children give evidence of heart disease. The seriousness of the condition depends upon the underlying pathology. Congenital heart disease is quite serious, frequently fatal before the child reaches adult life. Acquired heart disease in children of school age is usually associated with rheumatic fever, tonsillitis, or one of the acute communicable diseases. Almost invariably the lesion is in the mitral valve, with some degeneration of the heart muscle. Sometimes there is an accompanying adhesive pericarditis. It is quite difficult, in the ordinary school examination, to distinguish between transient and permanent cardiac disturbances. Many children have heart murmurs which disappear in later life. Again, the specialist is needed.

Limitations of School Examination. The ordinary school examination is not likely to detect such conditions as nephritis, syphilis, malaria, leukemia, or intestinal parasites, unless symptoms are quite marked and indicate the need for more intensive study. The routine examination does not include examination of urine, stools, or blood. The school examiner might very easily pass as apparently healthy a child with pyelitis, at that time under the care of a physician. Nor is the school examination likely to bring to light the primary phase of tuberculous infection, as it does not, in ordinary circumstances, produce sufficient physical signs to permit localization except by x-ray. Not infrequently the school physician, being struck with a marked and chronic malnourishment in a child, will refer him to a tuberculosis clinic for further examination: physical, tuberculin test, x-ray.

Nutrition and Malnutrition in School Children. Too much importance has been attached to height-weight ratio as an index of health. While one may say that of a certain number of children examined, the "average" child of such an age and height weighed about so much, one cannot say that a given child of a certain age and height must weigh a particular number of pounds. Consideration must be given to racial stock, familial characteristics, body type, and whether or not the child under consideration is in a period when body length tends sometimes to increase more greatly than does weight. The fact that a child is continuing to gain in weight, even though slowly, is of more importance than the height-weight ratio.

Where weight is used as an index of malnutrition, from 15 to 20 per cent of children are classified as malnourished. This type of diagnosis is quite unsound in that many true cases of malnutrition are missed, while many others who are not really undernourished are assumed to be. Further, poor nutrition may be secondary rather than primary, having arisen as the result of some acute or chronic infection or other basic disturbance.

It should be borne in mind that there are many types of malnutrition, different each from the other, as typhoid fever is different from pneumonia. Each of the deficiencies may vary in degree, and may or may not be in combination with others. The matter is exceedingly complex, and medical science has only recently gained an insight into some of the factors concerned. The laboratory tests involved in determining the nutritional status are not yet simplified to a point where they may be applied in school health examinations and, in the circumstances, the school health service may serve only as a rough screen through which children suspected of malnourishment may be sent for further expert examination.

In connection with nutrition of the school child it is well to remember that enthusiasm and sincerity cannot take the place of scientific knowledge. With the best intentions, many foolish things have been said and done.

Posture in School Children. In any discussion of posture in children of this age one must differentiate between mere slouchiness and poor posture. The former is quite frequent and is probably normal for that age when pride in appearance and consciousness of posture are largely lacking. Poor posture, on the other hand, is a habitual deviation, in carriage, from what is considered normal for that age.

Where from 25 to 30 per cent of school children are found guilty of slouchiness, not more than 5 to 10 per cent will be found to have poor posture, if judged by rational standards (see discussion, page 228). Posture enthusiasts are not likely to accept the distinction made above.

Somewhat related to posture is flatfoot. Findings as to this vary from place to place. Possibly, in about half the examinations of school children, the physician attempts to run the tips of his fingers under the inner edge of the feet and the examination is but a cursory one. Unless the examiner has special ability in orthopedics, this procedure is of but little value. Further, while some of the school children on detailed examination will show what appears to be some deviation from the normal in either the transverse or longitudinal arch of the foot, few complain of symptoms referable to the condition. The arches seem much shallower in Negroes than in other children, but this is due more to soft tissue than to bony structure.

To make a proper examination of the feet would require more time and equipment than the frequency and seriousness of the condition at this age justifies, especially as time so spent would be at the expense of that part of the examination designed to discover the more common, important, and easily correctible defects. Many parents and some school systems, however, demand that some sort of examination be made for "fallen arches."

The Correction of Physical Defects. Community provisions for correction of defects in children whose parents are unable to pay for private medical service are limited at best; in some places, particularly in many rural areas, they are completely lacking. It is unusual for either the health department or the school authorities to supply these services directly, though there is a gradually increasing tendency for one or the other to have special clinics for eye and ear conditions, for heart conditions, for orthopedic cases, for dental work, occasionally and intermittently, for tonsillectomy. Most "free" corrections are through the hospital dispensaries and unpaid service of private physicians. Many public health authorities think that special facilities should be provided at public expense; most physicians oppose this idea. They feel that it would result in pauperism of persons able to pay and in unfair competition with physicians in private practice.

It is neither honest nor safe to paint, for parents, glowing pictures of future scholastic accomplishment for their child if they will but have his tonsils removed or his teeth filled. Persuasions should be on the basis of the physical welfare of the child. Obviously, if the defect has caused considerable absence from school, better attendance may help progress in studies; or, if the child is so toxic or malnourished as to make both mental and physical effort a serious task, the removal of the handicap would make study and interest a possibility. However, it should always be borne in mind that a certain number of children are dull, tonsils or no tonsils, and the most complete correction of defects in a child with limited mental capacity will not put him at the head of the class.

There can be no doubt that in some instances removal of defects has made a remarkable difference in the school child's accomplishments in class, but these are exceptional cases. It may not be assumed that this would happen in all cases.

Health Records of School Children. Each school child should have a record kept of his physical condition from year to year.

The shape, color arrangement, and content of school health records vary, but the following items should be considered:

1. Identifying data (name, date of birth, parents' names, address, etc.).

2. Significant facts in past history.

3. Record of findings of each examination, with date.

4. Cumulative record of current services or contacts with child (home visits, exclusions from school, communicable diseases, correction of defects).

Records should be so filed that they are at all times available for reference and the use of the nurse and school physician. In understandable phraseology, teachers should be notified of the findings on each child. The size of the school record is usually 5 by 8 in. A larger size is better. A good grade of paper is even more satisfactory than cardboard.

Lunches for the School Child. A midmorning lunch may be given from 9:30 to 10:30 depending on the opening hour of school. It consists usually of crackers and milk, is provided (1) for markedly undernourished children, and (2) for those who come to school without adequate breakfast. This is not provided in all schools, the interest of the principal and teachers and the availability of funds being the deciding factors.

The hot lunch is designed, in winter, to replace or supplement sandwich or cake the child brings from home or the candy and crackers which he buys. In large urban schools, it is practicable to provide hot lunches through a cafeteria system. Undernourished children, unable to buy lunch at the cafeteria, are tactfully supplied with tickets. Governmental subsidies have made school lunch programs more practicable and popular.

In small rural schools, the hot lunch depends upon the teacher's interest and upon the support of individuals in the community. The pupils are fortunate if they can get one hot dish—soup, potatoes, stew, or hot chocolate—and this is cooked upon the top of the stove used to heat the room. If the teacher is clever, part of the ceremony in the rural hot lunch is cleaning up afterward.

Rest and Recreation in the School Day, and Special Classes. More and more, efforts are being made to relieve the tedium of the classroom and to obviate the fatigue incident to study through properly spaced rest and play periods. In the lower grades these periods are quite frequent. In the upper grades they come less often but last longer: outdoor games, gymnasium work, recesses.

When properly handled, these nonwork periods result in more alert, teachable children. As collateral benefits, the children gain experience in teamwork and in self-control. They learn that there is such a thing as sportsmanship and may come to practice it in later life. Many city children, with no home yards to play in, are taught games which may be played on the sidewalk.

Separate classes are provided for the handicapped, and special equipment and devices are maintained. Frequently, the seriously handicapped children are grouped in a specially equipped and arranged school building. Classes commonly provided are (1) for the hard of hearing, (2) for the totally deaf, (3) for the blind, (4) for the mentally retarded, (5) for the crippled, and (6) for cardiac cases. Specially trained instructors and medical service are necessary. Children may be transported from and to their homes by buses. It is an expensive procedure, seen mainly in the larger cities.

The Prevention of Communicable Diseases in School Children. In this connection, laws, regulations, and practices vary from place to place. The measures outlined below reflect the general practice.

1. Most cities and some states require smallpox vaccination for school attendance.

2. Efforts are made to have children protected against diphtheria before entrance to school, but this is not generally a requirement for school attendance.

3. Pupils suspected of being in the early stages of a communicable disease are immediately excluded from school.

4. Children known to have been recently exposed to communicable diseases are either put under observation or temporarily excluded from school.

5. Children who are known to have had a communicable disease recently are carefully examined before readmission to school; a physician's certificate or health department permit may be required.

6. Children with unexplained absences are routinely inspected before readmission to their classes.

7. The sanitary facilities of the school, theoretically at least, are such as to inhibit the spread of the intestinal type of communicable diseases.

When the school nurse suspects a child in school of having a communicable disease, the general procedure is as follows:

1. The child is immediately separated from his fellow students, and the principal is notified.

2. If the school physician is to arrive shortly, the child waits under the nurse's supervision, for the decision of the physician.

3. If the physician is not expected, the child is taken to his home. Getting him home is a problem. He should go with the least exposure to others. He should not be allowed to walk if he is acutely sick. It frequently ends up with the nurse accompanying him home, taking him in her automobile if she has one. He should not be permitted to go alone, or with an irresponsible person, or with a susceptible. When an older brother or sister is in school this helps solve the problem.

4. The parents are notified, preferably on a form provided for this purpose, why the child has been sent home. The parents are advised to call the physician of their choice. If they are unable to do this, a physician of the health department visits the child for the purpose of diagnosis. He does not ordinarily give treatment.

5. Children from the same home may or may not be excluded from school, depending upon the disease and regulations.

6. The class which the child attended is watched for new cases.

When a brother or sister or other child with home exposure to a communicable disease may return to school depends (1) upon the disease, (2) upon the immunity status of the exposed child as regards the disease in question, and (3) upon whether or not it is practicable and permissible for the child to change place of residence temporarily. Public health regulations differ in the various states and cities, but in general, if the fact of immunity can be established, if change of residence is practicable, and if freedom from causative organisms can be demonstrated, as in diphtheria, the child may return to school after complete change of clothing, a shampoo, and a "disinfecting" bath.

If the exposed child is not immune he may be allowed to change residence and return to school after remaining at a new residence for a length of time equal to the average period of incubation of the disease. If the child is not immune and remains at home, he must, in the more serious diseases, remain away from school during the time the case is under isolation, plus a time equivalent to the period of incubation of the disease. The latter part of the requirement is not always observed.

In some places, because of public fear of certain diseases, as meningitis, poliomyelitis, smallpox, sometimes diphtheria or scarlet fever, children from a family where the disease exists are not allowed to come to school during the time a member of the family has that disease, regardless of immunity, change of residence, or any other precaution. On the other hand, a number of health departments impose no restrictions, or little restriction, on contacts of measles, mumps, chickenpox, whooping cough, and German measles.

Teachers, living in families where a communicable disease exists, are required to observe the same precautions as pupils.

In connection with the control of communicable diseases in schools, there occasionally arises a question as to whether or not the schools should be closed during an epidemic. Theoretically, if the school group is the focus, closure of the schools would separate those who are spreading the disease from those who are susceptible. Practically, when schools are closed, children continue to play with one another, patronize the movies, and are generally uncontrolled. For these

reasons it is believed by most health authorities that regular attendance, and daily inspection before the entrance to classrooms, will do
more to detect early cases and prevent spread than will closure of the
school. It is entirely possible that in exceptional instances closing of
a school will result beneficially, but when schools are closed it is
seldom on the merits of the case but in response to a somewhat
hysterical public opinion. Sometimes in rural areas, parents, through
fear, keep their children at home and attendance is so depleted that
there are not enough pupils to carry on schools.

Minor Infections and Infestations Seen among School Children.
Those more commonly encountered are the following:

Impetigo contagiosa is spread by direct contact and tends to become epidemic, especially in the spring. Ammoniated mercury ointment, 5 per cent sulfathiazole ointment, or 2 per cent gentian violet
solution, or covering with adhesive plaster, usually results in recovery.

Ringworm spreads slowly from child to child by contact. Cases are
sometimes resistant to treatment, which must be careful, complete,
and continuing. This is especially the case with ringworm of the scalp.
This is a stubborn condition, cure seeming to depend upon preliminary epilation. Painting with mild tincture of iodine or tincture of
Metaphen (nitromersol) is reasonably effective.

Pediculosis of head is usually a family affection, spreading in the
classroom. Most of the older and messy forms of treatment have given
way to the more effective dusting powders containing DDT (chloro-
phenothane).

Scabies spreads rapidly from child to child and within the child's
family. The following procedure is usually effective: a hot, soaking,
soapy bath; thorough inunction with sulfur ointment; clean sleeping
clothes, bedclothes, and clean underclothes next morning. Repeat the
whole procedure for three consecutive nights. Repeat the three-night
series in every detail, beginning one week from the last preceding
treatment. All members of the family probably need treatment.

These minor infections and infestations carry problems peculiar to
themselves:

1. Whether or not to permit children so affected to continue in attendance at school. The usual procedure is to permit children under effective treatment to continue in school, otherwise to exclude them.

2. In absence of the school physician, may a nurse make a diagnosis of impetigo, scabies, etc., and prescribe treatment? This problem is particularly acute in rural areas, where it is difficult for the nurse to get the medical assistance needed. An attempt to solve the problem is made by authorizing the nurse, if she *suspects* a child of having one of these conditions, to advise treatment previously outlined by the school physician or health officer for such "suspects." This is, in a way, a subterfuge, but very practical. Doctors are inclined to oppose treatment by any health department personnel, and not infrequently and with occasional justification, feel that such a practice is unfair competition by the health department and unethical performance by the nurse. On the other hand, few of the cases would go to a physician, and something must be done to prevent the spread of these conditions to others.

3. Many parents cannot afford to buy the simple materials necessary for treatment. In these circumstances the only relief comes from a school or neighborhood fund or a welfare organization.

4. Some parents, especially of children with pediculosis and scabies, fail to give cooperation. Occasionally the parents themselves have the itch or are lousy and are not concerned over a similar condition in the child. Here treatments at school or the exclusion of the child may be resorted to. But if parents will not help, the situation is a difficult one to be met only by ingenuity.

One discovers children who have minor infections and infestations in different ways. It may be incidentally in dealing with the child for some other purpose, or in cases referred by a teacher who suspects something. Cases may be discovered in routine "morning inspection," or as the result of special inspection of classes or familial contacts of a known case.

Morning Inspection in Classes. This is designed for quick discovery of any minor infections, infestations, and for determination of individual status as to personal hygiene. It is done in an orderly, drill-like manner, teacher or nurse and pupils performing their respective parts. It is time consuming and is not done in all schools. The routine varies, but, in general, is as follows:

1. The teacher, or nurse, stands in such a position that good light will fall on the children as they pass.

2. At a given word, the children rise, stand in the aisle, roll up their sleeves, and sometimes loosen the necks of their shirts or dresses.

3. At a given word, and in order previously directed, the children proceed single file to the inspector, pausing.

4. Each child extends hands and forearms, pronating and supinating; pulls down lower lids; lifts hair from over ears and back of neck (girls); pulls open collar. Some inspections include teeth for cleanliness and throat for inflammation.

5. The inspector does not touch the children with his hands. Suspects are asked to step aside for further inspection.

6. Children whom the teacher believes to have some communicable condition or whom she thinks are ill are referred to the school physician or nurse, or may be sent home.

First Aid in Schools. This service is rendered in schools, occasionally by the school physician, but more frequently by the nurse or teacher. The nurse's service is essentially in the nature of first aid if she is present in the school when the accident occurs. Other demands on her time make it impracticable for her to respond to calls to the school for such service.

The treatment to be applied in these minor injuries should be covered in a standing order by the school physician. The usual equipment needed in the school first-aid kit will be: bandage, gauze, cotton, adhesive plaster, mild tincture of iodine, boric acid ointment, zinc oxide ointment, sulfathiazole ointment, possibly sulfur ointment, and ammoniated mercury ointment. Perhaps some smelling salts and aromatic spirits of ammonia, used in fainting attacks, will convey a good impression; no aspirin, no bicarbonate of soda.

There should be two or three day beds or cots in the "hospital suite" for children or teachers suddenly taken ill.

The Public Health Nurse in the School. Because the public health nurse plays such an important part in school health work, it seems desirable at this point to summarize her activities:

1. She assists the physician in examination of the pupils.

2. During the examinations she usually tests vision and hearing and takes height and weight.

3. She makes a routine inspection of groups of pupils and special inspections of those sent to her by the teachers.

4. She assists teachers in stimulating pupils' interest in health matters; to upper grades she gives demonstrations in home hygiene and care of the sick.

5. She passes upon readmissions after absences, referring questionable cases to the doctor.

6. She visits parents in connection with problems of their children: need for correction of defects, personal hygiene, food habits, etc.

7. She attempts to get children entered in free clinics when parents are unable to pay.

8. She gives first aid in minor injuries.

9. She assists parent-teacher groups in their health work and otherwise develops community understanding and participation in the school health program. Item (9) is not nearly so dramatic as item (8) but is far more important.

The Practice of Health Principles. There should be inculcated in school children an understanding and practice of personal hygiene and preventive measures. These include an annual physical examination by a physician of the parents' choice, correction of defects found, a yearly visit to the dentist with necessary remedial work, reasonably frequent bathing, washing hands after toilet and before meals, covering the mouth when coughing or sneezing, brushing teeth, drinking milk, the inclusion of green vegetables and fruit in the diet, sufficient sleep, and outdoor play.

The technique of arousing and sustaining the interest in children of various ages in health habits draws upon child psychology and demands common sense, precept, and example on the part of the teacher. See also chapter on "Health Education and Related Activities."

School Sanitation. The essentials for a healthful environment in the school are:

1. Adequate and clean toilet and lavatory facilities.
2. Ample quantities of pure drinking water, distributed in a sanitary manner.
3. Abundance of light without glare.
4. Glareproof blackboards, ceiling, and walls.
5. Ventilation without direct drafts.
6. Dustless chalk, waxed or oiled floors.
7. Desks and chairs suitable to respective ages.
8. Rest and play periods for pupils.
9. Wholesome, nourishing food at lunch period.
10. Efficient janitor and cleaning service.

The usually prescribed environmental standards for school are as follows:

Playgrounds should be reasonably level, well drained, not completely shaded, with minimum of 30 sq ft per child.

Classrooms should have dimensions approximately 30 ft in length, 24 ft in width, 12 to 14 ft in height. The number of pupils in a classroom should be so limited that each child is provided at least 300 cu ft of air space and 15 sq ft of floor space.

Lighting should be provided from a total window-glass area not less than 20 per cent of the area of the floor and properly placed relatively high from the floor, and mainly on the left of the pupils. Expressed in terms of measured light, illumination on top of the desks should be equivalent to not less than 15–20 foot candles (see page 235).

Ventilation should be about 1800 cu ft per person per hour. Air conditions will be satisfactory in a not overcrowded classroom with window deflectors when temperature, air motion, and humidity are properly adjusted.

Temperature should be from 65° to 68° F. Temperature must be supplemented by adjustment of moisture and air movement.

Water should be provided by at least one approved type of drinking fountain for every 50 children.

Toilet facilities should include one toilet and one urinal to every 40 boys; one toilet to every 25 girls; and special provision for ventilation and janitor service in toilets.

School Children Are Relatively Healthy. Table 4, page 41, shows that less than 1 per cent of the total deaths are in the age group 5 to 14 years. As this group constitutes about 17 per cent of the population, it is obvious that school children are not subject to a high death hazard. The school age, however, is one where the accident hazard, as from automobiles and drowning, is relatively high, where the attack rate from communicable diseases is quite high, and where physical defects are common.

REFERENCES

Swanson, Marie: *School Nursing in the Community Program.* The Macmillan Company, New York, 1953.

Wilson, Charles C.: *School Health Services.* National Education Association and the American Medical Association, Chicago, 1953.

Schlesinger, E. R.: *Health Services for the Child.* McGraw-Hill Book Co., Inc., New York, 1953.

chapter 14

Chronic Diseases

THERE ARE CERTAIN diseases largely noncommunicable in nature, which because of one aspect or another, have important bearings upon the public health. In these diseases, the attending physician sees their effect essentially as they relate to the individual: pathology, symptomatology, the problems of treatment in this case or that. The public health agencies see them in the mass: their possible preventability through mass action or information, their prevalence and tendency to increase or decrease, their relative importance as causes of incapacity or death, their economic burden in loss of efficiency or loss of life, or cost of care of those incapacitated. Only a few of the more outstanding diseases or conditions of this sort are presented below.

One must be cautious in interpreting the following data and discussions which generally indicate an increase in these chronic diseases. A number of collateral, but important, factors need to be taken into consideration in comparing older rates with those of recent years. Modern diagnosis is more sensitive and reaches a greater proportion of those who are ill; chronic diseases tend to occur at and after middle age, and there is now a greater proportion of old people than heretofore. Important, too, in interpreting the present place of any disease as a cause of death in relation to the place it occupied a generation ago, one must bear in mind the fact that a decrease in the death rates in one disease causes another death rate, in which there has been no change, to constitute a greater proportion of total deaths than was previously the case. Also to be remembered is the fact that from time to time there have been changes in the ways in which diseases are classified for statistical purposes: a category in 1959 might be more or less inclusive than the same title indicated twenty years ago. Finally, it must be recognized that human beings must eventually die of *something*. If medical science and public health can gradually increase life expectancy and bring an increasing proportion of those born into the period of old age, then the occurrence of, and deaths from, these so-called degenerative diseases may with equanimity be accepted as natural and inevitable phenomena.

Cancer as a Public Health Problem. In clinical work the word "cancer" is used to designate a pathological condition (carcinoma) with specific characteristics which differentiate it from other malignant tumors. In vital statistics, the term used is malignant neoplasm. This is a classification rather than a designation of a specific condition. So used, it includes other malignant tumors in addition to carcinoma: sarcoma, hypernephroma, etc. In figures thus lumped for malignant disease, it is fairly safe to assume that about 95 per cent represent carcinoma, about 5 per cent sarcoma. Hypernephroma causes less than 1 per cent of the total cancer deaths.

Cancer is a public health responsibility because it affects relatively large numbers of people; because its frequency as a cause of death appears to be on the increase; because in some forms, in certain locations and in particular stages, fatal extension is preventable; and because systematized social action seems necessary in approach to the problem.

The cause of cancer is not known. Various theories have been evolved: that it is an infectious disease, that it is a hereditary disease, that it is incident to the diet of modern life, that it is due to chronic irritation. Experiments and statistical studies have been made in connection with each of these theories, but no single one has displaced all others. Three things, however, stand out: (1) in many individuals cancer appears to arise in that area where a long-continued irritation has existed; (2) cancer occurs in some tissues more often than in others, and certain irritants appear more than others to contribute to the origin of cancer; and (3) in lower animals, and to some extent in human beings, there seems grounds for belief that a tendency to cancer may be truly inherited.

One may obtain an idea of the trend of mortality in cancer and other malignant tumors by comparing death rates from these conditions, and from tuberculosis, over a period of years. From the figures below it is evident that tuberculosis operates as a cause of death less frequently, and malignant conditions more frequently, than formerly. In 1900 the tuberculosis death rate was more than three times that of "cancer." The one has fallen and the other has risen, so that the malignant disease death rate is now about six times as great as the death rate from tuberculosis.

Of the 247,357 deaths reported caused by malignant tumors in the United States in 1956, the digestive tract was the seat of the disease in about 36 per cent, the female reproductive organs in 9 per cent, the breast in about 9 per cent, the buccal cavity and pharynx in some 2

TABLE 8

DEATH RATE FROM MALIGNANT NEOPLASMS AND FROM TUBERCULOSIS, IN THE UNITED STATES REGISTRATION AREA, FOR CERTAIN YEARS IN THE PERIOD 1900–1956*

	Number of Deaths per 100,000 Population	
Year	Malignant Neoplasms†	Tuberculosis (all forms)
1900	64.0	194.4
1920	83.4	113.1
1930	97.4	71.1
1940	120.3	45.9
1950	139.8	22.5
1951	140.5	20.1
1952	143.3	15.8
1953	144.7	12.3
1954	145.6	10.2
1955	146.5	9.1
1956	147.9	8.4

* National Office of Vital Statistics: *Vital Statistics of the United States,* 1956. Government Printing Office, Washington, D.C., 1958.

† Including neoplasms of lymphatic and hematopoietic tissues.

per cent. Malignant disease of the respiratory system caused 13 per cent of all of the deaths that occurred from malignant tumors.

Malignant Tumors and Age. Malignant disease is essentially a disease of middle life and old age. That this common observation is correct is borne out by the age distribution of deaths. Although only about 30 per cent of the population is 45 years of age and older, 86 per cent of all deaths from malignant neoplasms are in that age group. In connection with this question it should be remembered (Table 4, page 41) that of all deaths from all causes, at all ages, about 83 per cent occur in the age group 45 years and older.

Malignant Disease and Sex. What is generally designated as cancer has in the past been more frequent among women than men. In 1900 the male death rate was 47 deaths per 100,000 males in the population. The corresponding rate in females at that time was 81 per 100,000. However, in the past fifty years there has been a significant shift in the mortality rates in the two sexes until in 1950 there was actually a slightly higher mortality rate among males than among females, the rates being 117 per 100,000 for males and 113 per 100,000 for females. In 1956 these rates were, males 158, females 137.

Among males, malignant disease of the prostate is one of the most important causes of death, and in females, cancer of the uterus is the most important cause. In regard to organs common to both sexes, malignant disease of the stomach, rectum, pancreas, buccal cavity, and respiratory system is in general more common among males. Malignancy of the small intestines occurs slightly more often in females and cancer of the breast occurs almost exclusively among females. In the past two decades there has been a marked increase in primary cancer of the lung, particularly in males. There is increasing evidence of an association between smoking and the occurrence of primary cancer of the lung although there is general agreement that there probably are a number of factors.

Malignant Disease and Race. Fatal malignant disease is relatively more frequent in white persons than in Negroes, though this difference is growing less. Thus in 1940, death rates from malignant disease were 78 for Negroes and 125 for whites. In 1956 these rates, respectively, were about 118 and 151. Perhaps this change is due more to diagnosis than to change in innate racial reaction to malignancy.

Malignant Disease and Place of Residence. Place of residence appears to have some influence on the incidence of malignant tumors, but this may be more apparent than real. Generally, the death rate is higher in urban than in rural communities, and somewhat higher in northern than southern climates. On the other hand, the incidence of skin cancers is seen more frequently in those whose living keeps them in the sun, or those who, by work, are exposed continuously to chemicals and irritants that are considered to contribute to malignant conditions. As in the race difference in cancer, the availability of diagnostic facilities doubtless plays some part in the difference in death rate between urban and rural dwellers.

The Objectives in Cancer Control Programs. The ultimate objectives are, of course, to prevent illness and to decrease the death rate from cancer. These objectives, however, may be approached only through certain intermediate steps, the most important of which are the following:

1. To teach the public.

2. To influence the development of special cancer clinics, private and public, where there are ample provisions for diagnosis and treatment.

3. To influence the medical profession to make use of these special clinics in both diagnosis and treatment.

4. To encourage government and philanthropic support of institutes for cancer research, and to emphasize the need of experts in research.

What the Public Should Be Taught about Cancer. The particular points which should be impressed upon the public are:

1. The ordinary danger signals, such as lumps in breast, abnormal vaginal discharges or bleeding, unexplained indigestion and loss of weight, chronic ulcers, pigmented moles, etc.

2. That these danger signals are more likely to be significant in those about, and past, middle age.

3. That periodic and thorough examination of the adult is particularly worthwhile in this connection.

4. That any of the danger signals demands thorough examination by a competent physician.

5. That hope for recovery from cancer depends upon early diagnosis and appropriate treatment.

6. That quacks and persons who guarantee results should be avoided.

Difficulties in Obtaining Results. Results in programs for cancer control are not yet sufficient to have improved the situation. Among the difficulties are ignorance and lethargy of the public, human dread of learning that cancer is present, and the feeling that to have the disease is to be disgraced. It must be remembered, too, that in many instances none of the "danger signals" is seen until the condition is somewhat advanced; that many physicians are inadequately equipped, by knowledge, experience, and facilities, to make complete examination and diagnosis, or in certain types of cancer, for adequate treatment of the case; finally it must be admitted that even in the best circumstances, there are definite limitations in scientific knowledge and as to what can be done for the patient.

These are, perhaps, some of the reasons why "cancer control" programs were not much emphasized in this country until comparatively recently. Governments in many of the European countries, especially the Scandinavian, have undertaken this work seriously, as have some of the states and a few cities in the United States. However, clinics, institutes, radium, and other equipment are quite costly, and public opinion has not been such as to encourage legislatures and similar bodies to make large outlays of funds for these purposes.

The establishment of the National Cancer Institute as part of the U.S. Public Health Service indicates an interest in the problem and an acceptance of some responsibility on the part of the federal government; and the broadening and intensification of research and an increasing interest of the public are encouraging.

Heart Disease and Associated Conditions as Public Health Problems. The proportion and number of persons recorded as dying from heart disease is increasing. The trend of this mortality is shown in Table 9. In interpreting these data one must bear certain facts in mind: that the proportion of persons 45 years of age and older has increased greatly since 1900, that the term "heart disease" now includes diseases of the coronary arteries where formerly it did not; that diagnosis is now better, and diagnostic facilities more available. Further, it must be noted that the term "heart disease" is a somewhat inclusive term, like mental disease, and that much of the heart disease encountered in older persons arises as part of a general hypertension or arteriosclerosis. However, in spite of these cautions and qualifications, a rise in rate from 137 in 1900 to 360 in 1956 is definite and significant. More than one out of every three deaths is due to heart disease. The number of deaths is more than twice that due to any other single cause.

TABLE 9

DEATH RATES FROM HEART DISEASE IN THE UNITED STATES, OR
UNITED STATES REGISTRATION AREA, FOR CERTAIN YEARS
IN THE PERIOD 1900–1956*

Year	Number of Deaths per 100,000 Population
1900	137.4
1920	159.6
1930	214.2
1940	292.5
1950	355.5
1951	355.8
1952	356.4
1953	360.2
1954	347.5
1955	355.8
1956	360.5

* National Office of Vital Statistics: *Vital Statistics of the United States,* 1956. Government Printing Office, Washington, D.C., 1958.

Ninety-six per cent of all deaths from heart disease* in the United States in 1956 occurred in the approximately 30 per cent of the population 45 years of age and over. Death rates are higher in males than

* This term here used, relates to those conditions—Nos. 410–443—designated in the 1955 revision of the *Manual of the International Statistical Classification of Diseases, Injuries, and Causes of Death.* World Health Organization, Geneva, Switzerland 1957.

in females. No small part of this difference is due to the preponderance of deaths from diseases of the coronary arteries in males. In general, white rates are higher than those of nonwhites.

The Causes of Heart Disease. These may be listed as follows:

1. Congenital.
2. The acute communicable diseases, particularly diphtheria, scarlet fever, and pneumonia.
3. Acute rheumatic fever.
4. Syphilis.
5. Associated conditions.

Congenital heart disease, due essentially to a developmental defect in fetal life, usually produces "blue babies." Here not enough blood goes through the lungs for oxygenation. The more severe types usually result in early death. Modern surgery offers some promise, but prevention must depend upon new knowledge as to the true cause of the condition and why it develops in utero. Research and more research is, therefore, of prime importance.

Heart disease due to the communicable diseases is decreasing because the infections from which it arises are decreasing. Not only are diphtheria, streptococcal infection, etc., less frequent, but when cases of these diseases do occur, modern treatment ordinarily prevents extension of damage to the heart.

Acute rheumatic fever has long been the principal cause of heart disease in children and young adults, and most of the cardiac disabilities and deaths that occur before the age of forty are of rheumatic fever origin. Here, as in the acute communicable diseases, the antibiotics play an important role in prevention of extension. Cases thus treated have less ferquent attacks of rheumatic fever and less cardiac involvement. As a result, and because of other factors not completely understood, deaths from heart disease of rheumatic origin are decreasing markedly.

Thus less than a half century ago, in persons from 5 through 24 years of age, rheumatic fever, with its concomitant heart disabilities, was reported to have caused nearly 30 deaths per year in each 100,000 persons of that age group. As nearly as can be estimated at present, the similar rate is around 5 deaths per 100,000.

However, even though this decrease is gratifying, it does not affect the heart disease situation, as a whole, to any great extent, for deaths incident to rheumatic heart disease constitute only a small proportion (about 3 per cent) of the total deaths from heart disease.

Heart disease due to syphilis manifests itself in middle life and old age. It is part of a process which involves the cardiovascular system, particularly the aorta and heart. Inasmuch as syphilis can now be more satisfactorily treated than in the past, it is reasonable to believe that there will be a decided decrease in cardiac disabilities from this cause as the present younger generations move into middle and old age. Here, again, the action in controlling heart disease is preventive.

Conditions associated with heart disease are essentially hypertension, arteriosclerosis, and certain types of kidney disease. These conditions and heart disease are frequently grouped together as "cardiovascular-renal diseases." Because of their importance per se, as well as in connection with heart disease, they are discussed separately below.

Hypertension and Arteriosclerosis. These conditions, with heart disease and the degenerative kidney diseases, account for a little more than half the deaths from all causes. Of the deaths in this group of diseases more than 70 per cent are due to heart disease, about 25 per cent to hypertension and arteriosclerosis, and 4 per cent to chronic nephritis, and other cardiovascular diseases.

In considering the cardiovascular diseases, it is necessary to remember that, although the heart is involved to a greater or less degree whenever there is high blood pressure or arteriosclerosis, the manifestations of these conditions are not limited to the heart. Thus one may have a stroke (apoplexy) or mental disturbance as the blood vessels of the brain become seriously affected. At the other extreme, narrowed blood vessels may so interfere with circulation in the leg as to cause gangrene. This, however, is relatively a rare manifestation as compared with a brain lesion.

Inasmuch as hypertension, and particularly arteriosclerosis, occur mainly after early life, heart diseases associated with them are found more in the old than in the young.

Another organ involved in cardiovascular pathology is the kidney. Hence many deaths, recorded as due to disease of the kidney are really chargeable to this generalized disease of the blood vessels, and must be included as part of the picture.

Causative Factors in Hypertension and Arteriosclerosis. These two conditions are closely related. In the early stages of either, one might exist without the other but generally, as hypertension advances, some degree of arteriosclerosis occurs; and as the arteries become less elastic and narrower in arteriosclerosis, there is usually an increase in the blood pressure.

Hypertension, where there is no arteriosclerosis, appears to depend upon some imbalance in the endocrine glands, with the adrenal glands particularly involved. Abnormal impulses through the sympathetic nervous system appear also to play a role in the so-called "essential hypertension." Surgery is now employed, and reasonably successfully, in cutting some of these nerve fibers leading to the kidney. Recent research suggests that cholesterol, eaten as animal fat, may play an important part in the development of arteriosclerosis, but its true significance is not yet determined. Similarly, the cumulative effect on the heart and arteries from imbibing copiously of alcohol year after year, or of a life of marked and continuing muscular strain are not entirely known, although there are some firm opinions as to the former.

The Control of Heart and Arterial Diseases. As indicated previously, there has been an improvement in certain aspects of the heart and cardiovascular situation. Inasmuch as heart disease usually arises (except in the congenital type) secondary to some other condition, the key to control through prevention is to eliminate or reduce the contributing factors. This would leave for treatment only those not prevented.

Heart damage from the acute communicable diseases is definitely declining, as is that from rheumatic fever and syphilis. Not much of a preventive nature may be looked for in heart damage that arises from hypertension and arteriosclerosis until there is a better understanding as to cause and control of these conditions. It is known that disease of the vascular system is associated with certain conditions and situations, as referred to above, but there is a great need for more knowledge. The American Heart Association, the federal government, universities, and other research agencies are engaged in, or supporting, strong research programs in the search for this newer knowledge.

An important part of the movement for research and control of cardiovascular disease is public understanding and participation. This is coming, at an encouraging rate, from voluntary health associations. Through their vigor and foresightedness, more than through the official health agencies, community diagnostic facilities are being increased, rehabilitation programs are under way, and rather good health education programs are being carried on.

Diabetes as a Public Health Problem. Diabetes mellitus is not generally regarded as of public health significance, though it is estimated that about 1.0 per cent of the population has the disease, and in the United States in 1956 of those who died from all causes (1,564,476), nearly 2 per cent (26,000) were reported as dying from diabetes mellitus. The mortality rate in 1956 was 15.7 deaths per 100,000 population. It is largely a disease of midlife and after, being more frequent in females than in males, in white persons than in Negroes. Hebrews appear to be unusually susceptible (heredity seems a factor), and there is an association between diabetes mellitus and overweight.

This disease is one of those which regular medical examinations may bring to light in incipiency. It is, further, one where the individual with a tendency to high blood sugar, to overweight, may by a sensible regime hold the disease in abeyance. Fashion's demands that the well-dressed person remain slim, particularly women, may, if continued, make an antidiabetic contribution.

REFERENCES

Commission on Chronic Illness: *Chronic Illness in the United States.* Published for the Commonwealth Fund by the Harvard University Press, Cambridge, 1956.

chapter 15

Medical Care

ORDINARILY, WHEN ONE refers to measures which protect and maintain the public health, it is assumed that these measures are carried out by health departments and other public health agencies. This is only partly correct, for no small part of the preventive procedures of a modern public health program comes within the sphere of the practicing physician, and it is he, above all else, who attends the sick in home, clinic, and hospital. Even if the function of treatment were the only measure carried out by the private physician, it is well to remember that the prevention of death in the ill, and the return of the ill to as nearly normal as possible, are matters of vast importance in the health of the community and nation.

Consideration of these matters has led to a question of whether or not under the present private practitioner system, the people are receiving adequate medical care, and for more than a quarter of a century, this has been a highly controversial issue. As would be expected, extremists have been vocal, pro and con: some have maintained that the present system, from root to fruit, is without mar or blemish; their opponents have felt that the whole growth was diseased and should be uprooted and succeeded by a new planting of government-issued seed.

The student should be warned that not only is this a highly controversial subject, but one in which it is difficult to evaluate and interpret what seem to be pertinent facts and factors. It is difficult, too, to obtain an unbiased statement even from those who have given long thought to the matter.

The Private Practice System of Medical Care. The arrangement between the physician (or the dentist or nurse) and the patient is essentially a private one: the patient employs whatever physician he wishes or is able to employ, at such times and in such circumstances as the patient may feel the need of service and is able to pay for it. The physician attends the patients for as long as the arrangement is mutually satisfactory, has responsibility to no authority other than the patient, looks to him and him alone for payment.

Government does not at all enter into this private arrangement, except that the physician must be duly licensed to practice medicine in the state in which he is located, and must, of course, observe the laws of the state as to such practice. Should he exhibit what the patient regards as carelessness or neglect or incompetence, that patient may attempt to recover through the courts on a malpractice charge. Should the patient prove unable or unwilling to pay for service rendered, the physician may follow the usual civil procedure of creditor versus debtor in an attempt to collect. It may be said that malpractice suits are quite unusual, as is court action by the physician in an attempt to collect a bill.

This private system of practice safeguards individual liberty, permits competition, free enterprise, and freedom of choice in their most desirable forms. They leave the physician untrammeled in the exercise of his discretion, initiative, and skill. Assuming that in one way or another, those unable to pay regular fees would nevertheless be cared for, and assuming further an adequate supply of competent physicians and other medical resources, this basis should produce the most effective and satisfactory type of service and be particularly adapted to the unique and intimately personal relationship which is essential between physician and patient.

Supplements to Private Practice. Although physicians in private practice have always given care to many of the needy without charge, there have long been physicians for the poor. Thus in cities there were ward physicians, dispensary physicians, hospital externes, etc. The physicians employed, by salary or fee, for this office and home care were seldom the best in the community. Actually many of them obtained their appointments by political preference. This was rather markedly in contrast with the type of physician who gave medical care to the poor in hospitals. Here at the bedside and in operating room, the best of the medical profession labored, and continues to labor, without fee from the poor or charge to the city.

The more modern counterpart of the physician to the poor is the physician who cares for persons under the aegis of the department of welfare. In most places, such medical services are none too well organized.

Another supplement to private medical practice are the services extended to those employed by government, or for whom government is immediately responsible: armed forces, veterans services, certain civilian groups eligible for care by U.S. Public Health Service, state mental hospitals, and penal institutions. The physicians and other professional personnel concerned in this type of service are remunerated by government.

The workmen's compensation commissions of the various states are government-directed, and designed, among other things, to ensure medical care for those injured in employment, with fairness to employee and employer. Broadly speaking, it is an insurance scheme, the employer paying the fees. Physicians who serve are chosen in a number of different ways.

Some labor unions have developed strong and comprehensive medical care programs for their members and their families. Support is, in most cases, derived from what are usually called "fringe benefits" in the contract with the employers: for each unit manufactured or produced, a small amount of money goes into a welfare, health, or medical fund. This movement is of great significance, in that on the one hand it breaks away from private practice and, on the other, builds a wall against government medicine.

Industry has also set up schemes for medical care of its employees. In their simplest forms these are first-aid services as part of an industrial hygiene program. In the last two decades, the scope of some of these services has broadened into a nearly comprehensive medical care program: office, clinic, home, and hospital. The strongest of these undertakings are supported by employee and employer jointly, with prepayment and other elements of insurance against future risks.

A relatively small proportion of the population insures itself against the costs of illness through payment of premiums to commercial insurance companies. The coverage obtained through such policies varies: from rather complete, to those so circumscribed that one might receive benefits only if injured in most unusual and bizarre circumstances. In such policies, the person may choose his own physician, but with a provision for scrutiny of the claims as to disability by a physician of the insurance company's choice.

In a category somewhat different from the above which are designed to serve special groups rather than the general public, are the Blue Shield plans sponsored by medical societies and comparable plans, independent of medical societies but operated upon a nonprofit basis. In both of these, prepayment and the insurance principle are observed.

The Blue Shield plan is, in effect, the medical profession's attempt to meet the demand for a modernization of medical practice; a system wherein the insurance principles of pooled risks, with prepayment provision against sickness, is observed.

Blue Shield, while operating now in all states, is not a national organization. The undertaking, in any given state or county, is under the auspices of the concerned medical society. All Blue Shield groups observe basic requirements, ethics, and limitations broadly laid down by the American Medical Association, but fees and terms of membership and benefits vary from place to place. This variability has caused some difficulty. An industry may wish to give all its employees the benefits of Blue Shield. Perhaps this is a fringe benefit, negotiated under contract with a labor union. The industry, however, has employees in a number of states. The Blue Shield groups in these states have varying terms and benefits. It is impossible for the industry to give smaller benefits to different employees. Measures are now under way for resolution of this difficulty.

Another limitation in the Blue Shield plan is that coverage is concerned mainly with catastrophic illnesses, essentially where surgery is involved, but does include maternity cases. The patient has the choice of any physician who has indicated willingness to participate; and this being a medical society sponsored plan, most physicians cooperate. Further, there is a limitation on membership in that those in higher income brackets are not eligible.

Other voluntary, nonprofit schemes have developed, stemming from the old "cooperatives" in concept, but more formally organized and operated. Perhaps the outstanding of these is the Hospital Insurance Plan of Greater New York (HIP). This scheme observes the insurance principle, provides care in a wide variety of illnesses, in office, home, and in hospital. It does not itself undertake the hospital insurance element, but attempts to ensure this through coordination with the Blue Cross system. The Health Insurance Plan of New York serves employed groups, the employer acting as collecting agent, deducting from payrolls (on authorization of employee) and contributing half the cost. HIP operates through units of physicians organized into general-practitioner-specialist groups, paying the group so much per year per person carried by the group, regardless of whether he remains well throughout the year or is a chronic invalid.

Hospitals and Hospital Insurance. The American Medical Association makes a census of hospitals from time to time. In 1957, there were a little more than 7000 hospital "facilities"—hospitals, or hospital units within some institutions. These provided approximately 1,700,000 beds, plus a little more than 89,000 bassinets. Most of these hospitals were for general purposes, including the usual complementary special services. Hospitals for nervous or mental illness made up 9 per cent of the total, and 7 per cent were for tuberculosis. But because mental disease hospitals are usually quite large, nearly 50 per cent of all available hospital beds in the nation are for such cases. About 70 per cent of the hospital beds are in government institutions: local, state, federal, with state governments responsible for nearly 50 per cent of the total.

Voluntary hospitals occupy an important role in this field. Although numerous, they provide less than a third of the hospital beds. In general, the voluntary, nonprofit hospitals have exhibited the highest standards and performance, though with rising costs their future is not bright.

Of great influence in expanding and stabilizing hospital development is the Hill Burton Hospital program, under a federal law passed in 1946. This act, in effect, offered financial aid to the states in hospital construction. The plan required that, if a state wished to participate, it must study its hospital problem as a whole, lay down a state-wide plan, meet most urgent needs first, provide proper machinery for administration of the scheme, and for ensurance of high standards of operation. States received funds in proportion to population but also in a ratio inverse to per capita income. Not more than one half of costs could be placed against federal funds. Private nonprofit hospitals, as well as public hospitals, were made eligible.

Another constructive feature of this federal aid scheme is that many rural or small town areas, because the need was great, got priority in construction of hospitals. Further, state schemes provided for inter-relationships between hospitals of various sizes, from peripheral small hospitals to medical centers.

Hospital insurance, on a broad scale, is typified by the Blue Cross plan, a prepaid hospital insurance scheme. The public has responded quite remarkably to this method of offsetting most hospital costs by prepayment and at mid-century nearly half the population of the United States had insurance in Blue Cross or insurance companies. The movement is growing and is carried along in close coordination and cooperation with prepayment plans for medical care.

Medical and Allied Personnel Available. At mid-century, there were a little over 200,000 physicians in the United States. Nearly 90 per cent of these were engaged in community practice. The remainder were in federal service, other salaried positions, or inactive.

The proportion of physicians to population is increasing: in 1925 there were 125 physicians per 100,000 population; at present, it is approximately 135. These physicians are not, however, ideally distributed over the United States; there is a tendency to concentrate in urban areas. Such concentration is not so much a matter of better income in cities, for most young physicians in cities must go through a long period of lean living while their classmates who went to small towns have become prosperous and remain so. The lures of the city are facilities and associations: hospitals, clinics, libraries, participation in teaching and research, the stimulus of association with leaders. Better hospital facilities and an interrelationship between small and large hospital staffs are already carrying more competent young physicians into rural and small town practice.

Dentists in the United States number about 100,000, most of whom are in active practice: 59 per 100,000 population.

The American Nurses' Association shows that in 1951 there were something over 366,000 registered nurses in active civilian practice, exclusive of those retired or federally employed. About 25,000 nurses graduated that year. It is estimated that for civilian nursing work there are nearly 230 nurses per 100,000 population.

Dentists and nurses tend to concentrate in urban centers as do physicians. But in this matter of concentration, it should be remembered that rapid transportation, the telephone, etc., make it possible for much wider coverage of a geographic area by professional people than was formerly the case.

It is probably sound to say that the country could advantageously use more physicians and allied personnel. It is not true, however, that the supply of physicians is dwindling. It is proportionately higher than a quarter century ago, and this applies to other personnel. Medical schools, which graduated about 6,000 physicians a year in the 1930's, now graduate about 7,000.

Group Practice versus Solo Practice. Medicine, traditionally, has been practiced by the individual physician, utilizing his own knowledge, skill, and resources, calling a consultant from time to time, or sending the patient to the hospital to remain under his own care, or under a surgeon's care, or under care of the hospital staff.

The complexity of medicine, the fact that one person cannot encompass all the highly specialized knowledge or provide all the equipment necessary, has led first to specialization and an increasing tendency of physicians to practice in groups. Usually, the core of the group are general practitioners, with specialists associated in one office. Such an arrangement is economical in use of space, equipment, time, etc. When properly operated, the cost to the patient is less and the quality of service better.

It seems likely that group practice will become more and more the practice of the future. It is, however, somewhat more impersonal than the family doctor; it makes the physician a partner in a firm rather than privately a professional and, in most instances, brings him in less financial return than as an individual. One should not, therefore, look for too quick a change from solo to group practice as long as a considerable proportion of the public is satisfied to employ the physician practicing alone.

Free Choice of Physician. It is generally conceded that the individual should have the same freedom in choosing his physician as he would in choosing his grocery store or a new hat; that, actually, it would be less damaging to have an unbecoming hat forced on one's head than an unsatisfactory physician foisted on him. Nevertheless, freedom of choice of physician is a vague and somewhat tricky term. Very few now have such complete freedom of choice. First, the particular physician may not be able to serve them or not wish to. Second, the patient may be far removed geographically from the physician he would like to have. Third, the physician's fees may be outside the patient's financial reach. Among other deterrents to free choice, too, is that the physician desired may be the head of a large clinic, and persons attending the clinic because of his name might never come in contact with him. In the latter circumstances, of course, they have gone voluntarily to the clinic, consciously yielding the personal choice of physician.

Again, as an offset to the argument that each individual must have freedom of choice of physician are the facts that some of the best medicine in the nation is practiced in the large hospital clinic; that the public has no way of judging the competence of physicians; that it is better to get well in the hands of a strange doctor than to die under the care of a known one. But in spite of these arguments, there is a fundamental consideration that goes beyond the question of convenient administrative methods, efficiency, logic, and theory. It is this: the deprivation of the citizen of reasonable and practicable choice of his physician would be a dangerous procedure, leading toward a flaccid and subservient citizenship.

The Insurance Principle in Payment for Medical Service. It is only the quite well-to-do who can take a medical bill in their financial stride. This is particularly and distressingly so when the bill is for some devastating illness, of long duration or high cost. There has now been accumulated sufficient recorded experience to forecast, on a sound actuarial basis, about how much sickness may be expected per thousand persons, and risks can be translated into insurance premiums. There is thus a growing popularity for the prepayment medical programs.

But the mere fact that insurance programs are available did not lead promptly to action on the part of the public, for human nature is not such that all people will, month after month, pay such premiums. Further, to give protection to persons of all ages, the young and healthy as well as the half sick and old would have to pay premiums, for the expectancy of illness varies with age, sex, occupation, economic status, etc. Two solutions offered themselves: (a) compulsory insurance, under legal requirement, and (b) voluntary insurance, but with monthly payroll deductions authorized by the participant. The first of these alternatives is discussed under a separate heading, below.

Voluntary insurance, through payroll deductions, is gaining strong momentum in the United States. The arrangement is that the employer and employee each pay half of an amount necessary to insure the worker and his family against the cost of sickness, exclusive of hospital costs. The insured is usually encouraged to enter also into a hospital insurance scheme (Blue Cross) for which similar payroll deductions are made. The amount and diversity of medical care that one receives depends upon the group carrying the insurance. He may be insured against high surgical costs, or have an almost comprehensive coverage. In some instances, persons in the higher income brackets are not eligible or must pay a higher premium.

One of the drawbacks to this scheme is that it is limited largely to the employed in groups. The self-employed are not generally eligible. A second difficulty is that there must be some limitation on choice of physician for, obviously, one could not call upon a physician who is not a part of the scheme. A physician might remain outside because of choice on his part or on the part of the insuring organization.

The Growth of Hospital and Medical Care Insurance in the United

States. There has been a spectacular growth in hospital and medical care insurance in the United States particularly during the past 15 years. The increase in insurance against the costs of disease has been greatest in the program of insurance against hospital expense. Since 1940 the number of persons with hospital expense insurance has increased from 12,000,000 to 116,000,000. More people have hospital insurance than any other form of health insurance. There is considerable variation in the benefits provided by different types of insurance. For the most part the Blue Cross program of hospital insurance meets all or nearly all of the costs involved, whereas among the insurance companies the completeness of the coverage of hospital costs depends upon the kind of policy one has: they are not all the same. The rapid increase in this type of insurance, however, clearly demonstrates the interest of the American people in providing for the costs of hospitalization through insurance. There has been a general tendency in recent years to broaden the coverage under all types of hospital insurance; in keeping with rising costs these policies provide much larger payments toward all hospital charges than in the beginnings of the voluntary hospital insurance programs.

A markedly increasing number of people also have insurance against surgical expenses. In 1956, 101,000,000 Americans had surgical expense insurance. Here again there is a trend toward more liberal provision for the expenses of major surgery. This protection is provided by Blue Shield programs and by insurance companies. A new and growing type of health insurance is what is called regular medical expense protection. The extent of coverage under regular medical expense insurance differs markedly under differing plans. Under regular medical expense protection there is provision for payment toward doctor's fees, for visits in the hospital, home calls, or office visits. Other policies provide protection against only major medical expense, with usually some provision for a deductible amount paid by the individual. From the standpoint of the insured person, in both surgical expense protection and regular medical expense protection there is much to be desired insofar as the extent of coverage is concerned, but the rapid increase in coverage of the population is an indication of the popularity of this method of payment for medical services.

Medical Care as a Public Function. Until comparatively recently, the provision of medical care has been accepted as a responsibility of society or government only in those instances where the need for community or social action was dramatically obvious: in the care of the mentally ill, of lepers, of the tuberculous, of inmates of public institutions, and in emergency care of the pauper sick. Through a changing concept of social responsibility, because of the increased potentialities of medical science, because of a high specialization in medicine, because of the expense of elaborate diagnostic and therapeutic instruments and procedures, and perhaps because of a demand or a need on the part of the public for medical service at a cost lower than could be rendered by a physician in private practice, the problem of providing the public with high-grade medical service at low cost has become a sociological one, and may be taken over by government.

Whether or not the problem of providing medical care to the sick individual may best be solved by organized public action, through government, is a question on which there is much controversy. Many economists and sociologists regard a public medical service as sensible and inevitable, while the medical profession is against it. Neither has indicated a faith in the wisdom of the other. The latter express a belief that socialization of medicine would rob physicians of their personal and professional freedom, would discourage personal initiative, retard research, impair a desirable personal relation between physician and patient, put medical practice under the thumb of politicians, and in general be undesirable and undemocratic.

Those who are primarily concerned with assuring medical care to all levels of society believe that such care should be regarded as an essential right of the individual. They believe that private arrangements will never provide such rights, that they may be assured only by governmental action which would ensure for most of the population the necessary facilities, personnel, funds, and mechanisms.

Proposals for Government Medical Care. The attitude which in the past two decades crystallized in the minds of the proponents of a governmental medical care program is somewhat as follows:

As a part of social security, the federal government should provide a rather complete scheme of medical and hospital care, reaching the majority of the population. These medical benefits would be available to all who are eligible for the security scheme, and the medical service on a compulsory insurance plan would be supported by payroll deductions, contributed to on a per cent of pay basis by employees and employers. It would be a national medical and hospital service, controlled by the federal government. Physicians, including specialists, would be employed for providing medical care in hospitals and homes, the physician to be paid on salary, fee, or per capita basis. A physician would be free to participate or not in the scheme, and as long as he is on a part-time basis he retains the privilege of having private patients. Any patient could select any physician participating in the scheme, provided this suits the physician. The scheme would be sufficiently inclusive so that with few exceptions it would cover all employed persons and their families, but if one chose not to use the service he would not have to, though he would have to pay for it.

Some Deterrents to a Wise Course. Discussions of the merits and demerits of the present private arrangement for medical care, or of the advantages and disadvantages that might be expected to arise from a public medical service, are seldom approached objectively. On the one extreme, there is thrown into the argument the fervor of the reformer, who burns with a zeal for betterment of those whom he considers underprivileged. To him, all else than relief of their plight is of secondary importance; and the impracticability of a given measure, or that measure's implications of serious damage along other lines, are matters of less than passing interest. He is the kind of person who bleeds vicariously for humanity, and hurls terms like Bourbon, tory, and fascist at all who oppose him. He does not help his cause by comparing what he considers the backwardness of the United States along those lines, with the enlightenment of some other country; and not infrequently this type of person is a quite objectionable fellow.

On the other extreme in arguments as to state medicine and socialized medicine, is the extremely conservative physician who, by the tradition of his profession and by conviction, is honor bound to defend the private practice of medicine as it is. He seldom sees the economically distressed, except in an orderly hospital ward, or in the white cleanliness of the operating room; and so far as he is concerned, medical care of a high order is freely and amply available to all. He has himself won his position by hard work, and from his standpoint those who have not acquired a corresponding status in life are shiftless; and there should be no coddling of the shiftless. He reacts violently and emotionally to any suggestion that government operate a medical service, and seldom reads the bills which propose these changes. As is the case with his opposite number on the other extreme, those who oppose him are castigated as bureaucrats, communists, and troublemakers.

Summary. Obviously the above pictures of the extremes in proponents and opponents of public medical service are somewhat on the caricature side, but not nearly so much so as one might wish. And in all fairness it should be noted that each is usually sincere in his attitude. Fortunately, they are not indices of the public on the one hand or of physicians on the other; but, unfortunately, they are the most vocal, and to that extent appear as representative of their respective groups.

In the circumstances, it will be difficult to discover and put into practice a wise arrangement for medical care. Such a course would be one that damaged to a minimum the fine traditions and potentialities of the medical profession but which, at the same time, assured medical care of good quality to all citizens of the United States. At this time, there would appear to be a strong tendency toward voluntary prepayment for medical care on the insurance principle, an inclination toward group practice, and that by these provisions, plus the greater availability of hospitals and participation in hospital insurance, the American public is receiving as much and as high-grade medical care as anywhere in the world; perhaps the best.

It must be recognized, however, that in the United States there has been a strong current toward socialization. And one must not forget that a proposal to give ample and fine medical care to one's children, his wife, and himself carries a powerful appeal. It *should* carry such an appeal, for every decent person wants these safeguards for his family. Unfortunately, a medical care program adequate in quantity and of high standards cannot be assured merely by making it a governmental operation under an insurance scheme to which all must subscribe.

Doubtless, under such a scheme, more people would see more doctors more often. Thus all men would get a small piece of the medical care loaf, but the quality of the bread would not in any way be assured, nor would there be assurance that those who needed more than the average would get what they should at the time of need.

Obviously, this is an opinion, but it is based to some extent upon observation of situations where free medical care is offered to all. In such circumstances, the pressure of work and the requirements of regulations tend to cause the physician too much preoccupation with the filling out of forms of various numbers and colors, possibly at the expense of good medicine, and to the patient's detriment.

The survival of the independent practice of medicine, or the fortunes of the physicians, are not the real issues here. Actually, even the kind and amount of medical care that the present generations receive is probably not the paramount issue, for those who now live will be succeeded by others. What appears to be of fundamental importance is that a surrender to government of the vast undertaking of medical care for all people would carry a philosophical and social significance far greater than the health of those who at present constitute the United States. It could be the final overbalancing movement that would replace dependence on self by dependence on, and subservience to, government in all things.

There the situation rests for the moment. A contribution would be made if more levelheaded persons, representing physicians on the one hand and the public on the other, made themselves heard, to the exclusion of bitter and emotional voices.

No one is an expert in this field. One may be possessed of facts and figures, examples, references to what is being done, rightly or wrongly, in other places in the world. One further may be soundly experienced in the practice of medicine or in the administration of a particular plan of medical care. Within the limits of such respective fields he has the right to an authoritative position. But when such experience or knowledge is translated into what is best for the United States, in the future, competence in a limited field becomes but opinion in a larger one.

A good, though only partial, way to judge the soundness of a discusser of this subject is to grade him as good, in inverse proportion to the emotion he displays and the categorical statements he makes.

REFERENCES

The Annals of the American Academy of Political and Social Science, Vol. 273, Jan. 1951. (This is perhaps the best presentation for collateral reading.)

Bachman, George W., and associates: *Health Resources in the United States.* The Brookings Institution, Washington, D.C., 1952.

Britten, Rollo H. (The National Health Survey): "Receipt of Medical Service in Different Urban Population Groups," *Pub. Health Rep.,* **55**:2199–2224 (Nov. 29), 1940.

Britten, Rollo, H.; Collins, Selwyn D.; and Fitzgerald, J. S. (The National Health Survey): "Some General Findings as to Diseases, Accidents, and Impairments," *Pub. Health Rep.,* **55**:444–70, (Mar. 15) 1940.

Building America's Health; Report of the President's Commission on the Health Needs of the Nation, five volumes. Government Printing Office, Washington, D.C., 1953.

Falk, Isidore S.; Rorem, Clarence R.; and Ring, Martha D.: *The Cost of Medical Care.* University of Chicago Press, Chicago, 1933.

The Health Insurance Council: *The Extent of Voluntary Health Insurance in the United States.* New York, 1957.

Index

Abortion, 237, 238
Accidents, as cause of death, 39
  industrial, 212–14
  pregnancy, of, 237–38
Acquired immunity, 106
Active immunity, 107
Acute anterior poliomyelitis. *See* Polio-
  myelitis
Acute communicable diseases. *See*
  Communicable diseases, acute
Adenoids, 273
Aedes aegypti, 206
  breeding places of, 206
  dengue and, 206
  Finlay and, 9
  Reed and, 10
  yellow fever and, 206
Aesculapius, 5
Aesthetics, personal hygiene and, 223
Age-height-weight of, infants, 252
  preschool children, 253
  school children, 275
Agglutinins, 107
Air, 231. *See also* Ventilation
  disease transmission by, 93
  pollution of, and health, 220
Air Force Medical Corps, 52
Allergy, 110, 111
Alum, water purification and, 193–94
American Cancer Society, 63
American Epidemiological Society, 68
American Heart Association, 63, 298
American Medical Association, 68
  Blue Shield Plan and, 302
  census of hospitals and, 303
American Nurses' Association, 68, 305
American Public Health Association,
  30, 68
American Social Hygiene Association,
  63
American Society of Civil Engineers,
  68

American Society for the Control of
  Cancer, 63
American Society of Tropical Medi-
  cine, 68
American Statistical Association, 68
Anaphylaxis, 110, 111
Anopheles, 205–6
  breeding places of, 206
  control of, 206
Antenatal clinic, 242–43
  services rendered by, 243
Antenatal hazards, 249–52
Antepartum visits by nurse, purposes
  of, 243–47
  report to doctor, 245
Anthrax, Pasteur and, 8
Antibiotics, in communicable diseases,
  123–24
  Fleming and, 12
  treatment with. *See* disease con-
  cerned
Antibodies, 106
Antigens, 107, 109
Antisepsis, Pasteur and, 8
Antitoxin, 107
  action of, 108
  diphtheria, 114
    Biggs and, 11
    use of, 114
    von Behring and, 10
Army Medical Corps, 52
Arteriosclerosis, 296–97
  causative factors in, 297
  psychoses in, 173
Asepsis, Lister and, 8
Astigmatism, 269
Avenues of infection, 90–91, 92–93
Avian tuberculosis, 126

Bacillus, diphtheria, 9
  Ducrey, 156
  Klebs-Loeffler, 9

Bacillus (*cont.*)
  tubercle, 126
  typhoid, 9
Bacon, Roger, 5
Bacteria, as a cause of communicable
    diseases, 91
Bacterial action, sewage and, 189
Bacteriology, Klebs and, 9
  Koch and, 9
  Lister and, 8
  Pasteur and, 8
  of sewage, 189
Bathing, 222–23
  aesthetic effect of, 223
  physiological effect of, 222
  psychological effect of, 223
  public health and, 223
BCG vaccine, 128, 138, 140–41
  Calmette, 140
  Guerin, 140
Bedclothes, disinfection of, 98
Behring, Emil von, 10
Beriberi, 226
Biggs, Hermann M., 11
Biochemical oxygen demand, 189
Biological forces, 1
  operation of, 1
Birth certificates, certified copies of,
    33, 35
  delayed registration of, 28, 34–35
  federal government and, 22, 33
  filing of, 33
  local registrars and, 21, 32, 33
  midwives and, 21, 27
  physicians and, 21, 27, 32
  state government and, 21, 33
  statistics and, 26, 33
  transcript of, 26
  value of, 33
Birth control, 251
Birth-death ratio, 37
Birth rate, 41
  decline in, 251
  trend in U.S., 41
Birth Registration Area, U.S., 25, 26
Births, delayed registration of, 28, 34–
    35
  head circumference in, 252
  height in, 252
  laws as to reporting, 21
  midwives and, 239
  premature, 257, 258

Births (*cont.*)
  Registration Area in, 25, 26
  reporting of, head of family in, 21
    local registrar in, 21
    midwives and, 21
    physicians and, 21
    requirements as to, 21, 27, 28
    sequence in events in, 32, 33
    sex and, 257
    statistical reports of, 26
  stillbirths, and infant mortality
    statistics, publication of, 26
  weight in, 252
"Blue babies." *See* Congenital diseases,
    heart disease
Blue Cross, 304, 307, 308
Blue Shield plans, 302, 308
Boards of health, appointment of, 56
  authority of, 54
  local, 56
  members of, 54
  state, 53–54
Borax solution, treatment of manure
    with, 204
Botulism, 200
Bovine tuberculosis, 126, 127, 196
Box and can privies, 190
Boyle, Robert, 5
Bretonneau, Pierre, 6
Brucellosis, 197
Budd, William, 7
Bureau of the Census, 22, 27, 31, 35,
    36, 52
  grades of feeblemindedness and, 169
Bureau of Entomology and Plant
    Quarantine, 13
Bureau of Medical Services, 50
Bureau of Mines, 209
Bureau of State Services, 50
Burial permits, 21, 28, 29

Calmette, Albert, 140
  BCG and, 140
Cancer, 289–93. *See also* Carcinoma
  danger signals of, 292
  generic term, as a, 289
  mortality from, 290–91
  public health and, 289, 290
  public information and, 292–93
  theories as to cause of, 289–90

"Cancer control," limitations of, 293
objectives in, 292
other countries, in, 293
public and, 292–93
Carbon dioxide, 232
Carcinoma, cause of, 289
mortality rate, 290–91
age and, 291
comparison with tuberculosis, 290
place of residence, 292
race and, 291
sex and, 291
trend in U.S., 290
Cardiovascular-renal diseases, arteriosclerosis, 296–98
hypertension, 296–98
kidneys and, 296
Carriers, chronic, 104
classification of, 104
convalescent, 104
definition of, 103
incubationary, 104
precocious, 104
temporary, 104
typhoid fever, 104
Causes of communicable diseases, 90–
91
See also disease concerned
Causes of death, *International List of,*
31, 32
Manual of Joint, 31
natal, 257, 258
nomenclature as to, 31
prenatal, 257
ten most important, 39
Census, federal, 22. *See also* Bureau of
the Census
availability, 22
data obtained in, 22
frequency of, 22
importance of, 22
publication of, 22
Ceratophyllus fasciata, plague and, 205
Certificates, birth, 21
death, 21
delayed birth, 34, 35
stillbirth, 31
Certified copy of, birth certificate, 33,
35
documents in lieu of, 35
value of, 33–34

Certified copy of (*cont.*)
death certificate, 33
value of, 34
Certified milk, 198–99
definition of, 199
Cesspools, 179
Cestodes, as cause of communicable
diseases, 91
Chancre, 155
Chancroid, 155, 156
Chapin, Charles V., 11
Chemical privy, 191
Chemotherapy, in venereal diseases,
153, 155, 156
Chest x-ray surveys, 138–40
Chickenpox, communicability period
of, 101
incubation period of, 99
Childbearing, 236–47
contracted pelvis and, 238
deaths incident to, 236–37
heart disease and, 237, 238
liver disease and, 238
mental instability and, 238
nephritis and, 238
relation to public health and, 236–41
syphilis and, 239–40
tuberculosis and, 238
Child health conferences, 259–60
Child health programs, 258–61
clinics in, 259–60
health departments in, 260
hospitals in, 260
objectives in, 258–59
operated, by whom, 260
private physicians in, 259–60
voluntary agencies in, 260
welfare agencies in, 260
Childhood tuberculosis, 135
definition of, 135
Children's Bureau, 49, 51, 52
industrial hygiene and, 209
publications and, 80
Chloride of lime (chlorinated lime),
189
Semmelweis and, 8
Chlorine, 189, 193, 194
Choice of physician, 306
Cholera, John Snow and, 7
Chronic diseases, 288–98
age and, 288
factors in evaluating, 288–89

Chronic diseases (*cont.*)
   public health aspects of certain, 288–98
Chronicle of the World Health Organization, 74
Chrysops discalis, 204
Cities, sanitary measures in, 187–88
   excreta disposal, 188–89
   food control, 201–2
   garbage disposal, 202–3
   housing, 207–8
   milk control, 196–99
   rodent control, 187
   water supplies, 187, 193–95
Classes for handicapped, 279
Classrooms, essentials of, 286
Clinics, antenatal, 242–43
   child health, 259–60
   immunization, 57
   tuberculosis, 142
Clostridium botulinum, 200
Colds, common, communicability, period of, 101
   incubation period of, 99
Colon bacilli, 196
Communal living, 185
   modern urban, 186
   primitive settlements, 185
   problems incident to, 185–87
Communicability, period of, 100–102
   carriers and, 101, 103–4
   chickenpox, 101
   common colds, 101
   definition of, 100
   diphtheria, 101
   dysentery, amebic, 101
   dysentery, bacillary, 101
   gonorrhea, 101
   influenza, 101
   measles, 101
   meningococcus meningitis, 101
   mumps, 101
   pneumonia, 102
   poliomyelitis, 102
   rabies, in dogs, 102
   scarlet fever, 102
   smallpox, 102
   syphilis, 102, 151
   termination of, 101–2
   typhoid fever, 102
   use of knowledge of, 102–3
   whooping cough, 102

Communicable Disease Center, 52
Communicable diseases, acute, 89–124
   antibiotics and, 123–24
   carriers in, 103–4
   causes of, 90–91
   definition of, 89
   endemic, 89
   environment and spread of, 186
   epidemic, 89
   epidemiology and, 89
   factors in, 91–92
   heart disease and, 295
   immunity in, 105–8
   important points in, 112–13
   incidence of, 89
   incubation period in, 99–100. *See also* individual disease
   isolation in, 94–96
   legal requirements as to, 111–12
   pandemic, 89
   parasitism in, 90
   period of communicability of, 100–102. *See also* individual disease
   prevalence of, 89–90
   prevention of, 94
   protozoa in, 91
   public health and, 17, 90
   quarantine in, 94–96
   rickettsia in, 91
   in school children, 279–82
      exclusion from school, 280
      nurse and, 280
      prevention in, 279–82
   serum, 109
   spirochetes, 91
   sporadic, 89
   spread of, 91–96
   teachers and, 281
   virulence of organisms causing, 107
      resistant strains, 108
Compensation, workmen's laws, 211
Conferences, child health, 259–60
Confinements, 238
Congenital disease, definition of, 249
Congenital diseases, 249–52
   heart disease, 274, 295
   immunity, 105
   infection, 250
   transmission of, immunity, 105
      syphilis, 240
      tuberculosis, 126
Conjugal tuberculosis, 137

Conjunctivitis, 269
Constitution, authority for health work, 49
  intent of, 49
  United States, 48, 49
  "welfare clause" of, 49
Contact infection, 90
Copernicus, 5
Corneal opacities, 269
Correction of physical defects, 255
Corynebacterium diphtheriae, 9
Costs per capita, for local health service, 58
Croup, first tracheotomy by Bretonneau, 7
Culex, 206
  breeding places of, 206
  filariasis and, 206
Cyanogen chloride, 99

DDT, 99, 204, 206
  pediculosis and, 282
  Zeidler and, 13
Deafness, classes for, 279
  tests for, 269-70
Death certificates, autopsy and, 21, 32
  burial permits and, 21, 28, 29
  certified copies of, 33, 34
  completeness of, 28
  federal government and, 22, 29
  filing of, 33
  health officer and, 21
  local government and, 28, 29
  physician and, 21, 27, 28, 29
  state government and, 26, 29
  transcript of, 27, 33
  undertaker and, 21
  value of, 33
Death rates. *See* Mortality rates
Death Registration Area, U.S., 25, 26
Deaths, by age and sex, 40, 41
  from carcinoma, 290-91
  causes of, *International List of,* 31, 32
    Manual of Joint, 31
    nomenclature as to, 31
    ten most important, 39
  laws as to reporting, 21
  reporting of, 21
    coroner in, 21
    local registrar in, 21, 28
    physician in, 27

Deaths (*cont.*)
  requirements as to, 21
  sequence of events in, 28
  undertaker in, 21, 28
  statistical reports of, 29
Defects, physical, correction of, 277-78
  incidence of, in infants, 255
    preschool children, 255
    school children, 266
      adenoids, 273
      eyes, 268
      flat feet, 276, 277
      hearing, 269
      heart, 274-75
      malnutrition, 275-76
      mottled enamel, 272
      orthopedic, 274
      posture, 276-77
      skeletal, 274
      teeth, 270-73
      tonsils, 273-74
      vision, 268-69
Definitions, age-specific birth rate, 37
  age-specific death rate, 37
  allergy, 110
  anaphylaxis, 110
  antibodies, 107
  antigen, 109
  bacteria, 91
  birth-death ratio, 37
  carrier, 104, 105
  case fatality ratio, 37
  certified milk, 199
  childhood tuberculosis, 135
  communicability, period of, 100-102
  communicable disease, 89
  concurrent disinfection, 96
  congenital disease, 249
  contact, 90
  crazy, 166
  crude birth rate, 36
  crude death rate, 36
  death rate, standardized, 37
  disinfectants, 96-97
  endemic, 89
  endotoxin, 108
  epidemic, 89
  epidemiology, 89
  exotoxin, 108
  fecundity, 250
  fertility, 250

Definitions (*cont.*)
  foot candle, 234
  fumigation, 98
  health, 72
  health education, 75
  health problem, 15
  host, 89
  hygiene, 184
  immunity, 105
  incidence, 89
  incubation period, 99–100
  industry, 208
  infancy, 248
  infant mortality rate, 37
  inherited disease, 249
  insane, 166
  isolation, 94
  law, 53
  maternal mortality rate, 37
  missed cases, 104
  morbidity rate, 37
  neonatal mortality rate, 37
  neonatal period, 248
  neurosis, 166
  occupation, 208
  pandemic, 89
  parasites, 90
  pasteurization, 198
  preschool period, 248
  prevalence, 89
  preventable diseases, 17
  preventive medicine, 16
  psychiatry, 166
  psychoneurosis, 166
  psychosis, 166
  public health, 16
  public health nursing, 61
  public health responsibility, 15
  puerperal deaths, 236
  quarantine, 95
  rates, 36
  regulation, 53
  relative humidity, 232
  sanitation, 185
  serum, 109
  sewage, 188
  sewerage, 188
  social hygiene, 149
  specific-cause-of-death rate, 37
  sporadic, 89
  statistics, 22
  stillbirth ratio, 37
  stillbirths, 30–31

Definitions (*cont.*)
  subclinical cases, 104
  susceptible, 109
  terminal disinfection, 96
  venereal diseases, 148
  vital statistics, 20, 21
Deliveries, 238–39
Dementia praecox. *See* Schizophrenia
Dengue, 205
Density of populations, communicable
      diseases and, 186
    concentration of foci in, 186
    garbage and, 186
    problems in, 186
Dental caries, 272–73
Dental hygiene, 224
    diet and, 224–26
    fluoridation of water and, 225, 272
    schools and, 270–73
Dentists, child hygiene and, 264
    number of, in U.S., 305
Department of Health, Education, and
      Welfare, 49, 50
    establishment of, 49
    organization of, 50
De Paul, St. Vincent, 13
Dermacentor andersoni, 205
Dermacentor variabilis, 205
Descartes, 5
Diabetes mellitus, 298
    mortality from, 298
    public health problem, as a, 298
Dickens, Charles, 13
Diet, 226–28
    beriberi and, 226
    dental hygiene and, 224–26
    goiter and, 226
    mass effects of poor, 226–27
    mottled enamel and, 226
    night blindness and, 226
    pellagra and, 226
    rickets and, 226
    scurvy and, 226
    vitamins and, 226
Diphtheria, antitoxin, 114
      exposed children and, 114
      minimal lethal dose, 114
      preparation of, 114
      unit of, 114
      use of, 114
    bacillus, 9
      Klebs and, 9
    Biggs and, 11

Diphtheria (*cont.*)
  Bretonneau and, 6
  communicability, period of, 101
  incubation, period of, 99
  milk and, 196
  Schick test, 116
  Smith, Theobald, and, 12
  toxin, 114–16
  toxoid, 114–16
  von Behring and, 10
Disabilities, industrial, 212–15
Dishes, disinfection of, 98
Disinfectants, definition of, 96
  important considerations in, 97
  kinds of, 96–97
  phenol coefficient of, 97
  Semmelweis and, 8
  strength of, 97
  use of, 97
Disinfection, concurrent, 96
  in the home, 97–99
    dishes, 98
    floors and woodwork, 98
    hands of attendant, 98
    mattresses, 98
    soiled linen, 98
    sputum and nasal discharges, 98
    stools and urine, 98
    tuberculosis and, 144–45
  of sewage, 189
  terminal, 96
Drinking fountains, in schools, 286
Droplet infection, 93
Ducrey bacillus, 156
Dumping garbage, 202
  ocean, in, 203
Dusts, 214
Dysentery, amebic, communicability of, 101
  bacillary, communicability of, 101
  and milk, 196

Eberth, Karl Joseph, 9
Eberthella typhosa, 9
Ectoparasites, 90, 223
Ehrlich, Paul, 10
Encephalitis, mosquitoes and, 205, 206
  postvaccination, 119
Endemic, definition of, 97
Enders, John, 12
Endocrines, 227
Endoparasites, 90

Endotoxins, 108
Engineers and public health, 15
Entomologists and public health, 15
Environment, 1, 184. *See also* Sanitation
  adaptation to, 1
  modification of, 1
Environmental health, 184–220
Epidemic, definition of, 89
  school closure and, 281–82
  U.S. Public Health Service and, 51
Epidemiological Society, the American, 68
Epidemiology, definition of, 89
  Frost and, 12
  Sedgwick and, 10
Eugenics, 249
Excreta, human, 188
  diseases transmitted by, 192
  disposal of, 188–92
Excreta disposal, 188–92
  diseases and, 192
  privies and, 190–91
  sewered areas, in, 188–89
  unsewered areas, in, 189–92
  water-carriage systems, in, 188
Exercise, 229
Exotoxins, 108
Eyelids, diseases of, 269
Eyes, evidence of trauma, 269
  school children, 268–69
Eyestrain, glare and, 234

Factors in infection, 91–92. *See also* disease concerned
"Fallen arches." *See* Flat feet
Farr, William, 7
Fatigue, 228
  industrial work, in, 228
  industry, in, 210
  public health and, 228
Fecundity, 250
  definition of, 250
Federal Security Agency, 49
Feeblemindedness, determination of IQ, 168–69
  grades of, 169
Fermentation, Pasteur and, 8
Fertility, 250, 251
  definition of, 250
Fetal deaths. *See* Stillbirths
Filariasis, 205

Filters, water purification and, 194
Filtration, water, of, 193, 194
    sewage treatment in, 189
Finlay, Carlos Juan, 8
First aid, in school, 284
Flat feet, 276–77
Fleas, 204–5
    Ceratophyllus fasciata, 205
    plague and, 205
    rats and, 205
    typhus fever and, 205
    Xenopsylla cheopis, 205
Fleming, Alexander, 12
Fliedner of Kaiserswerth, 14
Flies, 204
    breeding places of, 204
    Chrysops discala, 204
    destruction of, 204
    dysentery and, 204
    Musca domestica, 204
    trachoma and, 204
    typhoid fever and, 204
Floors, disinfection of, 98
Fluoridation of water supplies, 225–26
Fluorine in drinking water, 272
Folliculosis, 269
Fontonelles, 252
Food, 199–202, 227–28
    deficiency diseases and, 227–28
    disease outbreaks from, 199, 200
    diseases transmitted by, 200–201
    fish poisoning, 201
    handlers, 111
    infection of, 200
    inspection of, 57, 201–2
    meat poisoning, 200
    mushroom poisoning, 200
    nutrition, 227
    plant poisoning, 200
    poisoning, 190–202
    "ptomaine" poisoning, 201
    rat contamination of, 200
    Salmonella group and, 200
    staphylococcus and, 200
Foot candle, 234
    definition, 234
    number needed, 234, 235
Fracastoro, Girolamo, 6
Francis, Thomas, Jr., 121
Frei test, 156
Fresh air, 231–32
Frost, Wade Hampton, 12

Fumes, 214
Fumigants, 98
    effectiveness of, 98
    hydrocyanic gas, 99
    sulfur, 99
    use of, 98–99
Fumigation, definition of, 98
    limitations of, 99
    use of, 98–99

Gafafer, W. M., 213
Galileo, 5
Gamma globulin, 117
Gamp, Sairy, 13
Garbage disposal, 202–3
    dumping, 202
    health hazard, as a, 202
    hogs and, 203
    incineration, by, 203
    ocean, in, 203
    reduction plants, 203
Gardner, Mary S., 15
Garrison, F. H., 5
Gases, 214
Geigy, J. R., Company, 13
Genetics, 249
    Mendel and, 8
Genitoinfectious diseases, 149
Goiter, 226, 268
Gonorrhea, 154–55
    blindness and, 154
    chemotherapy and, 155
    communicability, period of, 101
    diagnosis of, 155
    incubation period of, 99
    infectious material in, 154
    penicillin and, 155
    prevalence of, 154
    public health aspects of, 154–55
    sterility and, 154
    transmission of, 154
Gonorrheal ophthalmia, 154, 269
Gorgas, William C., 10
Government medical care, proposals
    for, 309–10
Government Printing Office, publica-
    tions available, 80
Granuloma inguinale, 156
Group medical practice, versus solo,
    305–6
Guerin, Alphonse, 140
    BCG and, 140

Handicapped, classes for, 279
Hands, disinfection of, 98
Hand washing, 206
    disease and, 206
Health departments, child hygiene
        and, 260
    federal, 49, 50
    local, 56–58
    state, 53–56
Health education, 75–88
    advertising and propaganda, 79, 82
    agencies conducting, 75, 79–80
    arts and letters, 79
    audiences in, 85
    community organization, 75
    definition of, 75
    educational processes, 79, 81
    essentials (five) in, 77–78
    growth of, 76–77
    maintenance of health, 76
        negative approach, 76
        positive aspect, 76
    materials used in, 82
    means of communication in, 82–85
    media available, 76, 82–85
    medicine and, 78
    methods of, 75, 81–82
    participants in, 86
    programs, kinds of, 80–81
    psychology and, 79
    publications available, 80
    public relations and, 75, 86
    purpose of, 75
    related activities and, 75–89
    results of, 87–88
    sciences and disciplines contributing
        to, 78–79
    speech techniques in, 82–84
    voluntary health associations, 79,
        80, 86
    written word, 84–85
Health educator, methodolgy and, 86
    trained, 78
Health principles, practice of, 285
Health problem, definition of, 15
Health publications, Government
        Printing Office, 80
Health records, school children and,
        278–79
Hearing, in school children, 269–70
Heart disease, 293–95
    causes of, 295–96

Heart disease (*cont.*)
    childbearing and, 237, 238
    conditions associated with, 296–97
    congenital, 274–95
    control of, 298
    mortality from, 293–95
    prevention of, 297, 298
    school children, in, 274–75
    trend in, 294
Height, at birth, 252
    infancy, gain during, 252
    preschool, gain during, 253
Hemophilus ducreyi, 156
Heredity, Mendel and, 8
Hill Burton Hospital program, 304
Hippocrates, 5, 6
Hogs, garbage and, 203
Holmes, Oliver Wendell, 7
Home, disinfection of, 97–99
Home deliveries, 239
    pamphlets listing materials needed,
        246
Hospital insurance, 303–4
Hospital Insurance Plan of Greater
        New York, 303
Hospital program, Hill Burton, 304
Hospitals in the U.S., 303–4
    availability of, 303
    beds in, 303–4
    child hygiene and, 260
    insurance and, 303–4, 308–9
    mental. *See* Mental Hospitals
    tuberculosis, 128, 146
    types and percentages, 303
Host, definitive, 89
    intermediate, 89
Hot lunch, 278–79
Housing, 15, 207–8
    need of program for, 208
    public health program, 207–8
Howe, Howard A., 12
Humidity, 233
    relative, 233
    ventilation in, 233
Hydrocyanic gas, 99
Hygeia, 5
Hygiene, background and associations,
        1–18
    definition of, 184
    dental, 224
    growth of, 4
    and the individual, 222–35

Hygiene (*cont.*)
  industrial, 210
  of infancy, 248–62
  maternal, 241–42
  social, 149
  of young childhood, 248–62
Hypermetropia, 268
Hypernephroma, 289
Hyperopia. *See* Hypermetropia
Hypertension, 296–97
  causative factors in, 296–97

Idiots, 169
Illness, employment and, 212
Imbeciles, 169
Immigrants, examination of, 51
Immunity, 105–8
  acquired, 106
  active, 107
  congenital, 105
  definition of, 105
  Ehrlich and, 10
  inherited, 105
  Jenner and, 6
  natural, 105
  passive, 106
  production of, 106, 107
Impetigo contagiosa, 282
Incineration, garbage and, 203
Incubation, period of, in carriers, 103–4
  chickenpox, 99
  common cold, 99
  definition of, 99
  diphtheria, 99
  gonorrhea, 99
  importance of, 100
  influenza, 99
  measles, 99
  meningcoccus meningitis, 99
  mumps, 99
  pneumonia, lobar, 99
  poliomyelitis, 100
  rabies, 100
  scarlet fever, 100
  smallpox, 100
  syphilis, 100
  typhoid fever, 100
  whooping cough, 100
Individual, personal hygiene and, 222–35

Industrial disabilities, 212–15
  data on, 213
  prevention of, 214–15
Industrial hazards, 214
  prevention of, 214–15
  special types, 215
Industrial health, 209–16
Industrial hygiene programs, costs of, 216
  development of, in the U.S., 209–10
  medical care and, 301
  purpose of, 210
  three main headings, 216
Industrial plant, medical staff in, 211–12
Industry, fatigue and, 210
  population concerned, 209
  women and, 215–16
Infant development, 252–54
Infant hygiene, accomplishments in, 262
Infant mortality, 248, 256–57
  rate, calculation of, 256
    definition of, 37
    race and, 257
    reduction in, 256–57
    sex and, 257
    syphilis, and, 257
    United States, 258
Infantile paralysis. *See* Poliomyelitis
Infection, avenues of, 90–91, 92–93
    carriers in, 103
    direct, 93
    droplet, 93
    factors in, 91–92
    indirect, 93
    insects in, 94, 203–7
  sources of, 103–5. *See also* disease concerned
    carriers as, 103–4
    difficulty in discovering, 103
    missed cases as, 104
    reported cases as, 96
    subclinical cases as, 104
Infections, minor, school children and, 282–83
Infectious abortion, in animals, 197
Infectious material, 92–93, 109. *See also* disease concerned
  disinfection of, 96
  exit from body, 92
  focus and, 92–97

Infectious material (*cont.*)
  intermediate agents and, 93
  portal of entry, 93
Infestations, 282–83
  detection of, 283
  school exclusion and, 283
Influenza, communicability, period of, 101
  incubation, period of, 99
Inherited disease, definition, 249
Inherited immunity, 105
Injuries, industrial, 212–14
Insanitary privies, 191
  dangers in, 191
  rural areas, in, 191
Insanity. *See* Mental diseases
Insect-borne diseases, 203–7
  control measures in, 203–4
  dengue, 205–6
  dysentery, 204
  encephalitis, 205–6
  filariasis, 205, 206
  malaria, 205
  rats and, 205
  Rocky Mountain spotted fever, 205
  trachoma, 204
  tularemia, 205
  typhoid fever, 204
  typhus fever, 204
  yellow fever, 206
Insecticides, 13, 50, 204, 206
Insects, 15, 204–7
  diseases transmitted by, 204–6
  ectoparasites, 203
  fleas, 204–5
  flies, 204
  as hosts, 203
  lice, 204
  mosquitoes, 205–7
  as parasites, 203
  sanitary measures against, 203–7
  ticks, 205
Insurance, compulsory, 307, 310
  medical care and, 302, 306–9
  voluntary, 307
Intelligence quotient, 168
International health, recognition of problems in, 69
International health agencies, more modern, 70
International health organization, 68
  first agreements for, 69

International health (*cont.*)
  International Office of Health, 70, 71
  League of Nations, health section, 70
  Pan American Sanitary Bureau, 70
  recognition of need for, 69
  World Health Organization, 68, 70, 71–74
International health program, early agreements, 69
  early history of, 69
  more recent developments, 70
International Institute of Statistics, 30
International Office of Health, 70
Interstate quarantine, 49
  U.S. Public Health Service and, 51
Iodine and simple goiter, 268
Ionizing radiation. *See* Radiation, ionizing
Isolation, definition of, 94
  limitations in, 94
  problems incident to, 95–96
  See also disease concerned

Jenner, Edward, 6

Kitasato, S., 10
Klebs, T. A. Edwin, 9
Klebs-Loeffler bacillus, 9
Knipling, E. F., 13
Koch, Robert, 9

Ladies Benevolent Society of Charleston, South Carolina, 14
Laennec, René T. H., 7
Laveran, C. L. Alphonse, 9
League of Nations, 30
  health section of, 70
Leeuwenhoek, Anton van, 6
Legal requirements, communicable diseases, 111–12
  enforcement of, 111–12
  food handlers, 111
  school children, 111
  teachers, 111
  midwives, 239
  premarital serologic tests, 240
  prenatal serologic tests, 240
  smallpox, 120

Legal requirements (*cont.*)
  tuberculosis, 143–44
  vaccination, smallpox, 120
  venereal diseases, 157–59
  vital statistics, 21, 27–28
Lice, 13, 99, 204, 282
Lighting, 234–35
  artificial, 235
  classroom, in, 286
  direct, 235
  indirect, 235
  industries, in, 234
  measurement of, 234
  natural, 234
  requirements in, 235
Linens, disinfection of, 98
Lister, Joseph, 8
Liver disease and childbearing, 238
Local health departments, costs of, 58
  functions of, 57–58
  organization and operation of, 56–58
  personnel, appointment of, 59
Local health officer, appointment of, 56
  salary of, 60
Lockjaw. *See* Tetanus
Locomotor ataxia. *See* Syphilis
Lunches, school children, 278–79
Lymphogranuloma venereum, 156–57
Lysins, 107

Malaria, mosquitoes and, 205
  Ross and, 11
Malarial parasites, Laveran's discovery of, 9
Malignant tumors, 291. *See also* Carcinoma
Malnutrition, 227–28
  determination of, 275
  disturbances in digestive tract, 227
  endocrines and, 227
  exercise and, 227
  food and, 227
  growth periods and, 227
  rest and, 227
  school children, 227, 275–76
  sleep and, 227
  toxemias and, 227
Malta fever. *See* Brucellosis

Malthus, Thomas Robert, 6
Manic-depressives, incidence of, 172
Mantoux test, 138
Manual of Industrial Hygiene, 213
Manual of Public Health Nursing, 61
Marine Hospital Service, 49
Maritime quarantine, 50, 51
  U.S. Public Health Service and, 50, 51
Massachusetts, Sanitary Survey of State of, 7
Maternal hygiene, 241–42
  program for, 241–42
  public health nurse and, 243–47
Maternal mortality, 240–41, 242
  causes of, 237
  decrease in, 241
  rate, basis of, 37
    calculation of, 240
    race and, 241
  by years, 237
Mathematics, vital statistics and, 19
Mattresses, disinfection of, 98
Measles, 117
  communicability, period of, 101
  incubation, period of, 99
  pooled blood in, 117
  treatment of, 117
Medical care, 299–313
  a controversial subject, 299
  deterrents to a wise course, 310–11
  group versus solo practice in, 305–6
  hospital insurance and, 303–4
  industry in, 301–2
  and private practice system, 399
  public function, as a, 309
  summary, 311–13
  supplements to private practice systems, 300–303
Medical care plans, Blue Cross, 304
  Blue Shield, 302, 308
  "cooperatives," 303
  Hospital Insurance Plan of Greater New York, 303
  insurance companies, 302
Medical care programs, labor unions and, 301
Medical institutions. *See* Hospitals in the U.S.
Medical personnel available, 304–5
Medical practice, private, 300, 301

Medical service, insurance principle, 306–7
Medical staff, in industrial plants, 211–12
Mendel, Gregor, 8
Meningcoccus meningitis, communicability, period of, 101
  incubation, period of, 99
Mental defectives, children, 254
Mental disease, public health and, 165
Mental diseases, causative factors of, 166–68
  classification of, 165–66
  definition of terms used, crazy, 166
    insane, 166
    neurosis, 166
    psychiatry, 166
    psychoneurosis, 166
    psychosis, 166
  epidemiology of, 171–72
  feeblemindedness, 168–69
    three grades of, 169
  government responsibility and, 178–79
  hospitalization and, 173–74
  hospitals for, commitments to, 176–77
    expenditures for, 175
  incidence of, 170, 174
  IQ and, 168
  manic-depressive psychoses, 172
    incidence of, 172
  other psychoses and related states, 172–73
    incidence of, 172
  present concept of, 168
  proposed model law and, 177
  psychoses with physical causes, 172–73
  schizophrenia, 171–72
    incidence of, 172
    prevalence of, 171
  social action and, 176–77
  terminology and classification of, 165–66
Mental health, 165–83
  advances in, 165
  community programs in, 182
  extent of problem of, 169–71
  federal government in, 178–79
    hospitals for narcotic addicts, 179
    mental health movement, 179

Mental health (*cont.*)
  National Mental Health Act and, 170, 179
  problems are many, 165
  state organization and administration for, 179–82
    board and state departments responsible, 179–80
    individual state laws vary, 180
  U.S. Public Health Service and, 177, 179
Mental hospitals, bed facilities, 173–74
  beds in, 303
  commitment to, emergency, 176
    involuntary, 176
    laws regarding, 176–77
    legal procedures for, 176–78
    observational, 177
    voluntary, 177
  cost of operating, 175
  hazards in populations of, 175
    gastrointestinal diseases, 175
    poor personal hygiene, 175
    tuberculosis, 175
  release of patients from, 177–78
    whose responsibility, 178
  state, 174
  treatment facilities in, 173
  types of, 173
Mental hygiene programs, difficulties in, 254
  public health nurse and, 254
  young children and, 254
Mental illness. *See also* Mental diseases
  epidemiological approach, 171, 173
  treatment facilities, 173
Mental instability, childbearing and, 238
Mental retardation, mild, children, 254
Merchant Marine, 209
Midwives, 239
  decline of, 239
  legal requirements as to, 239
  training of, 239
  vital statistics and, 21, 27
Milk, 196–99
  bacterial count of, 199
  certified, 198–99
  diseases transmitted by, 196–97
  essentials in sanitation of, 197

Milk (*cont.*)
  pasteurized, 198
  quality of, 199
  sanitary problem, as a, 196
Milk sickness, 196
Minor injuries, 284
  school children and, 284
Missed cases, 103
  definition of, 104
"Model Law" for vital statistics, 27
Moderately advanced tuberculosis, 136
Modes of infection, 90–94
Molars, six year, 253, 270
Molds, as cause of communicable diseases, 91
Morbidity statistics, 21
Morbus Gallicus, 6
Morning inspection, 283–84
Morons, 169
Mortality rates. *See also* disease concerned
  bases of, 36, 37
  calculation of, 37, 38
  general, 36
  infant, 37
  maternal, 37, 240–41
  most frequently used, 35
  specific age, 40, 41
  United States, in, 40, 41
Mosquitoes, *Aedes aegypti*, 9, 10, 206
  Anopheles, 205
  breeding of, 206
  control of, 206–7
  Culex, 206
  dengue and, 205
  diseases transmitted by, 205
  filariasis and, 205
  malaria and, 205
  Reed and, 9, 10
  Ross and, 11
  yellow fever and, 8, 10, 205
Mottled enamel, 272
Mouth hygiene, 224, 273
Mumps, communicability, period of, 101
  incubation, period of, 99
Musca domestica. See Flies
Muscular development, 229–30
  health and, 229
  longevity and, 229
Mushroom poisoning, 200
Myopia, 268

Narcotic addicts, hospitals, for, 179
Nasal discharges, disinfection of, 98
National Association for Mental Health, 63
National Foundation, 63, 65
National Foundation for Infantile Paralysis. *See* National Foundation
National Health Council, 67
National Institutes of Health, 50, 52, 293
  Communicable Disease Center and, 52
  National Cancer Institute, 293
  National Institute of Mental Health, 170, 179
  See also U.S. Public Health Service
National League for Nursing, 68
National Mental Health Act, 179, 181
National Office of Vital Statistics, 22, 29
National Research Council, 139
National Tuberculosis Association, 63, 65, 71, 133
Natural immunity, 105
Natural laws, 1
Navy Medical Corps, 52
Nematodes, as cause of communicable diseases, 91
Neonatal mortality, 256–57
Neonatal period, definition of, 248
Nephritis, childbearing and, 237
Newsholme, Arthur, 11
Newton, Sir Isaac, 5
New York City Mission, 14
Night blindness, 226
Nightingale, Florence, 14
Normal infant, figures on, 252–53
Notice to parents in school examinations, 267
Nurses, number of in the U.S., 305
  public health. *See* Public health nurses
Nursing, district, history of, 14
  public health, 14, 68
Nutrition, 226–28
  infancy, in, 253
  obesity and, 228
  pregnancy, in, 246
  school children, in, 265, 275–76, 286

Occupational diseases, 210
  physicians' report of, 210
Official agencies, 48
  approach to problems, 47
  duties of, 48
  government and, 47
  support of, 47
Opsonins, 107
Oral hygiene, 224, 273
Order of St. John of Jerusalem, 14
Orthopedic defects, 274
Orthotolidine test, 194
Oxygen, ventilation in, 232
  water, in, 192

Panacea, 5
Pan-American Sanitary Bureau,70
Pandemic, definition of, 89
Para-aminosalicylic acid (PAS), 108
Paralysis, infantile. *See* Poliomyelitis
Parasites, definition of, 90
  ectoparasites, 90
  endoparasites, 90
Parasitism, 90
  communicable diseases and, 90
Paratyphoid fevers, 197
Passive immunity, 106
Pasteur, Louis, 8
Pasteurization, 198
  definition, 198
  milk, of, 198
  Pasteur and, 8
Pasteurized milk, 198
  importance of, 198
  pathogenic organisms and, 198
  taste in, 198
"Patch test," 138
Pediatric clinic, 259–60
Pediatricians, infant hygiene and, 240–41
Pediculosis, 282
Pellagra, 226
Penicillin, Fleming and, 12
  gonorrhea and, 155
  syphilis and, 153–54
Periodic physical examination, 230–31
  diabetes and, 298
  limitations in, 230
  objectives of, 230
  prostitutes, of, 160
  public health and, 231
  school children, of, 266–68

Personal hygiene, 222–35
  aesthetics and, 223
  assumptions in, 222
  description of, 222
  effects of, 230
  limitations of, 230
  Newsholme and, 11
Personnel, in health agencies, 59
  public health, 59–61
  salaries of, 60, 61
  school work, in, 264–65
Phagocytosis, 107
Phenol coefficient, 97
Phlyctenular conjunctivitis, 269
Physical defects, correction of, 277
  incidence of, 255, 266–77
  infants, in, 255
  preschool children, of, 255
  school children, in, 266–68
Physical examinations, of adults, periodic, 230–31
  pre-employment, 212
  preplacement, 212
  preschool children, of, 255
  school children, in, 266–68
Physician-population ratio, 304
Physicians, distribution, in the U.S., 304–5
  free choice of, 306
  number of, in the U.S., 304
  school work, in, 264
Physicians' Handbook on Birth and Death Registration, 32
"Pink eye." *See* Conjunctivitis.
Pit type privy, 190
Planned parenthood, 251
Plant poisoning, 200
Playgrounds, 286
Pneumonia, lobar, communicability, period of, 102
  incubation, period of, 99
Poliomyelitis, communicability, period of, 102
  incubation, period of, 100
  Salk and, 12
  vaccination for, 121
Population, age, by, 22
  color, 22
  data, 22, 23
  enumeration of, 22
  estimation of, 23, 24
  importance of, 23

Population (*cont.*)
  industry, in, 209
  Malthus and, 6
  methods of estimating, 24–25
    arithmetic, 24
    census, 24
    geometric, 25
  problems in density of, 186–87
  race, by, 23
  rural, 24
  sex, by, in the U.S., 23
  urban, 24
Postpartum visits by nurse, purpose of,
  244
Posture, 228–29
  factors in poor, 228
  health and, 228
  school children, in, 276
Potato poisoning, 200
Practice, medical, group versus solo,
  305–6
Precipitins, 107
Pre-employment examination, 212
Pregnancy, accidents of, 237
  hemorrhage in, 237
  nonfatal complications of, 247
  nutrition in, 246
Premarital serological tests, 240
Premature birth, 257, 258
Prenatal care, 241–47
Prenatal serological tests, 240
Prepayment medical programs, 306–8
Preplacement examination, 212
Preschool hygiene, accomplishments in,
  262
Preschool period, 248
  definition of, 248
  hazards in, 248
Preventable diseases, definition of, 17
Preventive medicine, definition of, 16
  relation to public health, 17–18
Private medical practice, 299, 300
  advantages of, 300
  disadvantages of, 306
  medical care and, 300
  personnel engaged in, 304–5
  supplements to, 300–303
Private physicians, "cancer control"
  and, 292
  child hygiene and, 259, 260
  infant hygiene and, 259, 260
  maternal hygiene and, 241

Private physicians (*cont.*)
  public health work and, 16, 17
  school hygiene and, 264
  tuberculosis and, 143
  venereal diseases and, 158
  vital statistics and, 21, 28
Privies, 190–92
  box and can type, 190
  chemical type, 191
  essential requirements in, 191
  insanitary, 191
  pit type, 190
  rural areas, in, 190
  sanitary, 190–91
  septic tank type, 190
  vault type, 190
Prophylaxis, venereal disease and, 159–
  60
Prostitution, 160
Protein reaction, 110, 111
Protozoa, as cause of comunicable diseases, 91
Psychoses, causes of, 172, 173
  definition of, 166
Psychrometer, 233
"Ptomaine" poisoning, 201
Public health, acute communicable diseases and, 17
  associations, 68
  background and associations, 1–18
  barriers to promotion of, 3
  bathing and, 222–23
  childbearing and, 236–47
  chronic diseases and, 288–98
  communicable diseases and, 17
  contributing professions, 15
  contributors to, 4–16
  definition of, 16
  diabetes and, 298
  excreta disposal and, 188–92
  fatigue and, 228
  food and, 187, 199, 202, 226–28
  garbage and, 202–3
  hand washing and, 224
  heart disease and, 298
  housing and, 207–8
  insects and, 203–7
  malignant disease and, 292–93
  mental disease and, 165
  milk and, 196–99
  muscular development and, 229
  nurses, 13

Public health (*cont.*)
  nursing, 62
  personal hygiene and, 222
  physical examinations and, 230
  preventable disease and, 17
  problems, 15
  reports, 21
Public health associations, 68
Public health education, cancer and, 289–90
  personal hygiene, in, 222
  tuberculosis and, 142–43
  See also Health education
Public health nurses, 13
  antepartum visits, 243–44
  blood pressure, taken by, 243, 245
  child hygiene and, 261–64, 285
  infants and, 254–55, 261
  maternal hygiene and, 243–47
  maternity record and, 245, 247
  requirements for, 62
  salaries of, 62
  school health work and, 284–85
  tuberculosis program and, 145, 146
  urinalysis and, 243, 245
  venereal disease program and, 162–63
Public health nursing, definition of, 61
  development of, 13
  national organization for. *See* National League for Nursing
  objectives in, 61–62
Public health problems of significance, 15–17
Public health responsibility, definition of, 15
Public health work, administration of, 47–74
  antibiological aspects of, 2
  contributing professions, 15
  contributors to, 4–16
  costs of, 55, 58
  dentists and, 264
  engineers and, 15
  entomologists and, 15
  expenditures for, 55
  federal government, in, 48
  funds for, 55, 63–65
  health problems and, 14
  legal requirements and, 53
  mathematics and, 15
  medical care and, 17, 309

Public health work (*cont.*)
  nurses in, 13, 61
  official agencies in, 48
  organization of, 47–74
  personnel in, 59
  politics in, 56
  private physicians and, 16
  scope of, 16, 17
  society and, 2, 3
  state governments and, 49, 52, 55–56
  tendencies to limit, 17
  training for, 59, 60
  veterinarians and, 15
  voluntary agencies in, 16, 48, 63–67
Public medical care, 309–13
  advantages of, 309–10
  controversy as to, 310–13
  disadvantages of, 310–13
  federal government and, 309–10
  insurance and, 306–9
  proposals as to, 309–10
  sociologists and, 309
Puerperal deaths, and age, 237
  compared to other causes of death, 237
  definition of, 236
  rate of, 240–41
Puerperal sepsis, 237
  Holmes and, 7
  Semmelweis and, 8

Quarantine, definition of, 50, 51
  interstate, 51
  intrastate, 51
  maritime, 50, 51
  problems incident to, 95, 96
  stations, 50, 51
Queen's Institute, 14

Rabies, communicability in dogs, 102
  incubation, period of, 100
  Pasteur and, 8
Rachitic disturbances, 274
Radiation, ionizing, 139, 216–19
  genetic influence of, 217
  hazards of, 217–19
  health aspects of, 218–19
  protection from, 218
  public education program, 219

Radiation (*cont.*)
  public health program, 219
  use of, in medicine, 218
Radioactive substances, disposal of, 219
Rates, bases of, 36
  birth, 36, 37
  calculation of, 37–38
  caution as to drawing conclusions from, 38
  death, 36, 37
  definition of, 36
  infant mortality, 37
  maternal mortality, 37, 240, 241
  morbidity, 37
  neonatal mortality, 37
  stillbirth, 37
  types of, 36–37
  uses of, in vital statistics, 36
Rathbone, William, 14
Rats, destruction of, 205
  fleas and, 205
  food and, 205
  plague and, 205
Reaction, Schick, 116–17
  serum, 110
  tuberculin, 137–38
  Wassermann, 12
  Widal, 12
Recreation, 279
Red Cross, 65
Reduction plants, garbage and, 203
Reed, Walter, 9, 10
Registration Area, for births, 25, 26
  for deaths, 25, 26
  requirements for admission to, 25, 26
  United States, in, 26
Relative humidity, 233
  computation of, 233
  definition of, 233
  requirements, 233
Rheumatic fever, heart disease and, 295
Rickets, 226
Rickettsiae, as causes of communicable diseases, 91
Ringworm, 282
Ross, Ronald, 11
Rural areas, excreta disposal in, 190–92

Rural areas (*cont.*)
  insanitary privies in, 190–91
  sanitary measures in, 188, 190–92
  water supplies in, 195–96

St. John of Jerusalem, Order of, 14
St. Vincent de Paul, 13
Salaries, bureau chiefs, 60
  local health offices, 60
  public health nurses, 62
  state health officers, 60
Salk, Jonas E., 12, 121
Salmonella, 200
  S. enteritidis, 200
  S. typhimurium, 200
Salvarsan, 10, 153
Sanatoria, tuberculosis, 146
  maintenance, 146
  need for, 143
  public education and, 143
  ratio of beds to deaths, 146–47
Sanitary measures, in cities, 187–88
  excreta disposal, 188–89
  food control, 201–2
  garbage disposal, 202–3
  insect control, 203–7
  milk control, 187
  purpose of, 187
  rodent control, 205
  rural areas, in, 188, 190–92
  water supplies, 187, 192–96
Sanitary Survey of State of Massachusetts, 7
Sanitary type privy, 190–91
Sanitation, definition of, 185
  environmental, 185
  industrial hygiene and, 208–16
  school, 286–87
Sarcoma, 289
Scabies, 282
Scarlet fever, communicability, period of, 102
  incubation, period of, 100
  milk and, 196
Schaudinn, Fritz, 12
Schick test (reaction), 116–17
Schizophrenia, 171–72
  incidence of, 172
  prevalence of, 171
Science and medicine, 4
Scientific method, 4

School, first aid in, 284
School children, classes for handicapped, 279
  communicable diseases, in, 279–82
  defects in, 267–68, 269, 274, 277, 278
  health record of, 277, 287
  heart disease in, 274–75
  lunches and, 278–79
  minor infections and infestations, 282–83
  minor injuries, in, 284
  morning inspection, in, 284
  nutrition of, 275–76
  pediculosis in, 282
  posture and, 276–77
  recreation of, 279
  rest for, 279
  teeth in, 270–73
  tonsils and, 268, 273
School examinations, equipment for, 266
  frequency of, 266
  limitations of, 275
  procedure in, 266
School health services, 263–87
  grades served, 264
  personnel engaged in, 264
  physical examinations in, 266–68
  responsibility for, 265
  where done, 265
School sanitation, 286–87
  classrooms, 286
  essentials in, 286
  lighting, 286
  playgrounds, 286
  temperature, 286
  toilet facilities, 287
  ventilation, 286
Screening, against insects, 203
  sewage, 189
Scurvy, 226
Sedgwick, William T., 10
Sedimentation, of sewage, 189
  water purification and, 193
Semmelweis, Ignaz Philipp, 8
Septic tank privy, 190
Serum, 109
  antidiphtheritic, 114
  correct use of word, 109
  reaction, 110
  sickness, 110

Sewage, definition of, 188
  treatment of, 189–90
Sewerage, definition of, 188
Sex education, 161–62
Shattuck, Lemuel, 7
Silver salts, eyes of newborn, in, 157
  venereal disease prophylaxis, in, 159
Six year molars, 253, 270
Sixteenth century influences, 4
Skeletal defects, 274
Sling psychrometer, 233
Smallpox, communicability, period of, 102
  immunity in, 6
  incubation, period of, 100
  Jenner and, 6
  vaccination against, 117–18
Smith, Theobald, 11
Snellen test card, 268
Snow, John, 7
Social hygiene, 149
Social measures, operations of, 2
  relation to health, 3
Socialized medicine, 309
Society of American Bacteriologists, 68
Soiled linen, disinfection of, 98
Solo medical practice, versus group, 305–6
Sources of infection, 91, 103. *See also* disease concerned
  carriers as, 104
  difficulty in discovering, 103
  missed cases as, 104
  reported cases as, 95
  subclinical cases as, 104
Species, immunity in, 105
  problems of, 1
  survival efforts, 1
Spirochetes, as cause of venereal diseases, 91
Sporadic, definition of, 89
Sputum, disinfection of, 98
Staphylococcus, food poisoning and, 200
State departments of labor, and industrial hygiene, 209–11, 220
State health department, 53–56
  board of health and, 53, 54
  expenditures by, 55
  operation and organization of, 53–54
  personnel, appointment of, 54

State health department (*cont.*)
  politics and, 54
  relation to federal government, 56
  relation to local departments, 56
  services rendered by, 55, 56
  sources of funds, 54
  taxes, 54
  U.S. Public Health Service and, 55
State health officer, appointment of, 54
  salary of, 60
  tenure of office of, 54
Statistics, analysis of, 42–44
  birth, 21
  chance in, 44, 45
  divorce, 21
  interpretation of, 45
  marriage, 21
  morbidity, 21
  mortality, 37, 38
  population, 23
  presentation of, 19, 35–37
  public health work and, 19–20
    basic information, 20
    subdivisions of numbers, 19
Sterility, gonorrhea and, 154
Sterilization, germ life and, 98
Stillbirths, 30–31, 252
  causes of, 252
  certificate, 31
  collateral factors in, 252
  definition of, 30, 31
  ratio, 37
  reporting of, 31
Stools, disinfection of, 98
Strabismus, 269
Streams, 188
  protection of, 188
  self-purification of, 192–93
  sewage and, 188, 189
Streptomycin, 108, 123
Styes, 269
Subclinical cases, 103
  definition of, 104
  relation to carriers, 104
Sulfa drugs, gonorrhea and, 155
Sulfur, as a fumigant, 99
  ointment, 282
Superintendent of Documents, Washington, D.C., 32
Susceptibility, 109
Susceptibles, 109

Sydenham, Thomas, 6
Syphilis, 6, 150–54
  age and, 150
  case fatality of, 152
  cause of, 150
  childbearing and, 239–40
  communicability, period of, 102, 151
  congenital, 150, 151
  derivation of name, 6
  endemicity of, 152
  heart disease and, 295
  incubation period of, 100, 150
  infectious material in, 150–51
  intensive treatment of, 153
  mental disease in, 167, 173
  mortality rate, 153
  penicillin and, 153, 154
  prevalence of, 152
  recent advances in treatment of, 153–54
  recovery and, 151
  Schaudinn and, 12
  selective service examinations, found in, 152
  serologic tests, premarital and prenatal, 240
  treatment and, 153–54
Wassermann test, 12, 153

Tabes, dorsalis. *See* Syphilis
Tapeworm, 91
Teachers, mouth hygiene and, 273
  school health work, 264
Teeth, deciduous, 253
  defect incidence, 268, 271–72
  eruption of, 253, 270–71
  mottled enamel, 272
  nutrition and, 253
  permanent, 253
  school children, of, 270–71
  six year molars, 253, 270
Temperature, classrooms, in, 286
Terminal disinfection, 96
Tetanus, toxoid, 120
  vaccine, 120
Texas fever, Smith and, 12
Tick-borne diseases, 205
  Rocky Mountain spotted fever, 205
  tularemia, 205
Ticks, 205
  Dermacentor andersoni, 205
  Dermacentor variabilis, 205

Ticks (*cont.*)
  Rocky Mountain spotted fever and, 205
  tularemia and, 205
Toilet facilities in schools, 287
Tonsils, 273–74
  defect incidence, 268
  disease, diagnosis, 273
  heart disease and, 274
  school children, of, 273
  toxemia and, 274
Toxemia, 227
  puerperal, 237
  tonsils and, 274
Toxin, diphtheria, 113–14
  endotoxin, 108
  exotoxin, 108
Toxoid, action of, 116
  administration of, 115
  age and, 115
  alum-precipitated, 115
  dose of, 115
  preparation of, 114
  reaction after, 115
  tetanus, 120
  use of, 114
Tracheotomy for croup, Bretonneau and, 7
Trachoma, 269
  flies and, 204
Trematodes, as cause of communicable diseases, 91
"Trembles," 196
Treponema pallidum, 150
  discovery of, 12
  Schaudinn and, 12
  syphilis and, 150
Trichinosis, 200
Tsetse fly, 204
Tubercle bacillus, 126
  Koch's discovery of, 9
Tuberculin, 135, 137–38
Tuberculin test, 137–38
  BCG and, 128, 138, 140–41
  interpretations of, 137
  main schools in, 138
  Mantoux, 138
  materials for, 137
  "patch test," 138
  performance of, 138
  purified protein derivative (PPD), 137

Tuberculin test (*cont.*)
  utilization of, 138
Tuberculosis, 125–48
  active cases, 136
  adult type, 135
  age and, 126, 131–32
  age-specific death rate, 131–32
  arrested cases, 136
  beds available, 147
  Biggs and, 11
  birds and, 126
  calculation of death rate from, 129
  care at home, 144–45
  case finding, 138–39
  cases, 135–37
    children of, 137
    classification of, 135–37
    condition of, 136
    danger of, 136
    marital partners and, 137
  cattle and, 126, 127
  cause of, 126
  childbearing and, 238
  childhood type, 135
  classification of cases, 135–37
  clinics, 142
  communicability, period of, 126–29
  death rates, 19, 130
    causes of decline, 130
  disinfection in, 145
  drug therapy, 147
  endemicity of, 128
  endogenous reinfection, 136
  exogenous reinfection, 136
  health education in, 142–43
  health programs in, 141–42
  home care, 144–45
  hospitals and, 128, 146–47
  immunity in, 128
  important points in, 126–29
  inactive cases, 136
  incidence of, 132–33
  incubation, period of, 126
  infection, 126
  infectious material in, 127, 142
  inheritance and, 126
  laboratory and, 127
  legal requirements in, 143–44
  lesions, classification of, 136
  lymph drainage in, 136
  mass surveys, 138–40

Tuberculosis (*cont.*)
  milk and, 196
  mortality rate, 129, 130
    trend in, 129
  newer treatment of, 147
  open cases, 136
  prevalence of, 132–33
  probable cause of decline in death
    rate, 130
  program, objectives in, 142–43
  public health nurse in, 145–46
  public health problem, as a, 125–48
  public health program against, 141–
    43
  reinfective phase, 136
  reporting of, 11, 143–44
  sanatoria, 128, 146–47
    need for, 146
    public education and, 143
    ratio of beds to deaths, 147
  sex and, 131–32
  Smith and, 11
  sputum-positive cases, 128
  surgical treatment and, 147
  x-ray and, 138–40
Tuberculous infection, 134–35
  incidence, 132–33
  significance, 132
Typhoid bacillus, Eberth and, 8
  Klebs and, 9
Typhoid fever, Budd and, 7
  communicability, period of, 102
  incubation, period of, 100
  milk and, 197
  Widal reaction in, 12
Typhoid vaccine, 12, 120
  Wright and, 12
Typhus fever, 13, 205

Undertakers, vital statistics and, 21
Undulant fever, 197
Uniform Vital Statistics Law, pro-
    posed, 21
United States, birth rates in, 41
  Census Bureau. *See* Bureau of the
    Census
  death rates in, 40, 41. *See also* spe-
    cific diseases
  Department of Health, Education,
    and Welfare, 49, 50
  greatest causes of death in, 39

United States (*cont.*)
  population of, 23
  public health work in, 48
  Public Health Service. *See* U.S.
    Public Health Service
  Registration Areas of, 25, 26
United States government, Bureau of
    Census. *See* Bureau of the Cen-
    sus
  Bureau of Entomology and Plant
    Quarantine, 13
  Bureau of Medical Services, 50
  Bureau of Mines, 209
  Bureau of State Services, 50
  Children's Bureau, 49, 51, 52
  Department of Health, Education,
    and Welfare, 49, 50
  Federal Security Agency, 49
  grants to states, 51
  health department in, 49
  industrial hygiene and, 209–11
  National Institutes of Health, 50, 52
  Public Health Service. *See* U.S.
    Public Health Service
  public health work of, 48–52
    authority for, 48
  state grants, 51
U.S. Public Health Service, 26, 27, 31,
    49, 50, 51. *See also* National
    Office of Vital Statistics
  BCG vaccine and, 141
  Bureau of Medical Services, 50
  Bureau of State Services, 50
  duties of, 50, 51
  establishment of, 49
  funds available, 55
  industrial hygiene and, 209, 210
  and influenza vaccine, 121
  interstate spread of disease and, 51
  mental health grants and, 179
  National Institutes of Health, 50, 52
    Communicable Diseases Center
      and, 52
    National Cancer Institute, 293
    National Institute of Mental
      Health, 170, 179
  organization of, 49
  publications of, 80
  quarantine stations of, 50, 51
  relation to states, 51
  Surgeon General of, 50
Urine, disinfection of, 98

Vaccination, anthrax, 8
  diphtheria, 114
  influenza, 122
  against other diseases, 120–23
  poliomyelitis, 121
  smallpox, 117–20
    age and, 119
    course of, 118–19
    encephalitis and, 119
    exposure and, 119
    immune reaction, 118
    legal requirements, 120
    technique of, 117
    vaccine, 117
    vaccinoid, 118
  tissue response to, 106
  tuberculosis, 137–38, 140–41
  whooping cough, 121
Vaccine, influenza, 122
  poliomyelitis, 121
  smallpox, 117
  tetanus, 120
  typhoid fever, 120
  whooping cough, 120
Vaginitis, 154
Van Leeuwenhoek, Anton, 6
Vapors, 214
Variola. *See* Smallpox
Vault type privy, 190
Venereal disease programs, 157
  appropriations for, 157
  effectiveness of, 163
  public health nurse and, 162–63
Venereal diseases, 149–64
  chemotherapy and, 153, 155, 156
  control measures in, 157
  epidemiology and, 158
  laws and regulations, 157–59
    minimal requirements, 149
  no effective vaccine for, 158
  prophylaxis against, 159
  prostitutes and, 160–61
  public health problem, as a, 149
  recent advances in treatment of, 153–54
  sex education in, 161–62
  social hygiene, 149
  society and, 159–60
  sulfa drugs and, 155
Ventilation, 231–34
  air movement and, 232, 233
  carbon dioxide, 232

Ventilation (*cont.*)
  classrooms, in, 286
  fresh air and, 231
  humidity and, 233
  large buildings in, 234
  older conception of, 231
  oxygen, 232
  private homes, in, 234
  requirements in good, 233
  temperature and, 231
Veterans Administration, 52
Veterinarians and public health, 15
Virulence, 107–8
Viruses, as cause of communicable diseases, 91
Vision, defects in, 268–70
  expression of, 268
  school children, in, 268
  testing of, 268
Vision testing cards, 266, 268
Visiting nurse association, 67, 68
  how supported, 68
Vital Statistics, 19–45. *See also* Bureau of the Census
  chance in, 45
  collection of, 22
  comparison in, 20
  conclusions from, 45
  definition of, 20, 21
  Farr and, 7
  federal government and, 21, 22–23
  importance of, 19
  interpretations of, 20, 45
  local health departments and, 26
  local registrars and, 21, 29
  mathematics and, 19
  "Model Law" for, 27
  precautions in interpretation of, 45–46
  presentation of, 19, 35–36
  state government and, 21, 26, 27
  Uniform Vital Statistics Law, proposed, 21
  U.S. possessions and, 27
  "universe" in, 20
Vital Statistics in the United States, 22, 26
Vital statistics law(s), essentials in, 28
  function of states, 29
Vitiated air, 232
Voluntary health agencies, 16, 48, 62–67

Voluntary health agencies (*cont.*)
American Red Cross, 65
child hygiene and, 260
dangers of local, 67
financial support of, 63, 64
health education programs and, 80
interests of, 63
interrelations between national,
state, and local groups, 66
local, 63–66
National Foundation, 63, 64
national organization of, 65–66
National Tuberculosis Association,
63, 65
purpose of, 63
scope of, 63
value and disabilities of, 67
Von Behring, Emil, 10
Von Wassermann, August, 12
Vulvovaginitis, 154

Wassermann, August von, 12
Wassermann test, 12, 153
Biggs and, 11
Water supplies, 192–96
analysis, purpose of, 193
chlorine, disinfection of, 193, **194**
city, 193–95
cross connections and, 193
fluoridation of, 225–26
pollution of, 186
protection of, 191–93
rural, 195–96
treatment of, 193–95
Wedgwood, Josiah, 184
Weight, at birth, 252
gain in, during infancy, 252
Welch, William H., 9
Welfare agencies, child hygiene and,
260
Wells, 195
casing of, 195
curbing of, 195
depth of, 195
hazards of, 195
protection of, 195
pumps in, 195
rope and top of, 191, 195
top of, 195

Wesley, John, 184
Whooping cough, communicability,
period of, 102
incubation, period of, 100
vaccine, 120
Widal, G. Fernand, 12
reaction, 12
Women in industry, 215–16
Woodwork, disinfection of, 98
Workmen's compensation, costs paid
by, 211
federal, 211
laws, 211
state, 211, 301
World Health Organization, 30, 69, 70,
71–74
charter, 71
Chronicle of, 74
functions, 72, 73
headquarters, 72
health defined by, 72
organization of, the World Health
Assembly, 72
the executive board, 72
the secretariat, 72
principles, 71
regional offices, 72
scope, 72–74
Wright, Almroth, 12

Xenopsylla cheopis, 205
plague and, 205
typhus fever and, 205
X-ray. *See also* Radiation, ionizing
of chest, surveys, 138–40

Yeasts, as cause of communicable
diseases, 91
Yellow fever, 205
Finlay and, 8
first international health conference
and, 70
Gorgas and, 10
mosquitoes and, 8, 10, 205
Reed and, 10

Zeidler, Othmar, 13